All truth goes through 3 stages: First it is ridiculed. Then it is violently opposed. Finally, it is accepted as self evident.

— *Arthur Schopenhauer*

Masters points out that the 'track record' of the 'conventional wisdom' regarding Lyme disease is not very good: "First off, they said it was a new disease, which it wasn't. Then it was thought to be viral, but it isn't. Then it was thought that sero-negativity didn't exist, which it does. They thought it was easily treated by short courses of antibiotics, which sometimes it isn't. Then it was only the Ixodes dammini tick, which we now know is not even a separate valid tick species. If you look throughout the history, almost every time a major dogmatic statement has been made about what we 'know' about this disease, it was subsequently proven wrong or underwent major modifications."

—Quoted from the book *Bulls-Eye: Unraveling the Medical Mystery of Lyme Disease*, written by Jonathan A. Edlow (Professor of Medicine at Harvard Medical School), Yale University Press, 2003. The above quote from *Bulls-Eye* is a statement from Ed Masters, who discovered Southern tick-associated rash illness (STARI).

Zion, hear me! It is true, what many of you have heard. The machines have gathered an army, and as I speak, that army is drawing nearer to our home. Believe me when I say we have a difficult time ahead of us. But if we are to be prepared for it, we must first shed our fear of it. I stand here, before you now, truthfully unafraid. Why? Because I believe something you do not? No, I stand here without fear because I remember. I remember that I am here not because of the path that lies before me but because of the path that lies behind me. I remember that for 100 years we have fought these machines. I remember that for 100 years they have sent their armies to destroy us, and after a century of war I remember that which matters most... We are still here! Today, let us send a message to that army. Tonight, let us shake this cave. Tonight, let us tremble these halls of earth, steel, and stone, let us be heard from red core to black sky. Tonight, let us make them remember, this is Zion and we are not afraid!

—Speech given by Morpheus in the movie, The Matrix Reloaded, 2003, Village Roadshow Pictures & Silver Pictures.

i

Question: "Why do we need books on healing from Lyme disease? Won't a long Wikipedia article suffice?"

Answer: "Extensive books are needed because Lyme disease is such a bizarre disease, and the healing process so counter-intuitive, that one must literally learn a whole new approach to health, with its own new and unfamiliar rules and principles—rules and principles which are not found anywhere else in the discipline of medicine, or perhaps even the known universe. To make matters even more complicated, chronic Lyme disease is not yet recognized as a valid medical condition by the majority of mainstream medicine, making the already difficult learning process even more challenging. Successfully healing from Lyme requires the equivalent of a 4-year college education. You must literally learn to think about your life differently, because effective Lyme disease treatment requires a complete modification of your entire lifestyle. You can certainly accomplish this without books, but good Lyme disease books should pay for themselves 10-fold in the amount of time and energy they allow you to save by not having to re-invent the wheel. One of the biggest mistakes you can make when learning about Lyme disease treatment is to assume that this health condition is simple; instead, the more your recognize the complexity of Lyme disease, the better off you will be."

—Bryan Rosner

The Lyme patient's modern challenge isn't finding information (that was the challenge 10 years ago). Information is available as never before. The challenge now is to avoid drowning in endless information; the challenge is to determine which information is worth reading; the challenge is to organize that important information and figure out how to apply it to your own treatment plan. This challenge is the reason why I wrote this book: to organize and present the most useful information; not merely to bring you a 3-ring binder with 1500 pages which contain everything ever published on Lyme disease.

—Bryan Rosner

FREEDOM FROM
LYME DISEASE

New Treatments for a Complete Recovery

By Bryan Rosner

Foreword by Jon Sterngold, MD

Edited by Kim Junker

For related Lyme disease books, including Bryan's other Lyme disease books, please visit:
www.lymebook.com

Follow Bryan Rosner's updates on Facebook:
www.lymebook.com/facebook

BioMed Publishing Group
P.O. Box 550531
South Lake Tahoe, CA 96155
www.LymeBook.com

Copyright © 2014
by Bryan Rosner

ISBN: 978-0-9882437-4-3

Lyme disease books & DVDs: www.LymeBookStore.com

Disclaimer/Disclosure

The author is not a physician or doctor, and this book is not intended as medical advice. It is also not intended to prevent, diagnose, treat or cure disease. Instead, the book is intended only to share the author's research, as would an investigative journalist. The book is provided for informational and educational purposes only, not as treatment instructions for any disease.

Lyme Disease is a dangerous disease and requires treatment by a licensed physician; this book is not a substitute for professional medical care. Do not begin any new treatment program without full consent and supervision from a licensed physician. If you have a medical problem, consult a doctor, not this book. If you are pregnant or breastfeeding, consult a physician before using any treatment.

Many of the treatments presented in this book are experimental and not FDA approved. Some of the book's content is speculative and theoretical. The author and publisher assume no liability or responsibility for any action taken by a reader of this book—use of this book is at your own risk. The statements in this book have not been evaluated by the FDA.

The author offers no guarantee that the treatments in this book are the best Lyme Disease therapies; instead, they were simply the treatments that the author found (through research and experience) to be most helpful. Do not rely on this book as the final word.

DISCLOSURE: Some of the book titles mentioned throughout this book are published by BioMed Publishing Group which is owned by Bryan Rosner.

Acknowledgments

All the mentors who have given freely of their time to teach me what I know today. Too many names to list, but they know who they are.

My wife, who has walked beside me in love and support for over a decade.

My editor, Kim Junker, who is a true craftswoman and struck just the right balance on this project.

God, who offers us a life of purpose, value, and significance in an otherwise enormous, cold, and uncaring universe.

My readers, who have always inspired me with their perseverance and strength, and who spur me on to keep learning, growing, and writing.

Those who helped me prepare the book for publication, including Scott Forsgren, who has been a long-time friend and mentor; and other proofreaders.

Photo Credit: (mountain biking photo on cover): Christian Waskiewicz of Alpen Sierra Coffee Roasting Company (he took this photo of me while we were on a ride in the beautiful Sierra Nevada mountains).

Note to the Reader

There are many different viewpoints on how to treat Lyme disease. I want my readers to understand that this book presents only one of those viewpoints. The book should not be considered the final word on Lyme disease treatment, instead, it should be viewed as one of many pieces of the puzzle.

Also, I want my readers to understand that I am not a doctor. I am simply a person who has suffered from Lyme disease, and who has spent over a decade researching this disease. Please consult a licensed physician prior to making any treatment decisions.

—Bryan Rosner

A New Way to Keep Up With the Latest Lyme Disease Information

In the future, I plan to publish Lyme disease treatment updates more often, to get important information out to my readers in a more expeditious fashion than what books allow for.

Therefore, I am launching a new subscription-based newsletter. If you are interested in hearing from me and learning about new Lyme disease treatments, on a more frequent basis, please consider subscribing.

To learn more, please visit:

www.lymebook.com/updates

Also by Bryan Rosner

When Antibiotics Fail: Lyme Disease and Rife Machines, With Critical Evaluation of Leading Alternative Therapies

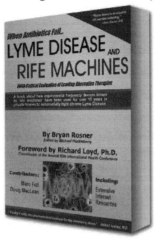

The Top 10 Lyme Disease Treatments: Defeat Lyme Disease With The Best Of Conventional and Alternative Medicine

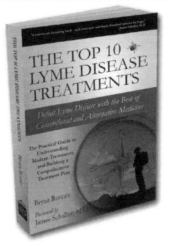

(No picture shown) The Lyme-Autism Connection: Unveiling the Shocking Link Between Lyme Disease and Childhood Developmental Disorders

Learn more about Bryan's books at www.LymeBook.com.

Table of Contents

Foreword by Jon Sterngold, MD 17

Preface: The Librarians of the Lyme Disease World 25

Before You Get Started: Information for the Reader 35

Please Read This First! 35

How This Book Is Organized.. 35

Treatment Protocols vs. Individual Treatments—What's the Difference? 36

About Part 1 and Why We Need "How-To" Information....................................... 37

Lyme Disease Terminology and Lyme Disease Beginners................................ 38

What You Can Expect To Get Out Of This Book... 38

"Peeling Layers Off the Onion" 39

Dosages.. 39

Should You Listen to Me? 39

My Opinion About Lyme Disease Testing, and Testing in General 41

Lyme Doctors: What Sets Them Apart? 43

How This Book Relates to the Past Lyme Disease Books I've Written................. 43

This Book's Strengths and Weaknesses... 44

With Lyme Disease, Problem-Solving Skills Beat Book Knowledge.................... 45

PART 1
Designing a Treatment Template

CHAPTER 1: Introduction: Taking Small Steps Toward a Cure ...51

Lyme Disease Treatment: A Work in Progress.. 51

CHAPTER 2: The Lessons of the Last 5 Years: Where We've Been and Where We Are Going 55

Which Category Do You Fall Into? 56

The Last 10% of Healing 68

The Co-Infections 71

Supporting the Body During Recovery 76

Why is It So Hard to Get Better? 77

The Rubber Band Principle 79

Chapter 3: The Antibiotic Rotation Protocol, Revamped and Revisited, with New Principles for Use 85

Introduction 86

Basic Concepts Underpinning the Antibiotic Rotation Protocol 88

Extending the Rotational Protocol Beyond Antimicrobial Therapies 90

Rotating Supportive Therapies: Further Discussion 93

How Over-Supplementation Can Retard the Body's Own Healing Energy 96

What About Rife Machine Therapy? 103

Three Ways to Feel Better Fast 105

Advanced Principles for Using the Antibiotic Rotation Protocol 106

Final Words on Building Your Treatment Template 122

PART 2
The New Treatment Protocols

Chapter 4: The Paleo Diet for Lyme Disease (and Other Nutrition Hacks) 127

Why the Paleo Diet? 127

Fat and Protein: The Foundation of the Paleo Food Pyramid 130

How Fat and Cholesterol Provide Specific Benefits to People Healing From Lyme Disease 132

Protein 134

Whey Protein & Dairy Products 136

But What About the Vegetables? 138

Fruit 138

Carbohydrates: Treating Them as Rocket Fuel 139

Saying Goodbye to Grains and Gluten 143

Putting It Into Practice: Meal and Snack Examples 146

Snack Ideas 148

The Marvelous Paleo Smoothie 148

Paleo Hot Chocolate 151

Paleo Ice Cream 151

The Green Smoothie 152

The Right Smoothie at the Right Time 154

Tips for Success with Your Healthy Eating Plan 155

Chapter 5: Adrenal Fatigue, Part I: Physical Symptoms and Physical Treatments..159

Adrenal Fatigue: A Condition That Affects Body, Mind, and Spirit 159

Introduction..160

Symptoms of Adrenal Fatigue 163

Emotional Symptoms...165

Treating Adrenal Fatigue 166

B Vitamins, Vitamin C, and Food Choices.......................................168

Adaptogenic Herbs..170

Hormone Supplementation and Glandulars 171

Tips for Recovery, with a Focus on Lyme Disease...........................173

Additional Resources 176

Chapter 6: Adrenal Fatigue, Part II: A New Worldview—Asking Basic Questions about Life as a Human Being 179

Moving from the Physical to the Non-Physical 179

Modern Life and Human Psychology 180

My Own Journey Out of That Deep, Dark Hole 184

Choosing Good Role Models..186

People Pleasing, Perfectionism, and Taking Care of Yourself 187

Managing Expectations 189

Choosing Financial Simplicity 191

Accepting Yourself 191

The Triangle of Emotional Distress 193

Help for the Burdened..199

Camping and the Outdoors: Medicine for the Soul.........................200

Essay: A Boring Camping Photo—More Than Meets the Eye? 202

Epilogue: The Word "Camping"...207

Chapter 7: Parasites and Worms: The New Lyme Disease Co-Infection? (Don't Skip This Chapter!) 209

A New Frontier in Lyme Disease Treatment 209

Profound Improvement Experienced with Parasite Treatment 213

The Subtleties of Synergism 215

Herbal vs. Pharmaceutical Treatments 216

The Anti-Parasite Protocols 218

The Basic Parasite Protocol 219

Notes on the Basic Parasite Protocol: 220

My Comments on the Drugs in the Basic Parasite Protocol 221

Other Useful Drugs 223

Non-Pharmaceutical Options 225

Tips for Success When Treating Parasites 226

Where to Purchase Anti-Parasitic (and Other) Drugs 228

Hints for Finding and Using Reliable Online Pharmacies 228

Climbing the Mountain of Victory and the End of Adrenal Fatigue ...231

Chapter 8: A Brief Update on Rife Therapy & Electromedicine 235

The Limitations of Rife Therapy 236

Rife Therapy in the Later Phases of Recovery 241

Which Infections Are Least Susceptible to Rife Therapy? 242

How Many Different Devices Do You Need? 243

An Important Revision to the Theory Presented in My Earlier Book 245

Where We Go From Here 249

Rife User Report by Jon Sterngold, MD 251

Chapter 9: The KPU Protocol and Heavy Metal Detoxification. 259

A Primer on Heavy Metals 260

What Is the KPU Protocol? 261

Heavy Metal Toxicity and the KPU Protocol 261

Zinc and the "Mother of All Detox Reactions" 262

Considerations in Heavy Metal Detox While Undergoing KPU Treatment 264

Cleaning Up the Body Prior to KPU Treatment 267

Why the Body Needs Help Detoxing Heavy Metals 268

Binders vs. Systemic Chelators..270

Other Supportive Supplements and Treatments.......................................277

Two Phases of Symptomology During KPU Treatment 278

Which Binders, Chelators, and Detox Supplements Should Be Used?..................280

The KPU Nutrients: Should They Be Taken Together or Separately?..................282

Copper Supplementation During the KPU Protocol 282

Side Effects of Arachidonic Acid 283

Do All Lyme Sufferers Have KPU Issues? 283

Conclusion 284

Chapter 10: Biophotons 285

The Powerful Immune System: Your Best Weapon in the Battle Against Lyme
Disease? 285

What Is Biophoton Therapy? 287

Is Biophoton Therapy Really a Legitimate Lyme Disease Treatment?..................288

What's Next for Biophoton Therapy?...290

Chapter 11: Tinidazole: New Research on an Old Drug 291

Recent Study Sheds New Light on Tinidazole..293

What If Tinidazole Works for a While, Then Stops Working?..............................296

What If Tinidazole Appears Not to Work at All? 299

Conclusion 300

Example of Tinidazole Use, With Consideration of the Above Discussion..........300

Chapter 12: Chlorine Dioxide 303

Chlorine Dioxide User Reports...309

Bryan Rosner's Chlorine Dioxide User Report......................................309

Other Chlorine Dioxide User Reports..313

Conclusion 316

Chapter 13: Medsonix® 317

Introduction...317

Can Medsonix® Actually Help Activate Dormant Layers of Infection?..............321

Other Benefits of Medsonix® Treatment..322

When Should This Treatment Be Used?..324

Additional Information 325

Chapter 14: Yeast and Candida 327

Don't Underestimate the Influence of Yeast in Your Current Symptom Picture ..328

You Can't Remove Yeast Without Clearing Out Mercury....................328

Helpful Tools for Killing Yeast..329

Probiotics and Repopulating the Gut With Good Bacteria..................330

Summary..331

Chapter 15: Liver Support... 333

Herbs and Supplements That Support The Liver.................................335

PART 3
The New Individual Treatments

Chapter 16: Introduction to the Individual Treatments 339

What are "Individual" Treatments? 339

Which Treatments Are Included in This Chapter, and Why?...............342

The Right Treatment at the Right Time..343

Chapter 17: The New Individual Treatments............................ 345

Neem 345

Alkaline Water..347

Immunocal®..348

IgG 2000 DF™..350

Boron and Related Compounds 351

Double Helix Water®..353

Moringa Oleifera 353

Liposomal Vitamin C 356

Eiro Super Antioxidant Juice...358

Resistant Microbes® by Herbs of Light 359

Stinging Nettle..359

Virapress®...360

Tart Cherry Extract 360

DMG & TMG 361

Supplemental Creatine 363

Low-Dose Naltrexone (LDN) 364

Pyloricin® by Pharmax® 365

Mild Hyperbaric Oxygen Therapy (MHBOT) 366

Earthing 369

Curcumin 372

Venus Fly Trap (Dionaea Muscipula) 374

EGCG and Green Tea Extract 374

Sarsaparilla Root 375

Haritaki Fruit (Terminalia Chebula) 377

Elderberry 380

Noni 381

Coptis 382

PART 4
Parting Words

Chapter 18: Tips for A Faster Recovery 387

How Lyme Doctors Can Help During the Recovery Process 387

Keep an Open Mind 389

Don't Become Hyper-Focused on Any Particular Infection or Health Problem 389

What to Expect When Treating Lyme Disease 390

Find a Healthy Balance Between Living Life and Treating Lyme Disease 391

Pharmaceutical Antibiotics Can Help You or Hurt You 392

The Yin and Yang of Lyme Disease Treatment 392

The Natural Approach to Lyme Disease May Delay Recovery 393

Keep Your Supplements Organized 394

There's No Silver Bullet Lyme Disease Treatment (at least, not yet) 394

When Infections Are Present, True Progress Won't Occur Until They Are Addressed 395

What is Energy Testing? 395

Focus on Sustainability in your Treatment Program 395

Don't Overlook the Importance of Exercise 397

Lyme Disease and Brain Healing 397

Why We Can't Find Simple Solutions to the Problem of Lyme Disease 400

Feeling Good Can be a Delicate Condition 404

Where to Buy Supplements 405

Who is the Best Lyme Doctor? What is the Best Lyme Treatment? 406

Keeping up with the Latest Lyme Disease Treatment Information 407

BIOMED PRODUCT CATALOG: Related Books & DVDs 409

INDEX 429

Foreword by
Jon Sterngold, MD

I t's very difficult for our Western minds to embrace the true complexity of Lyme disease and this limits our ability to effectively treat it.

We are driven to create order out of the seeming chaos of our existence. Using principles of data analysis and applying logic rules such as Occam's Razor, we're pretty good at figuring out how our universe works. Relentless application of critical thinking helps weed out extraneous factors that are not elements of the kernel of truth about a problem, a phenomenon, and a disease. This often works in modern medicine, though for many chronic diseases (conditions for which modern allopathic medicine is not very good), finding THE cause or a magic bullet that leads to wellness has become a winding path where many get lost. Is it the saturated fat or too much pasta? Cholesterol or inflammation? Is all bad cholesterol really bad? Which is causing what? And on and on. Lyme disease should be so simple!

I saw my first Lyme disease patient thirty-one years ago. Fortunately, she wasn't really sick yet—she just had a huge target rash on her chest. Having no idea what she had, my research consisted of a call to a dermatologist and discussion with the Public Health Department in our county. It was 1983 and news was just spreading about an emerging tick borne disease that could cause this type of rash. It was an infection and like most infectious diseases, all we had to do was choose the most appropriate antibiotic and a cure was almost guaranteed. I did that; she got well, and when I ran into her at a gathering in our small town about 25 years later, I was happy to hear that she remained well since treatment. Her case was reported to Public Health and this was the first report of Lyme disease ECM rash in Northern California.

And then, Lyme fell off my personal radar. I didn't see more cases—that I knew of—and was otherwise buried in the daily crush of emergency medicine cases at our small but very busy hospital emergency department. Only in retrospect I realized that my ignorance of the Lyme world kept me from being able to help some very sick patients. I will never forget the young woman who came in one summer morning about twenty years ago with a paralyzed face—she had bilateral Bell's Palsy—a completely disabling horrific condition and it never occurred to me that the number one diagnosis for her in our Lyme endemic community was Lyme disease. I didn't realize that antibiotics might have cured her. I referred her to ENT specialists but I doubt she was treated with anything other than steroids and to this day, I wonder what became of her. It leaves me with a pit in my stomach for what I now know. Too late for her, and almost too late for me.

I became a reluctant student of the realm because I had to. During my own eight-year battle with Lyme disease 'complex', I tenaciously resisted acceptance of the complexity of what I was up against. It just couldn't be as bad and as complicated as the picture many patients and treating doctors were painting. It must be that this bug had evolved survival techniques that required high doses and prolonged use of antibiotics and if I was just patient enough, I'd get my life back. As I was exposed to new information from respectable scientists—information that was troubling in both its complexity and implications for treatment—I clung to a simpler paradigm because that was less unsettling and disorienting. In retrospect, I can see that my attachment to simplicity—to the simple idea that antibiotics would be my salvation and that I didn't have to do anything else to get well—was no different than anyone blindly clinging to a belief for comfort. It's what we do as a species desperate for understanding in a very complicated and painful world. I like to think that I don't do that—but this is exactly what I did with my Lyme disease and I suffered longer, deeper, and lost more of my life than I might have if I'd been open to the complex reality others were showing me. I might have stopped doing what wasn't working sooner. But I'm hard headed and had spent so much time in the trenches of front line medicine that I trusted my judgment far beyond the point where it stopped serving me. My loss.

And then Bryan Rosner and I crossed paths. Not directly at first, but in the mysterious way that webs of information and influence travel and crisscross, the impact of his work (in particular, his book *Lyme Disease and Rife Machines*) on others eventually touched me and through a chance encounter with another Lyme patient-physician, at a time when it seemed to me that I was at the end of my rope, a light appeared in my darkness. At that moment when I experienced a Herx (die-off) reaction within minutes of my first Rife treatment, my simple paradigm fell apart and the game changed. The chink in my armor of rational reductionism was ripped open and I've never been the same.

But, I'm still me and I've had a tendency to apply my preference for simplicity to Rife therapy; I've viewed effective Lyme treatment through

Rife colored glasses. I got my life back using Rife machines, but I'm also aware that I'm not at 100%—yet. I figured that another year or two of coil sessions and I'd be there (the "coil machine" is one of the machines presented in Bryan's aforementioned book).

And then Bryan shared the manuscript of this new book with me. I thought that the armor protecting my reductionist tendencies had been opened up through my Rife journey, but clearly, I've still been up to my old ways—craving and embracing simplicity. My human nature, like nearly everyone else's, has kept me from a wider perspective. As of today, I'm surrendering. This is a disease that IS more complex than anything else I know of in medicine. Defeat of this miserable condition requires more tools, more medicines, and more knowledge than most people can imagine. How can a Lyme sufferer access these resources?

This is a critical problem in Lyme medicine. In his new book, *Freedom from Lyme Disease*, Bryan gives us a phenomenal amount of useful information about how to attack a disease that cannot be defeated by our own immune systems. We must act, often aggressively, to kill the bacteria and other organisms that conspire to take us over, but we can't do this without guidance, alliance, and medical care. Where do we get this medical care? Sadly, hardly anywhere. There are only a handful of 'Lyme literate MDs' in this country and most people cannot afford to see them. Care for Lyme disease is very expensive and most Lyme doctors do not accept medical insurances for payment. Even when a patient has the economic resources to see one of these physicians, their care does not guarantee a successful outcome. I don't know all the reasons why, but I do know some of them. Lyme doctors have a tendency to specialize their care—some using more detox approaches, others using herbals, and others using more pharmaceutical antibiotics. Certainly many use a combination but very few have (at least publically) embraced Rife treatment. This might be because it's not yet legal to promote Rife for treatment of disease, and this is understandable. It is only recently, and only in some states, that doctors aren't at risk with medical boards for prescribing long term antibiotics to those with Lyme. To include Rife machines and other cutting-edge yet experimental therapies in these practices would be pushing the envelope too far for most physicians' comfort.

Neither Bryan nor I can publically recommend Rife treatment for Lyme, but we can share our personal experience. At this point in the evolution of Lyme treatments, this is what we do and this is what this book does—with scores of pioneering treatment approaches in addition to Rife. It's a sharing of experience so that through the web and weave of information propagation, you—a fellow sufferer—might become empowered to use this to your advantage.

The evolution of the science of medicine begins with someone trying something. Doug MacLean, the first person ever to use Rife therapy to fight Lyme disease, tried a homemade coil device and saved his own life. Others experimented with herbs, supplements, different antibiotics, hyperbaric oxygen, and on and on.

And the story of trial and error extends far beyond Lyme. A physician from Australia tried using antibiotics for ulcer disease—long before it became the standard of practice. Word of success slowly but surely spreads until a critical mass occurs and it becomes more widely known and used. Eventually, it becomes part of medical practice, long before controlled clinical trials—the 'science' of medicine, prove efficacy. But before it is established 'science' it IS clinical medicine and some patients, including me, can be saved through judicious application of these new treatments. Anyone with an agenda to criticize clinical medicine BEFORE it has become accepted science has no sense of the 'on the ground' realities of Lyme disease. Not only is it unbelievably complex, impacting all body systems and requiring management of neurologic, hormonal, rheumatologic, orthopedic, psychological, ophthalmologic, cardiac, hepatic, gastrointestinal, urologic, dermatologic and other system complications, it produces a degree of suffering and disability that is un-paralleled in medicine. And this happens to hundreds of thousands of new victims every year. Good lord we need help! We need doctors trying new approaches in heroic efforts to snatch us from the jaws. Clinical trial based science will come, someday, but in the meantime, we need help. Bryan is offering us, as patients and practitioners, new things to try and a rational basis for these recommendations.

Bryan also makes the point that we, as patients, all need to become our own teachers. Doctors, even if available and affordable, don't know it all and cannot know what might work best for a given patient. Some Lyme patients do get better with nothing more than months or maybe a few years of antibiotics. Some seem to stay better. But many don't and now we understand more about why this is so. Biofilm, genetics, known and unknown co-infections, pre-existing deficits, hormonal degradation, and more—too many variables for anyone to compute are at play—so what do we do? We use trial and error. We attempt to base the trial part on reasons we know or suspect; that is, there's a rational basis for 'trying' this or that. It's plausible that it could work. And we see what happens. Does it induce a Herx? Does it relieve symptoms, eventually? That, then, becomes our own clinical trial. It has no statistical significance (n=1 in the language of statistics), but it has huge meaning for the subject—the patient—you, or me.

Many of us in the Lyme world know Bryan Rosner as the Lyme disease journalist, author, and lay researcher who exposed Rife technology to sufferers who could not get well with other treatments—mainly antibiotics. In the decade since the publication of *Lyme Disease and Rife Machines*, thousands of patients, including me, got their lives back through use of devices that produce an electromagnetic field at specific frequencies that disrupt and kill some forms of the Lyme bacteria: Borrelia burgdorferi. Some got well, some got better, some are still working on it, and some, as it too often is with this disease, are still struggling.

It's time to bring more approaches, and perhaps even to resurrect some of the prior approaches including antibiotics, to the table. Rife is an invaluable tool for killing mature spirochetes, but we know that there are many more types and forms of microorganisms that are at play making us ill, and that they might be susceptible to antibiotics and herbs we haven't considered, or to disruption of their nests—the biofilm. Even if a Lyme patient no longer feels ill, that doesn't mean that they don't or won't need more treatment. Bryan makes it clear that although the sky might be blue and cloudless, we must always be ready for the next storm. Why learn the hard way? That is, even if we feel well, it might be to our advantage to challenge our bodies with a treatment that might peel back a layer of the onion revealing smoldering infection that we've just made more accessible and susceptible to attack. Better to know that the "onion" is still there than to think we're home free. I don't know if we'll ever be home free, but it won't matter as much if we're properly armed, educated, and connected to others who can help us. This help might be a treating Lyme literate physician, the ear/heart/shoulder of an empathetic friend, or words of wisdom, experience, and breaking news from one of the great Lyme disease trackers of our era, Bryan Rosner.

—Jon Sterngold, MD

Dr. Sterngold was a board certified emergency medicine physician with 25 years experience as an emergency medicine doctor. He now practices preventative medicine as well as counseling/therapy/life coaching. He has been a licensed MD for 40 years, and he diagnosed the first reported case of Lyme ECM rash in Northern California in 1983.

Preface
The Librarians of the Lyme Disease World

Has the internet rendered librarians obsolete? Librarians used to help us find the information we were seeking amidst a sea of choices and chaos. While a librarian was never the source of information, he or she was certainly a critical part of our search for information.

Now, search engines like Google largely perform the role of a librarian automatically and almost instantly. While this has led to fantastic benefits, it also has drawbacks. If you are looking for an apple pie recipe, you can save yourself a trip to the library and grab a recipe online. However, what about more complex information with less obvious solutions? Google sorts information based on a very advanced algorithm, but Google can't provide expert guidance on the results it presents to you.

Many people hop on Google, search for *Lyme disease treatment*, and are faced with tens of thousands of resulting web pages. These people have two choices: simply read the first article in the search results and hope that it is the best approach to treating Lyme disease, or, feel completely over-whelmed by the many available treatment perspectives, therapies, and medical paradigms. In a sense, when it comes to treating Lyme disease, a person facing Google search results is a little bit like a person standing in a library without a librarian to help them: there is no shortage of infor-mation (thousands of websites and articles), but it is exceedingly difficult to discover which information is the most valuable, and, more important-ly, how to use that information.

In this day and age, we simply assume that we don't need a librarian to help guide us through. As a society, we have more information at our fingertips than ever before, but this information doesn't necessarily come with instructions—or strategies—that explain how to use it. When re-searching a simple topic, that may not be a problem. But, when research-ing more complex topics, the information is only as good as the instructions for putting it to good use.

Recently, social networks have entered the scene, and there are hun-dreds, even thousands, of Facebook pages and groups dedicated to Lyme disease. While these resources can be tremendously valuable, they also have drawbacks similar to those described in the previous paragraph. Lyme experts post to these groups and share tidbits of information. But the question remains: How does all of the information fit together? What strategies and wisdom should guide its use? Again, information abounds, but a cohesive model which ties it all together is elusive.

Therefore, I would argue that the problem facing Lyme disease pa-tients is not a shortage of information, but instead, a shortage of guide-lines on how to use that information. The information is available like never before, but how do we make sense of it? How do the hundreds of beneficial treatment protocols compare to one another, and when should they be used? Do they work for everyone? Are some more tried-and-true than others?

26

One of the best solutions to the problem of making sense of this abundance of information is to hire a knowledgeable Lyme doctor who can guide you through the treatment process based on his or her years of experience. And I certainly recommend doing just that; in fact, that is the first thing you should do. Lyme doctors are often the best librarians because they have vast experience in making sense of all the available information. Get a referral to a Lyme doctor via the International Lyme and Associated Diseases Society (ILADS) at www.ilads.org.

While having a Lyme doctor is important, as you know if you have read my past writing, I have observed that the patients who do the best are those who take control of their own recovery, become educated, and learn to be the captains of their healing ships. In other words, it's not enough to have a librarian helping you; you have to become a librarian yourself. The reasoning behind this assertion is sprinkled throughout my books and is essential to the approach I take to treating Lyme disease. Doctors can certainly help guide you, but they often don't have enough time to actually teach you how to guide yourself, nor will they have enough time to completely understand your body, your health history, and your unique response to treatments. You'll need to make many course adjustments along your healing journey, and sometimes, these adjustments may need to happen so frequently that no single doctor could keep up with them. While doctors typically adjust treatment programs monthly or even less frequently, in reality, your treatment program will probably need to be adjusted weekly, or even daily!

Do some people get well without ever becoming their own librarian? Yes! But I personally believe that they are the exception, not the rule. Healing from Lyme disease is such an individualized process that the individuals themselves are the ones who are best equipped to find the shortest path to their own healing. Without the tools and wisdom to make your own treatment decisions, you will be at a tremendous disadvantage, unless you are rich enough to afford a private Lyme doctor who can be at your beck and call and with whom you can consult daily. 99% of us do not have that luxury.

And that is where this book comes into the picture. In writing this book, I think of myself as a Lyme disease librarian who is teaching other Lyme sufferers how to be their own librarians. While this book does present many new and exciting treatment options, its primary purpose is not to simply list treatments for you; that is a secondary purpose. The primary purpose is to actually organize those treatment options into a logical structure and provide a framework, or paradigm, through which to view the options. In my opinion, this kind of structure and organization is much more important, and more difficult to establish, than simple information on the treatments themselves. The treatments themselves can be easily researched by using Google; you don't need to buy a book for that. But the strategies for their use cannot be found on Google. I like to refer to this organizational structure as the "Lyme disease treatment template." You'll hear me refer to this template many times throughout the book, and we will build the foundation for this template in Chapter 3.

If I'm going to give you a treatment template, then why do you need to become your own librarian? Can't I just give you the template, and we're done? While the treatment template I provide in this book may be very helpful to you, it will almost certainly need to be adjusted based on your individual situation and needs. If there's one thing we know, it is that Lyme disease affects people very differently, and there's no one-size-fits-all template. So, throughout this book, I'm not going to simply tell you how to use the treatment template; I am going to tell you about the logic behind the template, so you can gain a full understanding of it, and so you can adapt it to your own healing journey. In this way, you will become your own librarian, able to filter any new Lyme disease information that comes your way through your new-found understanding of how that information fits into the puzzle before you, just like a real librarian knows what section of the library to place new books. Accordingly, the usefulness of what this book teaches you should far outlive the time frame during which the treatments presented in this book are still considered cutting-edge. In a nutshell, becoming your own librarian means understanding Lyme disease so well that you can easily determine why certain treatments are needed at certain times, and how these treatments are related to other healing modalities you might choose to use. It also means being able to tell the difference between a new treatment that has the potential to be a breakthrough, and a new treatment which may provide little to no real, lasting value in your recovery. This knowledge will help you for years to come, long after this book has become obsolete.

Taking ownership of your own treatment template is where a doctor's expertise ends and your role begins. It is where my ability to help you ends and your need to help yourself starts. You are the one who will have to learn to interpret how treatments affect you and which ones are worth continuing. Unlike a normal research project, on, say, World War II, your research project is more like a "choose your own adventure" book, where the story will be different for each and every person who has Lyme disease.

So, this book will never replace Google, nor will it replace other Lyme disease books which have great treatment ideas. It will not replace your doctor. Likewise, it won't replace Lyme disease support groups, where you'll find fantastic ideas for recovering your health. What this book will hopefully accomplish is to help you learn how to apply the new information you discover from those various sources. Sifting through the onslaught of information and choosing which treatments might be beneficial becomes much easier when you know what you are looking for and why you are looking for it. And, in our information-rich era, learning how to assimilate and apply information is more important than ever.

I contend that understanding the overarching principles of Lyme disease treatment will benefit you much more than simply becoming an expert on a singular herb or treatment option. Don't misunderstand me. There is certainly a place for a master herbalist who can tell you everything you would ever want to know about a particular herb. However, for the Lyme disease patient, a different kind of challenge emerges: As the days, weeks, and years pass, you will be continuously bombarded by new information, new treatments, and new perspectives. There will be far too much information coming at you for you to become an expert in all areas. Instead, the tool you will need most will be the ability to rapidly assess the new treatments and decide if they are of benefit to you in your Lyme disease recovery, and, if so, how they should be integrated into your treatment program. While this book can't completely equip you with this ability, at the very least, it will make you aware that you actually need this skill, and it will get you started in developing it.

Here's a practical example: Let's take the herb known as Olive Leaf Extract. Anyone can Google this herb and learn everything there is to know about it: what species of plant it is, what the potential side effects may be, when it was discovered, and so on. Would it really be worth your time to read a book that contained this kind of information? Probably not! First of all, it would require thousands of pages to even come close to duplicating the fantastic information on all of the available treatments which can be found on the internet. And second, why even bother duplicating information that is already available? I am not saying this kind of information isn't important: you should fully understand any new treatment you will be using, so if you are planning to use Olive Leaf Extract, by all means, go read about it. Instead, I'm saying that this kind of information isn't worthy of a book in our modern, technologically wired world. And I'm also saying that this kind of information isn't what we are really lacking as a Lyme disease community.

In other words, we aren't missing the library; we are missing the librarians.

What we really need isn't a detailed description of Olive Leaf Extract. Instead, we need the following questions answered: Does this herb work for Lyme disease? Should it be taken continuously, or only once in awhile? How does it fit in with the rest of a Lyme disease treatment protocol?

What have been the experiences of Lyme patients who used this herb? What do Lyme doctors think of the herb? Is it better to be used alone or in combination with other treatments? How does it compare to pharmaceutical options? Which part of the Lyme disease complex is it targeting, and for which part is it ineffective? How can a person tell if it is working? Is it a really important treatment or just one that will provide a minor degree of healing? And ultimately, how can a person really understand the role that this particular treatment plays in the overall recovery process?

These are the most pressing questions, and these are precisely the types of questions which go unaddressed in most Lyme patients' research. Obviously, I won't have perfect answers to all of these questions. But, it is my goal to at least try to address these questions, where many Lyme disease resources either ignore them or don't know how to tackle them. And remember, the correct answers will differ for each person. My goal isn't to give you easy answers; it is to help you see the importance of the questions and give you some guidance on how to find your own unique answers.

So, now you can see what the primary purpose of the book is. It is not to compete with the internet on descriptions of available treatments (how could anyone possibly provide more information in a book than what is contained on the internet?), but to share my own perspective, as would a librarian, on how all that information should be conceptualized, organized, applied, and understood.

Let's get back to the treatment template I mentioned. I believe that the word "template" accurately describes the treatment plan that you will develop as you read and understand the information in this book. A template is, by definition, a structure which is not yet completed or filled in. Once you have the template, you can use it to determine how, when, and why to use various treatment options which come your way, and which you find via Google or Facebook. You'll be able to figure out why certain treatments are helpful and others are not, and you'll be able to decide how to integrate various treatments into a cohesive treatment plan. A template is flexible, but in order to benefit from that flexibility, the user of the template needs to understand how it works.

Here's an example of the timelessness and usefulness of good treatment templates: When I look back at the two Lyme disease books I published in 2005 and 2007, it is clear that many new treatments have become available since those dates. However, while some of the treatments in my prior books may be old and out-of-date, the treatment templates presented in those books are almost completely applicable, even today. Furthermore, a person who really grasped the ideas behind the templates I provided in those earlier books can quite easily assimilate the new information in this book, because the new template is only an incremental improvement over the old ones. Treatment templates are like the chassis on a car: Newer parts and technologies become available in the automobile industry almost daily, but they eventually all get plugged into the same frame. The frame itself, or the template, undergoes changes but not nearly as quickly as what is installed on the frame. Because of this, investing in a good understanding of your treatment template will pay dividends for many years.

To put it another way, the most important thing you can learn from my books isn't which treatments I've found to be most helpful, but instead, why I've found them to be helpful. If I do my job well and you understand the template (and the need for a template), you won't need me to write books anymore; you'll be able to evaluate new treatments for years to come, based on whether or not those treatments fit into your treatment template. Of course, your template itself will evolve and change as new information becomes available. And, there may even come a time when the template needs to be trashed in favor of a completely new way of thinking about Lyme disease treatment. However, based on what I've learned about Lyme disease, I believe that the more likely scenario is that the treatment template will need slight revising here and there, not replacing. And regardless of the degree to which the template will change, those who understand how it works will have a much easier time with any necessary transitions than those who mindlessly pop pills because their doctor told them to do so.

The concept of a treatment template is at the heart of this book, and I have divided the book up accordingly. The earlier chapters of the book focus on building and understanding the template itself, and these chapters serve as a foundation for the rest of the book. The later chapters of the book focus on the individual treatments and treatment protocols, which can be plugged into the template. I will describe in more detail how the book is divided and organized in the following section, entitled, *Information for the Reader*. To avoid frustration, it is important to note that when I talk about the "treatment template," I'm not referring to any one rigid, or defined, methodology. You won't find an easy summary of this template anywhere, and you won't find a page or chapter which fully describes it. Instead, the treatment template is better understood as the overarching direction of a person's Lyme disease treatment, or the foundational guidelines used to make decisions on which treatments to use and how to use them. The appropriate template will vary from person to person, and will be formed for each individual gradually as they read through the book.

Finally, please note that by reading this book, you are getting the opinion of only one librarian, and you are discovering only one librarian's treatment template. Others who have studied the same information may come to very different conclusions than I have. Such controversy isn't necessarily a bad thing. It is precisely this kind of tension that leads to progress in our understanding of Lyme disease. Still, though, please remember that my answers to the pressing questions should not be viewed as the final word in Lyme disease treatment. I encourage you to seek the guidance of many librarians.

OK—I'm sure by now you've heard enough of my philosophizing on treatment templates and librarians. Let's move on!

Before You Get Started
Information for the Reader

Please Read This First!

T his *Information for the Reader* section contains important details on how the book is structured and how to read it. Please don't skip over this information.

How This Book Is Organized

This book is organized with simplicity in mind and is divided into three sections:

PART 1: Designing a Treatment Template. This section provides general, overarching updates to my Lyme disease treatment paradigm. It doesn't list specific new treatments, but instead, provides guidelines for how to think about new treatments and how to integrate them into a treatment program. It provides the treatment template upon which the rest of the book is built.

PART 2: The New Treatment Protocols. This section explains the major new treatment protocols.

PART 3: The New Individual Treatments. This section provides a listing of the new individual treatments.

PART 4: Parting Words. This section covers topics that didn't fit into one of the above sections, and it provides generalized wisdom for healing.

Treatment Protocols vs. Individual Treatments—What's the Difference?

The naming of Parts 2 and 3 (described above) requires clarification. What is the difference between a "treatment protocol" (Part 2) and an "individual treatment" (Part 3)?

I created this distinction for the purpose of simply helping to distinguish between two general categories of Lyme disease treatments. Treatment protocols are therapies which have multiple components, or multiple steps. They are often more complex, involved methods for treating Lyme disease, and they may require numerous things, such as lifestyle changes, supplements, drugs, etc. They have more moving parts than other kinds of approaches.

On the other hand, individual treatments are singular items, such as herbs, drugs, or supplements, which can often be used in a stand-alone fashion, and can be "dragged and dropped" into your treatment program. They are less involved than the protocols, and typically simpler to use.

It must be emphasized that just because the treatment protocol sections are typically longer and more involved than the sections about individual treatments, this does not mean that the protocols are, themselves, more valuable or helpful than the individual treatments. Instead, it simply means that more ink and paper are required to explain them, and more time and planning may be involved for their use. Some of the individual treatments which may occupy only half a page can be just as beneficial as the longer treatment protocols, which occupy a couple dozen pages in the book. And since everyone responds differently to Lyme disease treatment, your results will vary.

About Part 1 and Why We Need "How-To" Information

The parts of the book which discuss the individual treatments and the treatment protocols won't necessarily tell you how, when, or why to use the various treatments. Instead, that kind of information is located in Part 1, especially in Chapter 3.

With many other diseases, especially simple diseases like strep throat, the kind of information contained in Part 1 (the "how-to" information) is largely unnecessary. With strep throat, once the correct treatment is identified, you simply use it for a period of time, and then discontinue it and move on with life. So, a book on strep throat might only list the ideal treatments but have very little information on the philosophy behind those treatments.

With Lyme disease, however, the recovery process will likely fail without a strong grasp of not just the best treatments and protocols, but also the appropriate ways in which they should be used. Therefore, the pattern I use to present information in this book is to first explain the strategy and philosophy which can be used to formulate a treatment plan (this is what Part 1 is about), and then describe the treatments themselves (this is the focus of Parts 2 and 3).

Lyme Disease Terminology and Lyme Disease Beginners

This book will use some specialized, vernacular terminology which is known to people who have already done some research on Lyme disease. The book is not intended as a beginner's guide. There are other available resources for people who find themselves lost in the terminology. For example, *The Beginner's Guide to Lyme Disease*, by Nicola McFadzean, ND, may be a good place to start.

What You Can Expect To Get Out Of This Book

Everyone who picks up this book will be in a different phase of the recovery process. If you already have a great treatment protocol that is working, you can use this book to gain new ideas which can be integrated with your current protocol. In this case, you may not need the information in Part 1, since you are already on a program that is working. Do not heavily modify your treatment program if it is achieving desired results.

On the other hand, if you do not have a protocol already and you are new to Lyme disease treatment, this book can help you establish some foundational components of your treatment protocol.

And then there's everyone in between these two scenarios. The point is that this book can and should be used differently by different people.

In any case, though, note that this book does not stand on its own. You'll need the help of other Lyme disease books and resources as well as the support of a trained physician to guide your recovery.

"Peeling Layers Off the Onion"

One of the most important phrases you will encounter throughout the book is, "peeling layers off the onion." This analogy is used to describe the healing process, and it will be defined and clarified in more detail throughout the book. If you haven't heard the phrase used before, it may seem confusing at first. Don't worry; keep reading. The more you read, the more it will begin to make sense.

Dosages

For most of the treatments discussed in this book, dosages will not be given. Because I am not a doctor, I will not tell you which dosages to use for the various herbs and drugs discussed. Please ask your doctor to help you if you decide to use these therapies. Any and all treatments you decide to use should only be undertaken under the care of a licensed physician.

Should You Listen to Me?

I am not a doctor or licensed health care practitioner, so when reading this book, please keep in mind that you are reading the work of a layperson.

Although I am not a doctor, I have spent thousands of hours researching Lyme disease. I am connected to numerous networks of Lyme disease patients, doctors and researchers. Much of my time over the last 10 years has been spent pouring over books, websites, and lectures on Lyme disease. I have battled Lyme personally.

Still, though, the reader must be made aware that this book is based on the research and conclusions of one person (me, Bryan Rosner). While I feel that my conclusions are logical and worth sharing, they are most certainly not the final word when it comes to Lyme disease treatment. A single individual's perspective is, by definition, an imperfect perspective. Furthermore, one of the most important principles with regard to Lyme disease recovery is that each individual responds differently (in some cases, dramatically differently) to various treatments. This book is biased toward the treatments that have worked well for me, and for those with whom I have communicated. There will be many people who read my book and find that my approach, perspective, and findings are not appropriate or correct for their own situation. Please view this book as one stop on your Lyme disease research journey, not the destination.

The obvious disadvantage of publishing imperfect information is that the reader may interpret it as perfect and complete, when in fact it is not. So, as you read this book, please be aware that its content is a constantly evolving work in progress. Some of the therapies described in this book are experimental and not well understood, even by top experts in the field. Therefore, much of the information about these therapies comes in the form of anecdotal results and conclusions reached via inductive reasoning. Please take note of this before reading this book.

Some people may wish to avoid using the kinds of treatments described in this book—that is, treatments which have not been clinically proven via double-blind, placebo controlled studies. While this is an admirable goal, it may mean that many treatments which have helped Lyme sufferers are off limits, because many such treatments have never undergone these trials and may not undergo them for years, or ever. I certainly respect the individual decisions made by Lyme sufferers, and the varying degrees of comfort each person has with each treatment. I recommend that you make decisions which you are comfortable with. Do not assume that my comfort with a particular treatment should automatically translate to you.

I must express the utmost humility in regard to my writing of this book. I have learned much of what I know from pioneers who are smarter and more experienced than me, and therefore, I do not take credit for the value contained inside the book.

While many of the ideas in this book didn't originate with me, my opinions about how to use the treatments are mine alone, and are not necessarily shared by Lyme disease doctors and experts. So, my book should not be seen as a representation of how Lyme doctors or experts feel about the treatment of Lyme disease. My opinions are mine alone.

Again, remember that your experiences and correct path to healing may differ from what is shared in this book. My intention for this book is that it will serve as one small piece of the Lyme disease puzzle, not the solution to the entire puzzle.

My Opinion About Lyme Disease Testing, and Testing in General

Some available tests may help you figure out what's going on inside your body and which infections are plaguing you. Other tests may provide misleading results, which point you in the wrong direction. In my opinion, whether you decide to use extensive testing or not, trial and error in your treatment program is still the key to finding out what works, regardless of what test results say. Even if a test accurately tells you which pathogen you have, it will likely not reveal which problem is the "top layer of your onion" (keep reading to learn more about the onion concept, we'll be talking about it a lot more). If you only go by test results, you may be missing out on fantastic treatments which have great potential to help you but which you would only discover through a willingness to experiment. The human body remains extremely complex and outside of the reach of modern science; sometimes cause and effect are not predictable using laboratory methods and analysis.

The only thing better than trial and error is energetic testing, or learning your body so well that you know which symptoms indicate which problems. So, while I'm not against laboratory testing, I am against using it as a substitute for getting to know your body and paying attention to how various treatments affect you. Here's a quick example: In my own personal recovery, all my Babesia tests were negative. Yet, when I experimented with Babesia treatments, I found great improvement. Had I only listened to the test results, I would have likely left my Babesia infection untreated!

Or, perhaps I never had Babesia; maybe I had some undiscovered and unknown infection which we don't currently know how to test for but which was susceptible to Babesia treatments. The medical community recognizes this possibility and has even come up with the phrase, "Bartonella Like Organism," or BLO, to indicate an awareness that the organisms we are fighting might be elusive and unidentified variations of the species which have been observed and identified in the laboratory.

I am not alone in my experience. Many people spend thousands of dollars on tests and still do not figure out what's going on. For these people, trial and error may yield telling results. Various supplements which cost a fraction of the cost of laboratory testing and which have helped other Lyme sufferers can be used as therapeutic trials. Then, a person can observe their response to these supplements, and conclusions can be drawn about what kinds of problems the body is dealing with. If an anti-Bartonella herb that cost $20 yields Herxheimer reactions and improvement even in the face of a negative Bartonella test result, a person may be able to conclude that they actually do have Bartonella (or BLO) and that Bartonella treatment might be useful. And, this particular lesson only cost $20, instead of hundreds or thousands of dollars for testing.

If you are one of those people who are really in tune with your body and can decipher treatment responses, trial and error may be even more useful. If you have no connection with your body and can never tell which treatment is working, you might need to rely more heavily on tests. Personally, I used more trial and error. In most cases, a combination of trial and error with some laboratory testing is probably ideal. However, in no case do I believe that laboratory testing can completely replace the need for trial and error, because most of the problems which face Lyme sufferers are not easy to test for. Don't allow tests to give you a false sense of comfort. Listening to your body and thinking about your situation analytically should always play a central role in your recovery process.

Lyme Doctors: What Sets Them Apart?

Specially trained physicians who understand the reality of chronic Lyme disease are available to help you navigate through the maze of Lyme disease treatment. These physicians are known as Lyme-literate Medical Doctors (LLMDs). Make sure you are under the care of an LLMD at all times during your Lyme disease recovery, and don't confuse an LLMD with a regular infectious disease doctor who isn't trained in, and doesn't believe in the existence of, chronic Lyme disease. Thousands of dollars and countless hours of frustration can be saved by choosing an LLMD to guide your Lyme disease treatment. You can get a referral to a LLMD in your area by communicating with the International Lyme and Associated Diseases Society (ILADS) at www.ilads.org.

I don't intend for this book to compete with the wisdom and experience of Lyme disease doctors. This book is based on my own research and experiences, and should not be used to replace the vast and authoritative knowledge base possessed by practitioners who treat Lyme disease.

How This Book Relates to the Past Lyme Disease Books I've Written

You will notice that throughout this book, I make references to the previous two Lyme disease books I've written. This book is built on the foundation of my prior books. Much of what I present in this book ties in directly with what I presented in those books. While this book can stand alone, it is certainly helpful if the reader is familiar with my past works and my general approach, or philosophy, to the treatment of Lyme disease.

If you've read my past books, you will find that this book emphasizes the importance of some suggestions in the older books and deemphasizes the importance of other suggestions. My understanding of Lyme disease has progressed and developed over the years. Still, though, you'll find that my overall treatment philosophy has remained largely unchanged.

This Book's Strengths and Weaknesses

Every author and researcher has their own slant, bias, area of study, and strengths and weaknesses of knowledge. My books have strengths and weaknesses; don't assume they are the only sources of good information. Even the top Lyme doctors have areas where they disagree. Furthermore, every person has a unique situation and set of problems. The bottom line is that no one source of information is the perfect resource, and no two Lyme patients will respond the same to a given treatment. Instead of passively relying on books to heal you, you must learn to be an active participant in your healing process, and you must begin to learn how to identify information that will be useful to you specifically as an individual, with your own unique situation. This point is so critical that you will hear me repeat it throughout the book.

One of this book's strengths, I believe, is the topic of aggressive, advanced, flexible anti-infective therapies targeted toward Lyme disease and co-infections. I believe that other Lyme books on the market do a wonderful job of filling in areas that this book doesn't cover, such as: diagnostic tools, testing, and labs; the history and politics of Lyme disease; and detailed information on pharmaceutical treatment options; etc. In this vein, I would never claim that this book is all you need. Instead, I believe this book is one piece of the puzzle.

As you read my book, take from it what is useful to you, and look to other resources when you find my book lacking the information you need.

With Lyme Disease, Problem-Solving Skills Beat Book Knowledge

As we saw in the Preface, there is one overarching, paramount concept which must be respected when fighting Lyme disease: learning how to think about, analyze, and understand Lyme disease and its related problems is as important, if not more important, than simply learning about the protocols and treatments that are available for treating the disease.

Below, I will share some tips which can help you to more effectively think about the problem of Lyme disease. These tips can aid in the acquisition of true problem-solving skills, rather than merely book knowledge, when it comes to Lyme disease recovery.

- Realize that Lyme disease and co-infections are problems which are highly dissimilar to anything you've ever learned about. Prepare yourself for a steep learning curve, and do what it takes to make time to learn what you need to know. Reprioritize your schedule, if necessary, building in sufficient time to read and study Lyme disease and co-infections. Without taking this step, it may be very hard for you to get well.

- Take ownership of the research you are doing. If you have a question about something as you are reading this book (or any other material), find the answer, even if it means you have to conduct additional research.

- Consult multiple sources for the best treatments for Lyme disease and co-infections. Talk to numerous doctors, read numerous books, and participate as much as possible on the available internet discussion groups. You must begin to create your own, unique path to wellness, since your body, biochemistry, and "infection soup" is different from anyone else's. Do not passively sit back and let one source of information dictate how you should proceed.

- Learn to keep track of your symptoms and your responses to various treatments. Are you dealing with heavy metal poisoning or infections? Or perhaps, hormonal imbalances? Or, all of the above? Laboratory testing can certainly help you to determine the answers to these questions, but laboratory testing isn't enough. You need to be a detective and investigate your own body. I have worked very hard over the years to be able to remember—to burn into my memory—how I respond to various treatments. If you record your response to a heavy metal detox protocol, for example, then next time you experience the same response, you can say "Aha! I must be moving heavy metals around in my body!" Sometimes, years after I use a given treatment, I can recall what that treatment did for me—or did not do for me—and that information becomes invaluable in making later treatment decisions. In fact, without this intimate knowledge of which symptoms indicate which problems in my own body, I am sure that I would have never been successful in my Lyme disease battle. Keep a treatment diary if that will help you to remember how you respond to the treatments you use. Only begin one new treatment at a time, so you can interpret how that treatment affects you. Remember, the goal is ultimately to figure out which problems you are dealing with, whether they be co-infections, heavy metals, hormonal imbalances, adrenal fatigue, or something else altogether. And, quite often, you may be dealing with all of these at the same time, since this particular grouping of problems usually goes hand-in-hand with a Borrelia infection. People who are only mildly ill may be able to get away with less of this detective work and simply "throw spaghetti at the wall to see what sticks," but the sicker you are, the more important it will be to understand your body.

- Do not be afraid of trial and error. Sometimes, when laboratory test results are ambiguous, trial and error is the only way to figure out what is really going on inside your body. You may need to just try different types of new treatments in order to find out whether or not they help you and to observe how your body responds to them. In past books, I have referred to this approach as a "therapeutic trial" or "therapeutic probe." There are various names for this approach, but they all lead to the same result—a better understanding of how your body responds to various treatment approaches. Of course, be careful when experimenting with new treatments, and do so only under the supervision of a qualified physician.

PART I
Designing a Treatment Template

In Part 1 we will be building a treatment template which will be used throughout the rest of the book. The treatments and protocols described in Parts 2 and 3 should be used according to the guidelines we establish here, in Part 1.

Note that Part 1 will not simply supply you with a one-size-fits all treatment template. Treating Lyme is unfortunately more complicated than that. Instead, it will give you the tools to build your own, unique treatment template, based on your own, unique situation. Tick-borne disease affects everyone differently, so your treatment template will be different from that of every other Lyme sufferer. This is an important concept, and one that is often ignored due to the burden it places on the patient to take control of their healing and determine how treatments should best be used in their own unique situations. Many doctors try to avoid placing this burden on their patients, which is a noble aim, but an aim which can severely short-circuit the recovery process as it results in one-size-fits-all protocols that don't work for real life individual human beings.

While doctors themselves can sometimes create truly unique treatment protocols for their patients, it is very difficult for them to do this due to time constraints during doctors' appointments and the fact that doctors cannot possibly know your body as well as you do. Your doctor will be much more successful in helping you if you are involved, too.

So, the responsibility lies on the patient to participate in the healing process and help develop and understand their treatment protocol.

Therefore, Part 1 is designed to equip you to build your own, unique treatment template, based on a deep understanding of how Lyme disease impacts the body.

CHAPTER 1
Introduction: Taking Small Steps Toward a Cure

When I first began sharing with researchers and colleagues that I was writing another book on Lyme disease, a common response I heard went something like this: "Haven't you already written a few books on Lyme disease? Why do your readers need yet another one?" These are good questions. If I am asking you to take a couple dozen hours of your time to read my book, I think it is fair for you to ask me why I wrote the book in the first place—especially considering the fact that I've already asked you to spend your time reading my previous books.

Lyme Disease Treatment: A Work in Progress

There is no known cure for Lyme disease. This does not mean that people do not get better; they do. Some even get cured, or at least, they get to a state of remission. What it means is that there is no single, silver bullet treatment that works for every person, every time.

There are many reasons for this variability in the success of assorted Lyme disease treatment approaches. Most obviously, the Lyme disease bacteria itself (and the host of co-infections that come with it) are simply too advanced, strong, and survival-oriented to be eliminated by the attacks we are able to stage against them, given our current medical knowledge and resources. The actual mechanisms utilized by Lyme disease and co-infections to accomplish such proficient survival are numerous and fascinating; some are discussed in my previous books—and this book—and in books by other authors.

Recently, Lyme disease patients and researchers have also learned that the infections themselves are only one piece of the puzzle. Co-conditions such as toxic mold, adrenal fatigue, heavy metal poisoning, hormonal imbalances, deranged energy metabolism, fungal overgrowth, chronic inflammation, biofilm, parasites, and other factors are now considered to be just as important as the infections in many people who suffer with Lyme disease. These factors provide additional roadblocks to getting well.

Due to all of the above hurdles, treating Lyme disease is complex, not simple, and information on the best available treatments is evolving rapidly. Furthermore, the multi-faceted nature of Lyme disease yields a very low probability that a single silver bullet treatment will ever be discovered. So, waiting for that silver bullet before publishing a new book might mean waiting forever, and never sharing new, useful information.

As I watched the developments over the last several years, I decided that I would only write another book if the new information I discovered reached a tipping point, that is, a point at which I believed the information would make a significant impact on my current view of Lyme disease treatment strategies and have a specific benefit for people beyond the benefit I believe that my prior books were able to provide. I waited more than five years to find the tipping point. It came in the year 2011. The tipping point was a result of several new, breakthrough treatments and also several big changes in what I believe an ideal treatment template looks like.

Utilizing the best available treatments to fight Lyme disease is always what makes the most sense for quality of life, whether or not they are the cure. Obviously the cure—the silver bullet—would be the ideal solution, but in the meantime, most patients appreciate the highest degree of quality of life that they can possibly attain. Those who are living at 50% recovered would very much appreciate the opportunity to live at 60% recovered. Those who are living at 80% recovered would very much appreciate the opportunity to live at 90% recovered. This is why I continue to write books on Lyme disease even when we don't yet have all the answers.

Of course, I could have waited a couple more years to publish this book, and there is no doubt that it would be a better book. But instead, I have chosen to make this information available now, as a result of the recent tipping point that I observed. I believe it is better to take small steps toward the cure for Lyme disease rather than wait until the final big step (the cure) is discovered, if ever that is to happen.

And, I'm confident that the book you now hold in your hands (or on your eReader) is indeed a great leap forward in Lyme disease treatment theory; it fills in many missing pieces of the puzzle, and I can't imagine fighting Lyme disease without the information contained within it.

CHAPTER 2
The Lessons of the Last 5 Years: Where We've Been and Where We Are Going

I'm going to use this section of the book to catch you up on what I've learned during the last five years or so. This section will take a birds-eye view of new lessons, concepts, and developments, and it will serve as a broad foundation for the rest of the book. For this section, just sit back and absorb as much as you can, and don't expect a lot of detailed explanation on any one subject; the details will come later in the book. This section begins to create the foundation for the treatment template we'll be using throughout the book. The following Chapter, Chapter 3, lays out the treatment template in detail. Then, in Parts 2 and 3 of the book, we'll learn about the specific treatments which can be plugged into the treatment template.

Which Category Do You Fall Into?

One of the most important lessons of the past five years is that every Lyme sufferer must realize that their own unique case is different from the cases of others suffering from this disease. Because Lyme disease affects people so uniquely, and each person is afflicted with different co-infections and co-conditions, it is important to identify the idiosyncrasies and distinctive aspects of your particular case of Lyme disease. The ways in which individual cases differ are too numerous to list. Your case of Lyme disease will be different from any other case on a number of different levels, including your symptomology, your most affected organs/body systems, the time it takes you to get well, the obstacles you encounter during recovery, the type and extent of Herx reactions you experience, the treatments that work best for you, the underlying causes of your chronic sickness, and many other aspects. While a book cannot help you identify all of the unique aspects of your disease, it can help you start to think about some of the broader categories of disease characteristics. Placing yourself into the proper category, or categories, is the first step in understanding your body and which treatments will be most beneficial to you.

Here we will look at just a few of the different categories dividing Lyme disease sufferers.

1. *Those whose symptoms are primarily caused by infections.*
   Lyme disease is, of course, a condition caused by infections. However, as you will read, one of the chief reasons that people get sick with Lyme disease is that, prior to the infection, their bodies were not functioning properly and were burdened by a plethora of toxins, nutritional deficiencies, and other types of challenges. So, which is the more important problem: the infections, or these other types of health problems? While these other conditions may set the stage for infection, and while they must be addressed in order to get well, for many people, the infections themselves eventually take center stage,

spiral out of control, and become the most pressing problem within the body. Admittedly, even for these people, non-infection conditions will need to be addressed in order to keep making progress in healing. But people who fall into this category—that is, people whose symptoms are primarily caused by infections—will experience the most profound and rapid improvement by the use of antimicrobial treatments. These people will get significant benefit by addressing toxicities, nutrient deficiency, and other non-infection conditions, but they will achieve more significant milestones if they focus on the infections. It is important to know whether or not this category describes you, because if it does, and you are unaware of that fact, you may spend far too much time pursuing non-infection treatments (such as hormone balancing, adrenal fatigue therapy, etc).

2. *Those whose symptoms are primarily caused by non-infectious problems.* Some people may, in fact, be suffering from one or more infections, but their biggest problems, and, hence, their real potential for improvement, lie elsewhere. These people may require significant anti-microbial therapy, but if they hyper-focus on infections, they may never recover. Often, this category of people can be identified by the occurrence of minimal improvement and minimal Herxheimer reactions during the use of antimicrobial therapy.[1] These people may have other problems in areas such as hormones, metabolic irregularities, allergies, and related conditions. During the final stages of healing, it is especially important to determine whether or not this category describes you. For example, maybe your infections have already been killed or rendered

---

[1] Note that there are other reasons why someone may not be responding to antimicrobial therapy. Even people whose primary problem is infections may not respond to antimicrobial therapy because their infection(s) may be dormant, or there may be an impenetrable layer of biofilm preventing the treatments from reaching their target.

dormant, yet you incorrectly continue to pursue only antimicrobial treatments when, in fact, you should be moving on to healing approaches which address non-infectious problems. For people in this category, their biggest leaps and bounds of improvement will occur not when they address infections, but when they address other kinds of health issues.

Of course, most people have a combination of the above two categories of problems. And, over time, you may find yourself switching back and forth between categories. The important thing is to recognize that the categories exist, and recognize that they are addressed differently. It is your job to be a detective and figure out what your current, most pressing need is.

A great way to think about this concept is to think about "peeling layers off an onion." This is an analogy we will be using throughout the book, because the act of peeling layers off an onion is very similar to the act of recovering from Lyme disease. In the beginning of the recovery process, we are trying to peel the outer layers off the onion. As we advance through the recovery process, we encounter and address deeper and deeper layers of the onion. In Lyme disease, the infections themselves can literally arrange themselves in layers, such that you encounter Infection A first, and then Infection B later, after Infection A is removed. But the layers of the onion do not stop with infections. Other, non-infectious health problems can be nested in the layers, too, and can come and go as you remove the infections. Layers can even alternate between infections and non-infectious problems, and some layers can include both infections and non-infectious problems. For example, as we will see in a later chapter, adrenal fatigue (which is a non-infectious problem) is often nested in the same layer as Bartonella (which is an infection).

Examples of other problems you may encounter within the layers of your onion include, but are not limited to, other co-infections, hormonal imbalances, nutrient deficiencies, and even emotional trauma which, if not addressed, will halt the peeling of the onion. Each layer may be different from the prior layer and may require a great deal of flexibility in your thinking patterns and treatment plan.

When all the layers of the onion have been removed, a person has achieved recovery.

Personally, I fell into the category of Lyme disease patients whose primary problem is infections. While I did experience benefit from addressing toxicities, hormonal imbalances, and nutritional deficiencies, these paled in comparison to the benefit I received from directly attacking the infections. For a long time, I did not realize that this was true of my case, and I wasted a lot of precious time and resources chasing down such things as thyroid hormone supplementation, mega-dose vitamin therapy, relaxation techniques, dietary changes, and even exercise. All of these therapies and activities helped me, but I didn't really get better until I started focusing on killing the infections. Hours of vigorous exercise and months of nutritional optimization did not provide nearly as much benefit to me as a 30-day course of powerful antimicrobial herbs or consistent use of rife machine therapy. Again, remember that the categories are not mutually exclusive. People generally fall into both categories at different times throughout the recovery process. The important question is: Which is the dominant category for you right now? And, are you paying close enough attention to your body to notice when the category shifts?

I present this information with the hope that you become aware of the many differences between Lyme disease sufferers, so that you spend your time, energy and money pursuing the most helpful courses of treatment for your specific situation, not for the average Lyme disease patient.

Before moving on to the next category, I would like to linger a bit longer on the discussion of infection vs. non-infectious causes of disease. Here, I will share a comment from a Lyme disease doctor who is arguably the most famous and influential of all Lyme disease doctors, Dr. Joseph J.

Burrascano, M.D. In his statement below, Dr. Burrascano shares his viewpoint on how treatments for non-infectious problems relate to treatments for infections:

> *While I do agree with the appropriate use of any and all reasonable supportive methods, I also believe that underlying it all, it is always the Lyme. I cannot tell you how many patients diagnosed as having CFIDS (Chronic Fatigue and Immune Dysfunction Syndrome) or known Lyme patients who are said to no longer be responding to (usually inappropriately weak) antibiotic regimens are now showing up with positive Borrelia blood cultures. This has been a real eye opener to many CFIDS practices and also to the patients themselves. As a corollary, I have also seen many patients who get treated with purely supportive methods, who actually do well as long as they receive this support, then go on to develop Borrelia disasters years later, due to untreated persisting infection. **I say, confirm the diagnosis as rigorously as possible, give appropriate supportive treatments (revised continually as patient status changes) and treat with as aggressive an antibiotic regimen as can be tolerated.***
>
> *—JJB*

The part of this excerpt I want to focus on is the last sentence, which I've added bold formatting to. Dr. Burrascano articulates my belief about this matter perfectly, and provides a fantastic model for us to follow. Let's take a look at what he says in that last sentence of the excerpt (note: the below discussion is my own opinion, not that of Dr. Burrascano). I will break down his sentence into several parts:

1. **"Confirm the diagnosis as rigorously as possible."** This first step is critical. Some people may believe their main problem is Lyme disease infections, but in fact, it is something else, possibly not related to infections at all. For example, mercury poisoning, nutritional deficiencies, mold exposure, and other similar issues can cause chronic illness similar to Lyme disease. It is important to decipher which problems are causing a

person's disease; Lyme disease may not be present at all. You must become a detective, and you and your physician must get to the bottom of the root causes of your health problems. If Lyme disease and co-infection tests do not produce reliable results (or if you cannot afford them), a therapeutic trial of Lyme disease treatment may be in order (that is, an empiric trial of anti-bacterial therapy[2] based on a suspected Lyme disease diagnosis). If improvement and Herxheimer reactions occur, then such a response can be used to clarify the diagnosis and possibly confirm a diagnosis of Lyme disease. Empiric treatment is advocated in some cases by numerous Lyme disease doctors, such as Burton Waisbren, MD, who writes about this type of treatment approach in many of the case reports that appear in his new book, *Treatment of Chronic Lyme Disease: Fifty-One Case Reports and Essays in Their Regard.* The point I believe Dr. Burrascano is making here is that the diagnosis is important. Everything hinges on whether or not Borrelia and co-infections are in fact present in the body. Someone with chronic fatigue syndrome shouldn't just assume that they have Lyme disease when they find out that Lyme disease is a sweeping, worldwide epidemic. While it may be likely that they have Lyme disease, they must keep in mind the importance of actually confirming this suspicion.

2. **"Give appropriate supportive treatments (revised continually as patient status changes)."** This is a very concise and articulate description of how supportive (non anti-microbial) treatments should be used, in my opinion. Dr. Burrascano addressed this perfectly with his use of the phrase, "as patient status changes." Good Lyme disease practitioners

---

[2] Throughout the book, the phrase "antibacterial treatment" will be used frequently, often in the place of phrases such as "antibiotics," "anti-bacterial herbs," "rife machine therapy," etc. The reason for this is that an individual Lyme disease sufferer may be the only one who knows which of the specific antibacterial therapies should be applied at any given time during the recovery process. Each of the specific therapies has value and may provide benefit, but they may be needed in differing levels at different times.

recognize that the supportive therapies that are needed throughout the recovery process are constantly changing, just as the patient's health and needs are dynamic and shift numerous times throughout the recovery process, depending on which layer of the onion is being addressed. Today's valid supportive treatment may be tomorrow's waste of time.

3. **"Treat with as aggressive an antibiotic regimen as can be tolerated."** This concept harkens back to Dr. Burrascano's original thought in the excerpt that, in those with confirmed Borrelia and co-infections, the infections are the primary cause of the chronic illness and associated symptoms. The two keywords in this phrase are "aggressive" and "tolerated." It has been observed that non-aggressive antibiotic treatment of Lyme disease is not just minimally ineffective, but entirely ineffective. "Monotherapy," or the use of only one antibiotic at a time, has been shown to be entirely ineffective in most cases of chronic Lyme disease. In fact, in my discussions with numerous Lyme disease sufferers since the publication of my previous books, I have heard it said more than a few times that real improvement does not begin until the right combination of antibiotics is used. For example, one woman told me, "With monotherapy, I would only Herx for a day or two, and I would plateau quickly … it wasn't until I began taking a combination of three antibiotics that I began to Herx continuously and make continuous progress." I believe this is an example of what Dr. Burrascano is referring to by his use of the word "aggressive." Some cases may, in fact, require intravenous antibiotics. Even if you reject the idea of using long-term antibiotics to treat Lyme disease, whichever alternative therapies you choose should still be applied aggressively. Lack of progress doesn't necessarily mean that there are no more infections left in the body; instead, lack of progress can indicate that the infections are present and that you simply aren't treating them effectively.

Now, let's look at the word "tolerated." It is important that any treatment regimen be well tolerated, not just from the standpoint of safety and toxicity to body organs and systems, but also from the standpoint of symptom exacerbations and intense Herxheimer reactions. Doctors and patients must understand the specific risks, side effects and interactions associated with all therapies used, even holistic and alternative therapies. Treatment must be administered only to a level that can be tolerated by the patient. Patient health must be monitored during many therapies, which includes the regular use of blood testing, especially liver function tests. Also, there are steps that can be taken to increase tolerability of many therapies, both from the standpoint of safety and toxicity, as well as the standpoint of patient symptoms and the intensity of Herxheimer reactions. Many such steps will be discussed in this book, and have been discussed in other books. Brief examples include the use of liver-supporting supplements to increase the body's ability to withstand potentially toxic drugs, and the use of appropriate detoxification therapies to increase the patient's ability to withstand Herxheimer reactions. And of course, the use of probiotics to protect the gut from the devastating effects of antibiotics. Other interventions will be required based on the specific side effects and reactions to particular treatments.

So, in conclusion to the discussion of these two categories (problems caused by infections and those caused by non-infectious issues), I believe that this question should be at the forefront of your mind, and your physician's mind, as you navigate through your Lyme disease treatment. Are your current, active problems caused by infections, or by other kinds of dysfunction in the body? Furthermore, it is entirely possible that even people whose primary problems are caused by infections would never have been susceptible to those problems had they not already been vulnerable to the infections as a result of some underlying weakness or predisposition, which must also be addressed in order to attain complete healing.

The key to placing yourself into the appropriate category is to discover which treatments are primary to your recovery. For some people, antibacterial therapies are necessary but nowhere near as helpful as balancing the hormones and getting their heavy metals under control. And for other people, the opposite will be true. Often, this determination is made via trial and error. And of course, we need to remember that the categories can flip-flop over time, and that you must stay alert. So, pay attention to your reactions to treatments to figure out which treatments are the most important ones for your recovery.

For now, let's assume that Dr. Burrascano's viewpoint is correct in most cases and that your primary problem is infections (a big assumption, I know). Don't worry, throughout the book, we will also be looking at many non-infectious treatments. But our general assumption in the book is that the infections are extremely dangerous and must be dealt with intelligently and aggressively.

There are two subcategories which must be evaluated, within the broader category of those whose primary problems are caused by infections:

1. *Those who benefit from sustained, long-term therapy using the same, unchanged antimicrobial protocol.* Some people get better when they use the same antibiotic (or the same combination of antibiotics) for a long period of time. In other words, a Lyme doctor may place a patient on one or more specific drugs (or herbs) for months at a time, and that person will continue to improve for the entire duration of the treatment. Treatment changes are not required, or if they are required, they are not needed very often—perhaps one change every 3-6 months. For example, I know a woman who took Rifampin (an anti-Bartonella drug) along with Flagyl (an anti-

Borrelia drug) for nine months. She took this drug combination and nothing else, and she got well. It was that simple.

2. *Those who benefit from frequent changes in their antimicrobial treatment protocols.* I believe this to be a much more prevalent category of Lyme disease sufferers. During the early phases of treatment, someone in this category may be able to get away with using the same treatment for long periods of time. However, as these people near the last 10% of healing, they quickly realize that any new anti-microbial treatment will rapidly lose its effect. The pattern goes like this: A new antimicrobial treatment is initiated. Herxheimer reactions are experienced shortly thereafter. A short period of improvement is noted, and then after a short period of time (possibly a few days or a few weeks), all reactions to the treatment cease, and continued use of the treatment is clearly not producing additional benefits. If people in this category are not aware of this, and, instead, believe or are told by their doctors that they are in the prior category, they may end up using the same antimicrobial treatment for months, when, in fact, it is only beneficial for the first several days or weeks of use. During the latter phases of use of an ineffective treatment, these people may misinterpret randomly shifting symptoms as "baby steps of improvement," and they may falsely believe that they are "somehow on the long road to recovery." However, when these people are treated effectively, with rapidly rotated antimicrobial therapy, they will instead experience dramatic, unmistakable, and steady Herx reactions and progress. So, what is the lesson here? In most cases, a lack of dramatic progress and improvement indicates that whichever treatments you are using are not working well enough to be continued, and that a new course of action should be sought.

Again, personally, I fell into Category #2, and I believe that many Lyme disease sufferers also fall into this category—but many believe they are in the first category (wherein antibiotic therapy with the same agent for extended periods is helpful). Incorrect categorization is a result of many factors. First and foremost, changing up a treatment protocol frequently is hard work, especially if you are under the care of a healthcare practitioner and required to communicate with him or her during protocol changes. It is much easier for the doctor to select a drug or two and tell you to stay on it for a long time, in comparison with frequent drug changes, which would require ongoing communication and evaluation. The modern medical paradigm is built around the idea of minimizing the time needed to care for each individual patient, and a rapidly rotating treatment protocol is much less efficient for doctors. Patients who don't fit the system are generally seen as high maintenance, and doctors' offices only have so much time and resources to deal with these types of patients. Furthermore, with regard to patient compliance, a long-term, unchanging protocol fits much more nicely into the routine of your daily life. Doctors prefer the simple approach because their patients are more likely to comply with that kind of approach.

Rotating treatments rapidly is quite inconvenient and requires a near-constant analysis of one's treatment protocol: Which treatment should be used next? When is it time to switch? How is it possible to cope with the ongoing Herxheimer reactions that are created by frequent switching of therapies? How can one pay for the additional supplements and/or drugs that must be purchased? What about unknown side effects of new treatments? And the list of disadvantages and inconveniences only goes on from there. But you must remember one point: If the goal is to eradicate the infections, then the proper course of treatment should not be dependent upon what we think of as easier, more affordable, or more convenient. It should be based on what is best at eradicating the infections. In other words, getting well is hard work. The easiest path may not be the best path.

This topic may feel familiar to you. If you're experiencing a strange sense of déjà vu, it is probably because you have read *The Top 10 Lyme Disease Treatments,* the last book I wrote on Lyme disease. In that book, I introduced what I refer to as "the Antibiotic Rotation Protocol," which is based on, more or less, the same principles we've just seen in the preceding paragraphs. So, why am I bothering to repeat myself?

The answer is that I did not take the Antibiotic Rotation Protocol far enough. Even I, the author of the book that contains the protocol, could never have foreseen just how far the protocol needed to be taken to facilitate recovery, especially in the final stages of healing.

In fact, in many cases, the closer one gets to 100%, the more aggressive one must be in using the Antibiotic Rotation Protocol: antimicrobial treatments must be rotated or switched more often, they must be selected with more precision, and the available arsenal of treatments must be expanded. I will spend a lot of time in this book examining why this is true and how it should impact your treatment decisions, but you will quickly see that the rotation protocol as described in my past book is a little too slow and incomplete to fully encompass what is required to successfully complete the journey from "feeling a lot better" to "feeling close to well," or "feeling completely well." The good news is that the new principles are not incredibly different from what I wrote in the older book; instead, they are simply more developed now.

And, by no means do I take the credit for discovering the Antibiotic Rotation Protocol or the extent to which it must be used during the last 10% of healing. In fact, as I continued to research, communicate with Lyme sufferers, and read new available information, it became more and more clear that this was the direction that was working for many Lyme disease sufferers. There are several people who I have considered mentors during this illness, and they have independently come up with the same conclusion that I have in regard to this matter.

Of course, the assumption here is that you are one of the people who will benefit most from rapidly rotating treatments, and that you are even one of the people whose primary problem is infections. These assumptions may or may not describe you accurately, but they will be the premise upon which much of this book is based. Your own unique situation may require you to modify the protocols presented in this book. The good news for you, if you are one of the few people who don't require rapidly rotating treatments, is that by learning how to rapidly rotate your available treatments, you'll be more than prepared for a milder, simpler treatment protocol. Rapid rotation is the most difficult and challenging approach, so if you understand how to do it, any other method for treatment which you require should seem relatively easy. In other words, if you are one of those people who can get well by staying on the same course of treatment for a long time, then you've got a much easier road ahead of you than most Lyme patients, and the information in this book will only serve to hone and sharpen your knowledge base.

Finally, what it means to "rapidly" rotate your treatments will vary from person to person. For some people, this may mean rotating treatments as frequently as twice a week; for others, it may mean rotating them less frequently. We'll talk more about this later.

The Last 10% of Healing

One of the themes in this book, which you will see again and again, is "the last 10% of healing." It could also be described as "the final phases of healing," or "the last steps of recovery." I believe my prior books do a good job of addressing the first 90% of healing, or the initial phases of recovery. But as we will see, the final phases of recovery are not only different than the first phases, but also more difficult to accomplish.

Over the last several years, I've heard a common theme over and over again: "I'm feeling much better, I'm even stabilized, but I just can't seem to get completely well." I hear this from people who use many different treatment modalities. This common theme has been the impetus for my continued research on Lyme disease, and I believe if one examines this theme thoroughly, one would find that it contains a complex, important, and relatively new principle (a principle which will be part of the governing theme of this entire book):

> *The last 10% of healing is more difficult than the first 90% of healing. Many people are able to attain 90% of healing but not the last 10%. There may be many reasons for this, but one of the primary reasons is simply that the "low hanging fruit" of healing has already been grabbed. In other words, the problems that the body has had the easiest time getting rid of are what you successfully eliminated during the first 90% of your healing journey. It is only the deeply entrenched, difficult, and resistant problems that remain.*[3]

What does this mean? It means that your expectation of being over the hump at 90% healed and having an easy ride into the finish line, during which you can coast and rest, is an unrealistic expectation. In fact, unfortunately, the opposite is true. The last 10% of healing is as difficult if not more difficult than the first 90%, and you must be prepared to redouble your efforts, become even more organized with your treatments, and continue aggressive research in order to finish the race. It may be very challenging to be vigilant in this phase, because you may feel well enough to go about normal life and ignore your treatment program. Don't fall into that trap. Complacency now could mean serious backsliding.

Your last 10% of healing may be mostly about infections, or it may be mostly about non-infection problems. Either way, the last 10% of your journey will likely be the most difficult.

---

[3] The metric of 90% is somewhat arbitrary. You may be 70% well (or perhaps even 95% well) and these principles will still apply to you. Most people hit a point in their treatment where all the usual approaches stop working, and it is difficult to break through the invisible wall and make it all the way to the finish line. It is this distinction we are talking about here, and it doesn't always happen when a person is exactly 90% well.

There is some good news, though. Even though the last 10% of healing is very difficult and can feel like a full-time job, you will find the motivation you need because you will be feeling more frequent and intense glimpses of your prior good health. This will drive you to continue the fight. Additionally, as you get better, you will have more energy to spend on healing, and your brain will start to work better, so organizing your treatments and staying on track will become easier.

The following observations result from the fact that the last 10% of healing is more difficult to achieve than the first 90%:

1. New treatments, new information, and new books are very important tools for Lyme sufferers to utilize in order to successfully attain the last 10% of healing. It is incorrect to assume that the last 10% will happen with minimal research and action on the part of the patient, let alone on autopilot doing the same old treatments that got the person to 90% well. In fact, you may even spend more time, money and effort to attain the last 10% than you did the first 90%.

2. There are fewer guarantees in the last 10%. Since this territory of recovery often involves the most deeply entrenched problems in the body—the problems that have not yet responded to all of the many treatments someone has presumably used to get to 90% well—it can be concluded that the corrective measures necessary to get to 100% are more difficult to undertake and must be more precise, effective, and targeted than what was necessary for the first 90% of recovery. This leads to a brutal fact: those who are more resourceful, dedicated, and persistent will finish the race, while others may never achieve full health.

3. Chronic inflammation is often one of the final problems keeping people sick. Pay particular attention to chronic inflamma-

tion during the final 10% of healing. Watch for inflammatory foods, like sugar, refined carbohydrates, and foods which you are allergic to, as these can contribute to the vicious cycle of inflammation. Many of the pesky problems that won't go away during the final phases of healing can be solved or at least greatly improved if chronic inflammation is addressed rigorously.

The last 10% of healing is largely about experimenting to find out what supplements and treatments your body needs to correct subtle, underlying, damaging imbalances that have accrued over the years. Like a ship that is one degree off course and ends up hundreds of miles from its intended destination, so are the tiny imbalances in your body which, after years, result in huge problems. Similarly, if your final remaining problems are infections, these are sure to be the more entrenched, resistant, difficult-to-treat infections, so killing them will require some new strategies.

The Co-Infections

As mentioned previously, the Antibiotic Rotation Protocol, which was first described in my prior book, is still a central part of the recovery process. However, one big topic area which was incomplete in that book was the problem of co-infections. I greatly underestimated the importance of co-infections, and my previous books suffered from a complete vacuum of information on the topic. The rotation of anti-microbial therapies described in my past books did not include therapies targeted at the co-infections. The co-infections include Babesia, Bartonella, Mycoplasma, and others. Interestingly, they also include completely different kinds of organisms, such as nematode worms, yeast and fungal infections, intestinal parasites, and even other parasites which can exit the intestinal tract and infect other organs in the body—including the brain! All of these co-infections can play a huge and important role in the disease process, and ignoring them can cause a halt in recovery.

There were various reasons why I underestimated the co-infections. I just found it impossible to actually believe that thousands of people who are infected with Borrelia also, coincidentally, just happen to have the same set of rare and strange "co-infections" that all the Lyme doctors talk about. And it seemed equally as improbable that these co-infections were just as elusive, treatment-resistant, systemic, and unrecognized by conventional medicine as Borrelia. To believe that Borrelia alone fit that bill was a stretch of the imagination; but to also swallow the idea that there were all these "buddy" infections that come along with Borrelia in most or all Lyme disease sufferers? It seemed like blatant science fiction—highly unlikely at best.

I was wrong. The science fiction is true! The fact is that most Lyme disease sufferers do have co-infections and must address these infections in order to get well. In fact, I discovered that it is quite common for these co-infections to rear their heads during the last phases of healing, after Borrelia has been sufficiently weakened. When co-infections are present and untreated, an infinite amount of Borrelia-targeted treatment will be ineffective. In other words, finishing off Borrelia is impossible unless and until co-infections are addressed.

My realization of how important the co-infections are was further catalyzed by my recent study of scientific literature, which proves that many ticks do in fact harbor what researchers call "polymicrobial infections" (multiple infections). Numerous studies are available on PubMed that document this phenomenon, studies which weren't published yet when I wrote my first books. One of my mentors put it like this: "You should assume you have co-infections, even if you don't test positive for them and even if you don't now, and have never, experienced symptoms attributable to them. They will likely show up at some point during the recovery process, and while now may or may not be the right time to go after them, you should start researching them and preparing yourself for the eventuality that they will become a large part of your recovery process. They often rear their heads in the final phases of recovery." A different mentor said, "Many people who think they are over Lyme disease often experience a rude interruption in their remission, experienced as a mini-relapse, punctuated by never-before-experienced symptoms of co-infections like Babesia and Bartonella."

When Lyme disease and co-infections are all present together in your body, they work with each other synergistically for survival, and you end up with a "pathogen soup" that is very hard to eliminate. When one pathogen is attacked and its numbers are reduced, another is waiting in the wings to come out and take its place on center stage. Again, this collaboration between brainless bugs may seem like science fiction, but it is, instead, solid science. The scientific literature presents dozens of examples of bacterial colonies filled with different kinds of organisms that all work together for survival. It would be one of the most grave and dangerous mistakes to underestimate this phenomenon during the recovery process.

But there's more. We now know that all of the different kinds of bacteria and organisms within the infective colonies hide behind a protective shield, or slime layer, called "biofilm." This impenetrable membrane prevents antibacterial treatments from reaching the infections, and can even block human blood from getting into the infected areas, thus short-circuiting the healing that blood normally accomplishes. We will look more at these "biofilm communities" throughout the book. Some organisms are capable of actually producing the biofilm, while others take refuge in the shelter created by the biofilm. Organisms inside the biofilm communities all work together to perpetuate their survival. Toxins and debris can also exist inside the biofilm communities, creating an even bigger mess and a more robust enemy terrain.

The pathogen "merry go round" (as a friend and fellow researcher refers to it) occurs when you successfully suppress one type of infection, only to have another infection surface and become dominant. This is one of the reasons that rapid and continuous treatment rotation is required. Your rotation of treatments must always account for which infection is presently the most active. Strangely, it is typically the case that only one infection at a time is highly active. It is almost as if they take turns doing their damage to the body. One Lyme doctor refers to this active infection as the infection that is "on top." If you think of healing from Lyme disease as peeling layers off of an onion, you can visualize the exposed layer of the onion as the one that is "on top," and once that layer is peeled off, another layer (or type of infection) will take the position of being "on top." The amount of time it takes to peel a layer off the onion can vary greatly, and any given infection can be "on top" for anywhere between a day or two to several months or years. Whether brief or long-term, the dominant infection can change rapidly at any time. Also, the same infection can become active and "on top" multiple times before it is eliminated. The later in the recovery process you are, the faster this rotation seems to take place. One top Lyme doctor made the following statement:

> *My patients commonly experience what they perceive as "relapses." But in actuality, these are not relapses, but instead co-infections rearing their ugly heads toward the final stages of recovery, after Borrelia has been considerably weakened. These occurrences can result in violent and extreme symptom changes. The co-infections often cause more intense, extreme, and rapidly changing symptoms than does Borrelia itself. Studious patients can distinguish between their Borrelia, Bartonella, and Babesia symptoms, and in some cases, the differences between symptoms can be quite obvious and pronounced. Since the treatments needed for each infection are completely different, it is important to know which infection is dominant and which treatments target that infection. Otherwise, improvement will come to an immediate halt.*

Often, co-infection symptoms do not emerge and become distinct until the background noise of Borrelia itself is turned down low enough to be able to pick out the peculiar and unique symptoms associated with co-infections. Of course, some people experience the distinct symptoms of co-infections early on in their sickness. Everyone is different, and there is no one-size-fits-all rule. One thing is for sure, though: co-infections, like

Babesia and Bartonella, can often be identified by their unique symptom sets; for example, Babesia is typically associated with dizziness, night sweats, "air hunger," low-grade fever, and a feeling of being detached from reality.

Some Lyme disease sufferers know how to effectively fight one kind of infection, but when another surfaces, they may spend weeks, months, or even years, in a stalemate (or even getting worse), because they aren't equipped to deal with that particular infection. Therefore, as the infections take their turns on center stage, you have to be ever-ready, waiting with just the right, targeted antimicrobial treatment for the particular infection that might surface next. You also have to have studied the available treatments enough to know which therapy works for which infection. I wasn't kidding when I told you that the last 10% of healing is complex and difficult!

But there's more to this true science fiction. When co-infections are attacked, particularly Babesia and Bartonella, any remaining Borrelia becomes immediately weakened and susceptible to treatment with regular anti-Borrelia therapies. This may be experienced in the following way: A person may have been successfully targeting Borrelia and feeling better and better, and then, all of a sudden, plateau in their progress. Old Borrelia treatments will stop working, and improvement will slow or halt. At this point, if a co-infection has taken center stage, symptoms will likely begin to shift and feel very unlike Borrelia symptoms. If that co-infection is successfully treated, and the person returns to attacking Borrelia, all of a sudden, the anti-Borrelia treatments that were used previously will have renewed usefulness, and the person may notice accelerated killing of, and improvement from, Borrelia. In a sense, the co-infections help to hide Borrelia, and when they are removed, Borrelia is again vulnerable. It is important to know this; otherwise, you may be confused when you experience big Herxheimer reactions to anti-Borrelia treatments immediately following co-infection therapy. And the most important lesson to learn here is that the perfect time to attack any remaining Borrelia is immediately following a campaign against co-infections.

In summary, co-infection treatment is very important during Lyme disease recovery. Additionally, the vast majority of Lyme disease sufferers are infected with co-infections, so this is something that shouldn't be ignored. We will be looking more at co-infection treatment throughout the book.

Supporting the Body During Recovery

I know I said that people whose problems are primarily caused by infections shouldn't get too sidetracked by supportive treatments like nutrition, detoxification, hormonal balancing, and other ancillary aspects of treatment. I am remiss to pile more on your already full to-do list for treating Lyme disease, but these other areas of treatment must be addressed more thoroughly during the last 10% of healing. Although infections may be your primary problem, there are likely also many deeply entrenched health problems that you may finally need to face at this point in the journey. Hopefully, you've already begun to address things like past emotional trauma, heavy metal toxicity, diet and nutritional optimization, physical exercise, and nutrient supplementation by this point in your healing. If not, it is time to address these things. We will look at many of these items in this book, or at least provide some references on where you can go for important information.

A great example of this kind of health issue is gluten sensitivity. One well-known Lyme doctor has said that upwards of 95% of his patients improve rapidly when they eliminate gluten from their diets. During the first 90% of healing, gluten removal may not result in much noticeable symptom improvement, because the body is completely overwhelmed and overburdened by a dozen other problems. However, during the last phases of healing, gluten avoidance may produce profound benefits. If someone ignored this issue and kept their focus on just the infections, their tunnel vision would be preventing them from a huge leap in improvement. Of course, gluten avoidance, even before the final phases of recovery, would be very beneficial. But the point is that the benefits from these kinds of fine-tuning supportive therapies are particularly pronounced during the last 10% of healing.

So, if you are currently in the final phases of recovery, make sure you leave no stone unturned. Supportive therapies, which may have provided minimal benefit earlier in your recovery process, may now begin to have profound impact.

Why is It So Hard to Get Better?

Let's take a look at the tangled mess that is Lyme disease and find out why it is so difficult to get better.

Lyme disease is characterized by a peculiarity: the sickest people, with the most deeply entrenched infections, may not actually be exhibiting extreme symptoms. This is because, once the infections establish their colonies and presence within the body, they can become walled off within their biofilm communities, living in a separate, enemy-occupied space, unreachable by the immune system and antibacterial treatments. If your infections and toxicities are left alone without treatment for long enough, the body reaches a sort of homeostasis, or equilibrium, wherein you may feel a lot better than you actually are.

In other words, a person who has not yet treated their infective colonies aggressively may only be experiencing symptoms which are the tip of the iceberg. The infections can become established in a stealthy and quiet fashion, and it is only when you begin to remove them that you realize how bad they really are. This is quite different from most other kinds of health problems, wherein your feeling of how sick you are is pretty closely tied to the reality of how sick you are.

This leads us to a very important principle: At all times, you are either adding layers to the onion or peeling them off, and, unfortunately, adding them is often a rather comfortable process while peeling them away is highly uncomfortable and painful. Removing them is painful because as they are removed, we experience inflammation and toxicity as a result of our immune systems killing the infections and as a result of the toxins which are released when they are killed. Therefore the natural tendency is to allow the layers to pile up rather than keep toiling to remove them. Because we generally prefer comfort over pain, this is, unfortunately, the case.

To make matters even more complex, the process of removing the layers from the onion may be irreversible, and you may find that there's no turning back. This wouldn't be a problem, except that with the removal of each layer, there is a new battle to be fought, whether you are ready or not. When you effectively penetrate the biofilm, start killing the infections, and start "mixing the pot," you may ignite a process that takes on a life of its own. The happily protected infections may come out, go berserk, and begin to multiply and proliferate if you don't kill them. Dormant infections and hidden toxicities may rear their ugly heads and demand attention. When this happens, you will be required to engage in aggressive treatments—if you don't, new layers may begin to form and strengthen, causing more and more havoc. The released infections and toxicities will not simply go away on their own. Instability may become the new normal. Once you make the decision to attack the infectious colonies and peel layers, there may be no turning back. So you are faced with a paradox, of sorts: allow the infections to happily exist behind biofilm and abandon your mission to completely eradicate them, or attack them and risk getting sicker? Of course, the correct course of action is to attack the layers of the infection—but only when you are ready, and only when you have the appropriate tools and treatments lined up and ready to go.

The above observations allow us to glean a lot of useful information about Lyme disease. One of the things we can see is just how hard it is to actually get better from this affliction. Because Lyme disease symptoms are typically not disabling or life-threatening, but instead more chronic and persistent, no urgency is felt by the patient, medical establishment, or family and friends, at least not the same kind of urgency one experiences when presented with a heart attack, broken leg, seizure, or similar acute emergency. Yet, if nothing is done, a person with Lyme disease will get progressively worse, and their infections and toxicities will become increasingly entrenched. And, ironically, even the sickest Lyme sufferers can feel much healthier than they actually are.

So, patients typically don't get the natural support circle that forms for someone with, say, cancer—instead, you are left to get worse and feel increasingly helpless, and even question the validity of your condition. In my view this is the main causative factor behind Lyme-related suicides. Yes, Lyme infection itself causes psychiatric manifestations which include suicidal ideation and severe depression, but these symptoms are only compounded by the lack of support most Lyme sufferers are faced with.

There you have it—some of the reasons why Lyme disease is so difficult to heal from. I don't introduce this discussion to discourage you, but instead to help you better understand this disease, so you will be more prepared to handle the challenges that you will be faced with. If you are a caretaker or loved one reading this book, I hope you will use this information to provide needed support for the person suffering from Lyme disease, even if this whole subject is new to you, and it doesn't make complete sense to you.

The Rubber Band Principle

One of the realities of writing another Lyme disease book is the requirement for me to correct or update statements which were made in my previous books. In some cases, this correction may be only a slight modification to a previous statement; in other cases, it may be a complete do-over. The Rubber Band Principle is one such area where a do-over is needed; a belief I held in the past has been turned on its head by recent research and new information.

In my prior book, *Lyme Disease & Rife Machines* (page 46), the following statement is made:

> Additionally, the ideal treatment must not rely on an intricate and delicate protocol that requires the user to take dozens of supplements and conform to dozens of lifestyle restrictions. These protocols, with regard to Lyme disease, are almost always ineffective because they are typically an attempt to control the symptoms of disease instead of restoring the body's ability to eliminate the disease. Although taking supplements and rebalancing the body is important, over-complicated treatment protocols are a strong indication that the root cause of the problem has been missed. If the root cause of the disease was effectively treated, dozens of supplements would not be necessary to correct disturbances and imbalances in the body because the root problem would no longer be present to cause those disturbances and imbalances.

While many parts of this statement still reflect my current view of Lyme disease treatment, at the time I wrote that book, I was not aware of what I now refer to as the Rubber Band Principle.

Rubber bands like to rest. They don't like being stretched. You can stretch a rubber band if you apply force to it, but if you release the force, the rubber band will predictably condense back into its smaller, resting position. The further you stretch it, the more energy is required to hold it there. In essence, rubber bands want to be in a resting state, and they exert a great deal of energy in opposition to any effort you apply against this state.

The human body is like a rubber band. It can experience some conditions, or states, that it likes to maintain, and others that it exerts energy to prevent. For example, let's consider the condition of health; this is like the "resting" rubber band. When the body is healthy, it wants to stay that way, and it will exert effort and energy to ensure that the state of health isn't changed. The healthy, or resting state, is a state of homeostasis when "all is well" within the body. If you try to "stretch" the body into a disease condition, the body will fight back, similarly to how a rubber band will resist you if you try to stretch it.

When all internal and external circumstances are ideal, not much energy is needed in order for the body to maintain health (to maintain homeostasis). For healthy people, the simple acts of eating nutritious food, sleeping, and drinking water will allow the body to maintain its basic state of health. Healthy people who get an acute illness, such as the common cold, become stretched rubber bands—the body (or rubber band) will begin doing everything in its power to get back to a state of health, or a state of homeostasis. The body of someone with a common cold wants to return to health so badly that it begins to fight the cold using various methods: You may experience a fever; you may experience fatigue; you may experience loss of appetite; and you may experience greater-than-normal thirst. Getting well becomes the body's primary priority, and a great deal of energy is expended by the body to allow it to return to its relaxed, or healthy state. When you have the common cold and your rubber band is stretched, the body will experience a tension until the cold is resolved and the rubber band is again resting.

Here's where we run into a problem. The situation changes when we talk about chronic illnesses. People with chronic illnesses have bodies that were, for whatever reason, unable to win the fight against the disease when it was in its acute stage. The body did everything it could to thwart the attack, but eventually lost the battle. The new homeostasis then became a sick state. The body learns to accept the diseased state, and the rubber band (or human body) is in its resting position not when healthy, but when sick! This is exactly what happens with Lyme disease. Consequently, for people with chronic illness, in order to get healthy, you have to stretch the rubber band—that is, apply energy to it when it is in its resting state. Coercing the body back to health will actually require you to stretch the rubber band; otherwise, the resting state will remain as a sick state. In this way, chronic illness has the opposite effect that acute illness has.

So how does this connect with the above-quoted excerpt from *Lyme Disease & Rife Machines*? In that book, I made the statement that we shouldn't need overly complex treatment protocols to recover from chronic disease, because the body will want to recover on its own, and it will do everything it can to achieve recovery. And, this would have been true had we been talking about acute illnesses. However, based on the Rubber Band Principle, and because we are talking about chronic, not acute, illness, it is clear that we must expend a great deal of energy to coerce the body out of its natural sickly homeostasis and into a new homeostasis of health. I wish I could tell you that this is an easy process. It is not. We may need to address many factors in order to get back to health, including, for example, gluten sensitivity, food allergies, various kinds of toxins, mold exposure, sleep disturbances, infections, hormonal problems, inflammation, nutrition, genetic weaknesses and predispositions, and various other things. We must make a conscious effort to support the body in just about every area of our lives in order to reverse the sickly homeostasis which has become the norm for our body. We must stretch the rubber band away from its resting position and maintain that tension, or pressure, until a new state of health can be achieved, sustained, and perpetuated.

Of course, the Rubber Band Principle isn't a perfect analogy and doesn't completely describe every aspect of Lyme disease recovery. It is simply an illustration intended to show you that hard work is required to beat Lyme disease, whereas hard work is not required to beat a common cold.

The hardest thing about getting well from Lyme disease is that you have to keep pushing in a lot of directions. It's totally counterintuitive in comparison to how the body heals almost any other sickness, injury, or health problem. When you have the common cold, you don't really need to do anything at all. Just sit back, relax, and you'll get well. But, if your body is perfectly happy living in harmony with millions of invasive Lyme and co-infection bacteria in all your organs, you will have to be the one to change that; it will not happen automatically.

This new perspective on healing is very important. If you assume the body will get better all by itself, you might end up foregoing important treatments that can help you to get well. If, on the other hand, you realize that the battle is yours to fight, and that many action steps are required, you will properly focus energy, attention, and resources into the recovery process, and you will get better much faster.

Fortunately, as one gets better and better and closer to recovery, the amount of work required to maintain health decreases. The body will again find its correct, healthy state of homeostasis. So, the battle isn't infinite. But, the initial stages of the battle are quite rough, and it will take a lot of work to get past those initial stages.

Now that we've covered some of the lessons of the last five years, let's turn our attention to some of the nuts and bolts required in building our treatment template.

Chapter 3
The Antibiotic Rotation Protocol, Revamped and Revisited, with New Principles for Use

"The underlying causes of Lyme disease are diverse and complex. Therefore, a multifaceted healing approach is necessary. You won't find any single silver bullet treatment, because there is no single underlying cause in the Lyme disease complex."

Important Notes About This Chapter

This chapter is one of the most important chapters in the book. It will serve as the foundation for our treatment template. This treatment template will dictate how most of the treatments in the book should be used. This chapter will not list or describe specific treatments; instead, the chapter will provide the outline which governs how to use the treatment protocols and individual treatments described in Part 2 and Part 3 of the book.

Also, the title "Antibiotic Rotation Protocol" is a bit inaccurate. In actuality, this chapter talks about rotating all kinds of treatments, not just antimicrobial treatments. However, I decided not to change the name of the chapter because my past books refer to this treatment philosophy as the "Antibiotic Rotation Protocol," and I feel that maintaining this consistency is valuable in providing a cohesive transition from my past books to this one. Simply note, though, that this concept of rotating treatments is not limited to antibiotics, nor is it limited to other kinds of antimicrobial treatments. It can also be applied to other areas of the recovery process, including supportive and nutritional therapies (its use for these other purposes will be discussed).

Introduction

As years pass and more research is conducted on Lyme disease, top experts are beginning to agree on one key point: "Lyme disease," as we call it, isn't caused by a single factor; Borrelia burgdorferi is only one of the underlying problems in people with Lyme disease. For this reason, it is more accurate to refer to Lyme disease as the "Lyme disease complex," or, perhaps, by the phrase coined by now-famous Lyme doctor Richard Horowitz, MD: "Multiple Systemic Infectious Diseases Syndrome," or "MSIDS" for short. Regardless of what you prefer to call it, the Lyme disease complex involves multiple infections and multiple dysfunctions within the body. It is for this reason that I don't see the invention or discovery of any single silver bullet cure on the horizon. It is also for this reason that modern medicine will likely be greatly delayed in finding a cure for Lyme disease, since modern medicine is dependent upon clinical trials, and clinical trials usually aim to only evaluate one single variable at a time. Because Lyme disease has so many variables, clinical trials are likely not the best vehicle by which to study the disease; we need a holistic, all-encompassing approach. Grasping this multifaceted nature of Lyme disease is a good jumping off point to begin our discussion of the Antibiotic Rotation Protocol.

In a prior Lyme disease book I wrote, *The Top 10 Lyme Disease Treatments,* I introduced a method for using antibiotics (both pharmaceutical and herbal) that I call the "Antibiotic Rotation Protocol." The basic logic for use of this protocol is that the infection(s) inside the body quickly become resistant to any given antimicrobial treatment, so the treatment in use must be changed often in order to stay ahead of the infection(s) (we will soon see that "resistance" doesn't quite describe what is happening, though). When a particular antimicrobial treatment is used, it catches the infections off guard, but they quickly adapt to the treatment. Using the same treatment for too long not only results in decreased effectiveness, but also increased side effects, since most treatments become less and less tolerable the longer they are used.

With the addition of modern research and patient experiences that have become available since I first wrote about the protocol, it is now clear that the Antibiotic Rotation Protocol is even more important than I had believed when I wrote about it several years ago. It is especially important during the last 10% of healing. In fact, the strategy of rotating treatment methods should be at the core of most Lyme disease treatment protocols, and, accordingly, it is at the core of this book. I will not make the claim that this methodology will work for everyone; it likely will not, but based on my research, it is one of the best methodologies available at the time this book was written.

In simplified terms, there are two opposing camps of Lyme physicians: those who advocate staying on the same treatment protocol for months or even years, and those who recognize that treatments should be rotated immediately after a "plateau"[4] is reached. As time passes, I'm finding that more and more Lyme doctors are moving to the latter camp.

---

[4] The word "plateau" refers to the cessation of benefit and Herxheimer reactions attained from any given treatment. When killing Lyme disease organisms, the pattern is generally as follows: When a given treatment is first initiated, Herxheimer reactions will occur as Lyme organisms are dying. After the Herxheimer reactions fade, a patient will experience improvement in their symptoms. Finally, the last phase in the cycle is the "plateau," which occurs when the infection becomes resistant to the treatment in use, and improve-

The term "rotate" in the context of the Antibiotic Rotation Protocol simply means to change over to a new treatment or protocol once a plateau in progress is reached. In this chapter, you'll see that I've made some significant improvements and modifications to the original Antibiotic Rotation Protocol which I set forth in my past writings. For the purposes of our discussion here, we are talking about all different kinds of antibacterial treatments, including pharmaceutical antibiotics, herbal antibiotics, and other anti-infective interventions. We'll also look at the Antibiotic Rotation Protocol as applied to therapies that aren't targeted toward infections.

Basic Concepts Underpinning the Antibiotic Rotation Protocol

We will now look at a few basic concepts which underpin the Antibiotic Rotation Protocol. If these concepts look familiar, that is because many of them were presented in *The Top 10 Lyme Disease Treatments*. I do not see this repetition as a waste of your time. Instead, I see it as good news that the treatment strategy I presented in that book needs only to be refined here, instead of replaced.

1. When we talk about "peeling layers off of the onion" as an analogy for understanding Lyme disease treatment, we aren't just speaking metaphorically. The infection actually does have layers, and deeper layers of the infectious colonies do not get hit by the antibiotics or antimicrobial herbs you are currently using. Visit the following website and scroll down toward the bottom of the page to see a picture of a Lyme disease bacterial

---

ment in symptoms ceases. Backsliding of symptoms or even a relapse of symptoms may occur at this point. The topic of the plateau, and what to do about it, is one of the main themes of this book. Experiencing a plateau (that is, a cessation of both Herxheimer reactions and improvement) should be the trigger to rotate, or switch, to a new Lyme disease treatment.

colony: http://www.lymebook.com/top10forms—this picture will demonstrate the layered appearance and configuration of Lyme disease colonies.

2. Old treatments that stopped working may again become effective as previously sheltered layers of the infection eventually get exposed and become reachable by new rounds of treatment. I can't emphasize enough how important this point is, and how important it is to revisit treatments you haven't used in a long time. As new layers of infection become exposed, old treatments can be critically useful and can take on a whole new life in your treatment program.

3. The majority of available treatments will have the most benefit immediately after they are begun, and benefit will decrease the longer they are used. Similarly, their side effects will be at their lowest point immediately after they are begun, and side effects will increase the longer the treatment is used. Therefore, the most favorable ratio of side effects to benefits will be experienced early during the course of their use, and that same cost-to-benefit ratio will become less and less desirable over time. This provides an additional reason to favor rotating treatments instead of using the same treatments continuously.

4. In most cases, when a treatment stops working, it is not because the organisms you were targeting have become resistant to the treatment. Instead, it is likely that a different type of microbe (or co-infection) has become the dominant layer of the infection, and whichever treatment you were just using doesn't effectively target that microbe. This changing of dominant microbes has been called "the merry-go-round effect," or "musical chairs," as each species of pathogen takes its turn in the spotlight. Although I have sometimes referred to the decreasing effectiveness of a given treatment as "resistance," that explanation is only used for the sake of simplicity. In real-

ity, it is very important to understand what is actually happening here, as described in this paragraph. Because true bacterial resistance isn't occurring, most treatments will still have usefulness again, later in the recovery process.

5. Rotating treatments is even more important during the last 10% of the recovery process. As has been noted earlier in the book, the last 10% of the recovery process can be much more difficult than the first 90%. The stalemate you experience with the infections will be more intense, more difficult to overcome, and more frustrating. You will need to mix things up even more than you have in the past, and when you think you've done all the mixing you can, you'll have to mix it up some more. It is encouraging to remember that the stalemate isn't permanent, and the bacteria are not completely resilient in the face of your treatments. The infections can be killed, but only if you get more aggressive and rotate more new treatments than ever before. This is what gets you over the hump for the last 10% of healing.

The above points serve as the foundation for our discussion of the Antibiotic Rotation Protocol.

Extending the Rotational Protocol Beyond Antimicrobial Therapies

So, by now we can see the logic in rotating antimicrobial treatments. But here, I will introduce a completely new concept which I haven't written about to date, but which I think is accurate under many circumstances: Anti-infective treatments aren't the only treatments which may need to be rotated. Supportive therapies, too, can also be rotated according to the current symptoms/problems being experienced. As you unpeel layers of infections from the onion, you will find that each different infectious layer can occupy different body tissues, organs, and systems, so the collateral damage to bodily functions will vary greatly depending on which locations contain the active infections. This is a profound realization. In the past, we've just sort of assumed that the supportive treatments we use during Lyme disease recovery should be roughly the same throughout the entire healing journey. We've always thought that supportive interventions should just be continued in an ongoing fashion, regardless of which layer of the onion we were currently fighting. While it may be true that some kinds of supportive treatments—like detoxification, hormone balancing, and nutritional supplementation—are, in fact, needed continuously, there will be other supportive interventions that are desperately needed at certain times throughout the recovery process, but which are unneeded and can even be burdensome during other times.

For example, one particular layer of the onion may uncover adrenal issues, while another layer may uncover heart or circulatory issues. As a result, both antimicrobial as well as supportive therapies should be tailored and customized to the specific layer being addressed. We will look more closely at this concept throughout the book, but it is a very important building block for a complete understanding of the recovery process. Why is it important? Because the variability in affected organs and body locations explains the confusing experience of having certain kinds of symptoms wax and wane, and come and go. Also, understanding the transient nature of collateral damage relieves us of the burdensome feeling that we should be taking every different kind of supplement at all times throughout the recovery process.

I spoke with one Lyme disease sufferer who began to have severe adrenal fatigue issues right when he started treating his Bartonella infection. He had to take extreme measures to address the adrenal fatigue, utilizing treatments which have nothing to do with antimicrobials. So, he was treating Bartonella, and, at the same time, using supportive therapies which address adrenal fatigue, because both of these problems were part of the same layer of the onion. It turns out that many Lyme disease sufferers notice that Bartonella, in particular, can activate adrenal issues. Accordingly, when dealing with Bartonella infection, adrenal support is often greatly needed. However, at later times throughout the recovery process, when Bartonella isn't front and center, adrenal issues may fade into the background and be replaced with the need to support other organ systems. Let me tell you: The experience of fighting Lyme disease can be completely overwhelming and confusing if you aren't aware that this kind of scenario can take place. When adrenal support is needed, you had better use it; otherwise, your recovery will be greatly stalled. However, when adrenal support is not needed, focusing heavily on the adrenals will take your time, attention, and money away from other areas that have a greater need for attention.

You can now begin to see a theme emerging: we should be deciding which antimicrobial treatments are needed at each given time throughout the recovery process, and at the same time, asking ourselves which supportive therapies should be paired with those antimicrobial treatments. As you read about the protocols and treatments in Part 2 and Part 3, keep this in mind, and try to select both the best antimicrobial therapy as well as the best supportive therapy for the particular issues you happen to be dealing with today. And remember, the picture will soon change and you will soon need to reevaluate.

Your physiological responses to the infections in your body will be unique, so the supportive therapies you require may be different from those required by other Lyme sufferers. You may have certain kinds of organ dysfunction that persist throughout the entire recovery process, and other kinds which come and go according to which infections you are addressing. The key lesson here is to stay in tune with your body, so you can determine which organs are most stressed.

Rotating Supportive Therapies: Further Discussion

We've established that antimicrobial therapies aren't the only kinds of treatments which should be rotated—supportive treatments, too, may also have the best effect when rotated instead of used continuously. Now let's look at some questions which are a bit more challenging.

What about supportive therapies that don't necessarily correspond to any given layer of the onion? What about general supportive therapies, like immune-stimulating supplements, hormone balancing protocols, adaptogenic herbs, and anti-inflammatory substances? Should all of these types of therapies be rotated, too? It is easy to see why some supportive treatments should only be used when they are needed for specific layers of the onion, but what about treatments which just can't be assigned to a specific kind of organ dysfunction?

There is no shortage of information on beneficial supplements and how they can help you, but there is a scarcity of information on how, when and how often these supplements should be used.

While many doctors and researchers advocate continuously using various supportive therapies, I would like to make an argument for using even these more general treatments on a rotational basis. As you will see, my reasons here are different than my reasons for rotating antimicrobial therapies, and even different than my reasons for rotating supportive therapies targeted to specific layers of the onion.

Please note that the following information is theoretical, and people may respond differently to various supportive protocols, so a "one-size-fits-all" approach should never be adopted. Your job in reading this information will be to decide, often via trial and error, which approach is most helpful for your individual and unique needs and situation. Also note that my own results and my own interpretation of information will not be accurate for everyone.

Personally, I have responded more favorably to the rotation of not just antibacterial therapies, but also general supportive therapies, such as nutrient supplementation, herbal immune boosters, anti-inflammatory compounds, and even therapies like the KPU protocol (the KPU protocol is composed of several different vitamins and minerals, see Chapter 9 for more information). You, too, may have noticed a pattern in your own recovery process wherein you find yourself moving through protocols and not sticking with all of them forever.

We must ask the question: If general supportive therapies are providing benefit, why not continue them forever? What are the disadvantages of doing so? If we establish some disadvantages of continuous use of supportive modalities, it will set the stage for us to examine the advantages of rotating them.

Let's start with an important statement: Some types of nutritional supplements, including nutrients which become deficient in Lyme disease sufferers, might need to be taken continuously. Examples may include vitamin C, B vitamins, Coenzyme Q-10, omega fatty acids, a multivitamin product, probiotics, and others. I am by no means implying that such core supplements should always be rotated. Likewise, certain herbs such as milk thistle may also best be taken continuously due to the ongoing stress experienced by the liver throughout the healing process.

However, here's the key point: The list of supplements proven to be helpful to Lyme sufferers is much, much longer than these few items. Hundreds, if not thousands, of different herbs, supplements, and products have been found to be useful during the recovery process. When you read the section of the book on liver support (see Chapter 15), you will see that when the liver is strained, you have a dozen proven supplement options for liver support. There are dozens of supplements that may be used for immune system support. There are dozens of supplements available for other aspects of healing, such as detoxification, hormone balancing, fatigue, intestinal flora balancing, etc. And we haven't even scratched the surface yet! There are adaptogenic herbs, homeopathic remedies, Chinese formulas, and so much more! When you add them all up, the list of helpful supplements available to you can be mind-boggling and extensive, even when we are talking about generalized supportive therapies.

I have spoken with many Lyme disease sufferers, and a majority of them feel a sense of angst and anxiety about which supplements to take, and when. Many people feel like they won't get well unless they take as many supplements as possible. The inconvenience and financial cost of taking so many pills can be overwhelming. So, the primary reason why continuous use of supportive treatments may not be optimal is the simple reality that there are literally hundreds of beneficial products, but using them all continuously can be incredibly impractical, even impossible. If you have limited money and limited time to organize your supplements— limitations which apply to most of us—then the discussion could end right here, since it is quite simply impossible to take hundreds of supplements at once.

But let's look even deeper into the issue. I would like to make the argument that, even if you had unlimited financial resources, and even if you had your own personal assistant to manage and administer your supplementation program, it would still be inadvisable to take huge amounts of supplements for extended periods of time. Some readers may intuitively agree with my position yet be unable to articulate the reasons why they agree with me, so I will present the logic behind this position.

How Over-Supplementation Can Retard the Body's Own Healing Energy

The Rubber Band principle in the previous chapter illustrates how the human body naturally and automatically attempts to maintain equilibrium, but in the case of chronic illness, this equilibrium may, unfortunately, be a sick state, instead of a healthy state. It is our goal, then, to provide the body with the tools and resources necessary to cause a shift from an unhealthy equilibrium back to a healthy equilibrium.

Let's look at why supplements should be used only temporarily and only a few supplements at a time.

1. The argument for **temporary use** of supplements: The purpose of most supplementation should be to provide the body with a temporary boost in resources in order to re-attain healthy equilibrium. Once the body has successfully utilized those resources (or supplements) and healthy equilibrium has been attained, the supplements can be discontinued. Ongoing use of the supplements after healthy equilibrium is attained will not strengthen that equilibrium but will, instead, threaten it. One way to understand this is to think about a person with a broken leg. When you have a broken leg, a cast is necessary to provide support while the bones are healing. But, if you never took the cast off after the leg healed, you would be causing damage, not healing. The cast needs to come off so the leg can be strengthened and regain its natural, healthy flexibility and utility. The same is true with the human body: ongoing, unending supplementation prevents the body from engaging its own healing energy and blocks the body from regaining its natural equilibrium.

2. The argument for using only **a few supplements at a time:** As the body journeys back to a healthy equilibrium, it cannot

deal simultaneously with all of the obstacles in its way. The body has a limited capacity for healing specific health problems. A healthcare practitioner who I have come to respect for his vast wisdom and insight explains it as follows: The body is typically only dealing with one major problem at a time. This may be an infection, a toxicity, or an imbalance of some kind. This primary problem can be thought of as the "top," or outermost, layer of the onion which we must help the body remove using supportive therapies (remember, the onion we are unpeeling contains not only infections, but also many other kinds of non-infectious dysfunctions). Ideally, we can become aware of which problems the body is currently dealing with and use supplements and treatments to support the body in the healing of those particular problems. Knowing which symptoms are associated with which health problems can aid in identifying the layer of the onion with which the body is currently dealing. If you are taking dozens of supplements for dozens of different health problems, the body may become overwhelmed and have difficulty dealing with whichever problem is currently the primary problem. In fact, the superfluous supplements may actually start to impede the body instead of help it—they can have not just a neutral effect, but a negative effect. So, instead of the "shotgun" approach where we are trying to address all problems at the same time, it is much better to figure out which problem the body is working on and provide focused, targeted, specific support for that particular battle. In other words, it is much more beneficial to take a few of the most needed supplements rather than many of the potentially beneficial supplements.

Now that we understand the importance of using supplements temporarily and only a few at a time, the next question we must address is the following: How does one know when—or even if—a given supplement has succeeded in helping the body re-attain equilibrium, and consequently, when that supplement should be discontinued? There is no easy answer to this question. Some people are able to perceive when a given supplement is helping them. If you are one of these people, the task will be easier for you; the supplement can be discontinued after that perceived help is no longer experienced. If you are unable to perceive or feel what a supplement is doing inside your body, it will be your job, along with your trusted physician (and possibly with the help of lab work), to figure out how long a given supplement is useful. Energetic testing and muscle testing can be very helpful when making this determination. I cannot provide an easy step-by-step guide for this topic here, as the correct path is influenced by individual differences among the Lyme disease population.

At this point, many skeptics will be silently (or audibly) yelling at me: "This advice you are giving here is dangerous… if helpful supplements are discontinued, won't the problems they solved just return?" My answer is that yes, perhaps some problems will return. But my goal here is to address a real problem which demands a solution: there are literally thousands of beneficial supplements out there, and we can't use them all at the same time!

If problems do recur at a later date, you can always return to the supplements which helped you in the past. If the body was unable to maintain equilibrium without the help of supplements, those supplements may be needed intermittently to maintain progress. Still, though, it is best in most cases to avoid using supportive interventions continuously and to, instead, only use them as needed. The body should be left alone as much as possible to use its own healing energy to maintain equilibrium. As a general rule, the fewer supplements you are taking, the better. Only the most helpful supplements should be used at any given time, and less helpful supplements should be discontinued until they are truly needed.

By now you've read a lot about the logic behind rotating supportive therapies—both specific supportive therapies targeted at particular organ systems as well as general supportive therapies which provide multi-organ support. Please keep in mind that the correct course of action with regard to this topic in your own healing journey may be different from what is presented here. This information is not one-size-fits all; it must be customized to your own unique situation and needs. I can't give you all the answers, but I can give you tools and strategies for addressing the very challenging question of which supplements to take and for how long to take them.

Before moving on, let's take a look at a few final reasons why the rotation of supportive therapies may be beneficial:

1. Many supplements have side effects, interactions, and other undesirable effects—especially when they are combined with other supplements and used for extended periods. I have spoken with people who are taking dozens of supplements and only begin to actually feel better when they reduce the number of supplements that they are consuming. The more supplements and products you are taking at one time, the more likely it is that you will suffer from interactions or side effects from those products. Remember, everything you swallow must be processed by and eliminated from the body. Heavy supplementation can place a great deal of strain on organs like the liver, kidneys, and intestinal tract.

2. Various doctors and researchers have documented the phenomenon in which the body becomes "resistant" to all kinds of supplements. This is not the same kind of resistance displayed by infections that are treated with antibacterial therapies. Instead, the body simply adjusts to a given supplement and the supplement no longer has a positive effect. If the supplement is continued past the point at which this occurs, no benefit will be realized, yet the financial costs, inconvenience, and possible side effects/interactions will continue. On the other hand, if the supplement is

discontinued for a period of time and then restarted, these problems will be avoided. This concept is similar to the strategy that athletes use during training, in which workouts are switched up and varied so the body does not adjust to a stagnant training schedule. The phenomenon of supplements having decreasing benefit over time appears to be true with the majority of supplements Lyme sufferers use, including some nutrients, detox agents, herbs, and other treatments. Discontinuing supplements when the body becomes "resistant" will give the body a chance to engage its own healing energy to get back on its feet and maintain a healthy equilibrium. This concept boils down to the very simple fact that the body will only temporarily need the helping hand provided by most kinds of supplements. After the body gets what it needs from the supplement in question, the body is ready to move on to attack a different problem.

3. After the body has utilized supplements to attain equilibrium, the very supplements that aided in this process may actually start to cause an imbalance in the opposite direction from the original problem. For example, in the case of nutrient deficiency, the body may have a genuine need for supplementation with a given nutrient. Yet, if too much supplementation is given, a nutrient imbalance may begin to occur in the other direction; that is, the supplemented nutrient may begin to block the absorption of other needed nutrients, and a secondary imbalance might be the result. This scenario can be seen when supplementing with zinc during the KPU protocol (see Chapter 9). In the initial phases of zinc supplementation, the body is desperate for the zinc, and the added zinc is very helpful. But if too much zinc is consumed, a secondary imbalance of copper can occur, and copper deficiency has been documented in the scientific literature to be dangerous and even life-threatening.

4. A fascinating and rarely discussed reason for avoiding continuous nutrient supplementation, especially with regard to chronic infections, is the principle that the infections themselves may be thrown off guard by supplementation of various kinds—not just antibacterial supplementation. It is well documented that Lyme disease and co-infections contribute to, and even cause, various nutrient deficiencies. It is believed that this is done by the infections in order to compromise host immunity and create a more favorable living environment for the infection(s). As a result, nutrient supplementation may have the indirect effect of weakening the infections by restoring nutrients which bolster immune function. However, after immune function is restored, the infections quickly adapt to the new, stronger immune system by going dormant or activating other bacterial defense mechanisms. By rotating supplements that impact differing body systems, the infections are constantly kept off guard by having to deal with rising and falling levels of different nutrients, which, in turn, activates different host immune mechanisms. In a sense, this concept is similar to the rotation of actual antibacterial herbs and drugs, but instead of the treatments themselves impacting the infections, the body's own defenses are weakening the infections.

5. Finally, be aware that taking many supplements all at once can mask what is truly going on inside your body. Perhaps your fatigue and headaches aren't caused by Lyme disease, but they are instead caused by interactions among the dozens of supplements you are taking? The only way to know how you truly feel and how your recovery process is truly progressing is to observe how your body feels when it is left alone to take care of itself.

In summary, there are three basic categories of treatments which Lyme disease sufferers use: antibacterial treatments, supportive treatments targeted at specific organ dysfunction, and supportive treatments which have a general, broad impact on the body. I've presented my arguments for using each of these kinds of treatments on an intermittent or rotational basis. The logic substantiating a rotational approach differs for each type of treatment, so it is important to read the above section carefully in order to understand how these kinds of treatments differ from each other, and under what circumstances they are best used.

While I believe that I've presented some interesting arguments against using most kinds of treatments continuously, ultimately, I suggest that each individual work with their doctor and listen to their body to determine which therapies should be rotated and which should be used without breaks. Also note that a healthy diet is critical for the body to take in the nutrients necessary to remain in equilibrium.

Finally, a word on how this information fits into the bigger picture in the book. The purpose of this chapter is to give you a template, or framework, through which you can think about the various treatments discussed later in the book in Parts 2 & 3. So, as you read Parts 2 & 3, you can think back to this chapter and ask yourself questions such as: "Let's see. Which kind of treatment am I currently reading about? Is this treatment an antibacterial treatment, a targeted supportive treatment, or a general supportive treatment?" Ultimately, this chapter should equip you with some decision-making tools that can help you determine when and for how long each particular treatment should be used. It is not a perfect science, so you'll have to do the best you can to adapt the information in this chapter to fit your own unique needs and circumstances. Our treatment template isn't a roadmap. Instead, it is a way of thinking, or a philosophy. Your own template will be unique and personalized.

Now, I would like to turn our attention to another question which I believe many people will be asking (at least, those who've read my past books). This question brings us back to the topic of antimicrobial treatments, specifically, rife machine therapy. We've already seen that many kinds of antimicrobial treatments, and even supportive therapies, should be rotated during the recovery process. But how should rife therapy be used?

What About Rife Machine Therapy?

What about rife machine therapy? Isn't rife machine therapy an important approach to healing from Lyme disease? After all, my first book, *Lyme Disease and Rife Machines*, advocated rife machine therapy as a primary treatment. How does rife machine therapy fit into the Antibiotic Rotation Protocol?

My current position on this topic is that rife machine therapy is still the single best therapy for a certain part of the recovery process, specifically, killing mature, free-swimming spirochetes. Most people experience a dominance of these kinds of spirochetes during the early phases of their infection and before they are 90% recovered. And, rife machine therapy may be one of the only treatments which can remove these spirochetes without causing them to convert into more dangerous, defensive bacterial forms. So, if a person is just starting off in their Lyme disease treatment, rife therapy may be one of the most useful treatments they can use.

However, later in the recovery process, it seems to be the case that these spirochetes fade into the background and are replaced by other forms of Borrelia and co-infections, such as Bartonella, Babesia, and parasites, and these infections become more entrenched and sequestered behind biofilm in tightly-packed colonies. Based on the available research, rife machine therapy in its current forms may provide some help here, but it is not adequate to completely address these kinds of issues. Furthermore, many other problems unrelated to infections also appear to punctuate the final phases of recovery—problems such as mold exposure, adrenal fatigue, hormonal imbalances, etc. These other problems cannot be addressed by rife therapy alone.

This does not mean that rife machine therapy should be abandoned after a person reaches their final phases of healing. Rife therapy probably has some effect (the degree to which is unknown) on co-infections. Also, up until the very end, spirochetes will spontaneously emerge from the colonies, and great improvement will be felt when rife machine therapy is applied at the right time. As noted, this anti-spirochete effect may be needed less often toward the end of recovery, but when it is needed, rife therapy is absolutely indispensible.

And there's one more thing. There are still a lot of unknowns surrounding rife therapy, so it may provide benefits we don't yet understand, and we can't yet quantify. For example, I believe that for both known and unknown reasons at various points in the recovery process, rife machine therapy exerts a powerful, spontaneous, and tremendously useful effect which can greatly weaken entire infective colonies—including Borrelia, co-infections, and even biofilm. This spontaneous effect may be different from the other effects that rife has; it may be an unknown benefit which hasn't been studied or well-documented. So, it's not easy for us to quantify exactly what rife therapy is doing and how useful it can be during the final phases of healing. Much of this area of study remains experimental.

In conclusion, I don't believe there's any substitute for what rife therapy can accomplish, even up until the very last part of the recovery process. If I had to summarize my view on rife machine therapy during the final phases of healing, I would say that it may be important less often, but when it is important, it is very important. This bears repeating: when rife therapy is needed, it is a treatment which has no good substitute.

Rife machine therapy and how it fits into the Antibiotic Rotation Protocol was discussed in detail in my prior books, and I still believe that those guidelines are applicable today. One of the core principles described was that rife machine therapy should be used during breaks from other antimicrobial therapies, and that during these breaks, rife therapy is exceedingly effective, because it targets forms of the infection which are only vulnerable during periods when other types of antimicrobial treatments are avoided.

We will explore additional updates on rife machine therapy later in Chapter 8.

Three Ways to Feel Better Fast

Regardless of which treatments you happen to use at any given time as part of your Antibiotic Rotation Protocol, I want to provide you with a lifeline. There are three simple, broadly applicable tools that you can employ at virtually any point in the recovery process, which, in most circumstances, will provide you with reliable relief of symptoms almost immediately:

1. <u>Detoxification therapies</u>. Many of the symptoms associated with Lyme disease and co-infections are a result of the toxicities that build up in the body faster than the body's ability to eliminate them. Using various detoxification treatments described in this book and other books can provide immediate relief of symptoms. If you feel badly, think "detox."

2. <u>Anti-inflammatory therapies</u>. Over-activity of the immune system and chronic inflammation account for a large percentage of the symptoms you will experience. Anti-inflammatory substances and protocols will rapidly help to alleviate symptoms in most cases.

3. <u>Supportive therapies which take into account the particular organ or body system being affected by the current active layer</u>

<u>of the onion</u>. Remember, each layer of the infection is located in a different body tissue, and hence, symptoms will vary throughout the recovery process. Make sure to use supportive therapies that address whichever body system is currently being affected.

Regardless of what else is going on in your healing journey, using the above three tools is sure to provide relief from symptoms when you aren't feeling well.

Advanced Principles for Using the Antibiotic Rotation Protocol

Now that we've looked at the foundational logic behind rotating antimicrobial therapies (and even rotating some types of supportive therapies), let's examine some specific tips and strategies for putting this philosophy into day-to-day practice.

The following principles aren't presented in any particular order, and they cover a wide range of topics related to making decisions during use of the Antibiotic Rotation Protocol. They are also not intended to give you a complete, easy-to-follow outline. Since everyone is different, you will need to be the one to fine-tune these principles to your own unique needs. There's no one-size-fits-all approach to getting well. As you read the principles, don't worry too much about exactly how they can be used in your protocol; instead, read this section with an open mind and absorb the information, and it will become evident to you over time where and when these principles apply to your recovery. The following principles are at the heart of designing a treatment template.

Principle #1: **Co-infections almost always prevent healing. Until co-infections are addressed, treatments for Borrelia are largely futile.** This is a principle which applies to many, not few, Lyme disease sufferers.

In the event that you are not experiencing progress, it may very likely be due to an untreated co-infection, especially Babesia or Bartonella. Therefore, most rotational protocols should begin with therapy for these co-infections. Typically, Bartonella and Babesia are treated for separately. Borrelia treatment may be combined with the treatment for either co-infection. Other co-infections, including Ehrlichia, mycoplasma, and parasites may also be holding back your recovery.

Principle #2: **The whole is greater than the sum of the parts.** What I mean is, when you are using any given antimicrobial treatment and it is causing Herxheimer reactions and improvements, what you are experiencing isn't merely benefitting you in the present moment. While the treatment you are using certainly is killing infections and helping you on your path to wellness, there's also a lot going on behind the scenes. By disrupting the infective colonies with that single treatment at that single moment in time, you are actually weakening the colonies and making them more susceptible to all of the future treatments you use. So, when the particular treatment you are using stops working and you move on, the next treatment in your queue will have increased effectiveness as a result of the prior treatment. This is a very encouraging realization, as it means that the investment you are making now will pay dividends for a long time to come. Sometimes, there is one pesky infection that is blocking the treatment of many other infections, and when you target that one pesky infection effectively, you are opening the door for dozens of other, subsequent therapies to be highly effective. This is why it can be so important to find new treatments and use new therapies you haven't previously used. These new therapies will pack a punch that will render all future treatments (even ones you've used previously) much more effective.

Principle #3: **Any stagnation in symptoms is usually a sign that you need to change up your treatment plan.** This can extend beyond simply choosing a different antimicrobial. In fact, it may mean shifting gears entirely from an antimicrobial campaign to a detox campaign or from a detox campaign to an adrenal support campaign. If you are stuck, think outside the box. Think outside your normal patterns of treatment planning. Try something new.

Principle #4: **Research has shown that treating for nearly any problem will result in mobilization and release of toxic heavy metals, to some degree**. Therefore, heavy metal detox should be addressed throughout the recovery process. Each time microbes are killed, heavy metals are released. In my opinion, the most proven, safe, and effective methodologies for removing heavy metals are those described by Andrew Cutler, Ph.D., in his book, *Amalgam Illness: Diagnosis and Treatment*. However, everyone will respond to heavy metal treatments differently, so you might need to experiment to find what works for you. Heavy metal detox is a very involved and complex process, and you should conduct as much additional research on this subject as you possibly can.

Principle #5: **Some people can discern the differences between Borrelia, Bartonella, and Babesia symptoms.** Or, if they can't discern these differences, they may be able to learn to discern them over time. Furthermore, it has been noted that the distinction between symptoms becomes clearer and more apparent the further one is into the treatment process. For example, in the last 10% of healing, the symptoms of the respective infections may be much more easily identified. It is helpful to review publicly available symptom lists for the different infections. If and when you learn to discern which symptoms belong to which infections, you can use this information to determine which therapy should be used next in your rotational protocol, as you assess your dominant symptoms. One clue which can help you learn how to match symptoms with their corresponding infections is to experiment with specific treatments intended for a specific infection and then observe your Herxheimer symptoms. For example, if you take Rifampin, which is a drug specifically targeted toward Bartonella, the resulting flare-up of symptoms likely includes Bartonella symptoms. But even if you never figure out which symptoms belong to which infections, you can still succeed in recovering by using trial and error—try treatments for various infections and keep moving on until you get a "hit"—that is, Herxes and improvement. When you get a "hit," you've found a beneficial treatment which is killing the top layer of the microbial onion.

Principle #6: **The strongest Herxheimer reactions often indicate the most potential for progress.** Herxheimer reactions that cause you to think, "I'm sure I'm making the infections worse. This can't be right. I feel horrible," are often the most productive reactions. Hang in there during these reactions, as you are likely making great progress against the infections! Note: it is possible for you to mistake drug side effects or adverse reactions for Herxheimer reactions. Be sure you are experiencing an actual Herxheimer reaction and not a drug side effect before you assume that the reaction is beneficial. Over time, you will learn to tell the difference between the two kinds of reactions. Again, detective work on your part plays a huge role in the recovery process. Lastly, remember that actual worsening of the infections can also make you feel worse.

Principle #7: **There will be times when one dominant infection is all you feel for weeks, months, or years, and other times when they alternate rapidly, even daily or weekly.** This is a very interesting principle. You might literally experience Bartonella as your dominant infection for years, and then, suddenly, the dominant infection might switch to Borrelia, and subsequently, might continue to switch rapidly to other infections. Stay alert; yesterday's wisdom won't necessarily apply to today's problems.

Principle #8: **Different antimicrobial therapies target different infections.** This may seem obvious, but it is important to understand that different kinds of herbs, drugs, energetic therapies, and other substances target different infections. Some herbs and drugs are highly effective for one infection but do nothing to kill another. There are also some substances which have broad-spectrum activity. It is important to learn which antimicrobial treatments work for which infections, if you are to successfully integrate them into your rotational protocol.

Principle #9: **As you begin to treat for the co-infections Babesia and Bartonella, the Borrelia infection will become more active and susceptible to treatment.** Experts believe that co-infections hide or protect Borrelia from anti-Borrelia treatment. As you treat for co-infections, and Borrelia is exposed, you may find yourself in somewhat urgent need of anti-Borrelia treatments (due to burgeoning Borrelia symptoms), and the use of anti-Borrelia treatments may yield much more productive results than were achieved prior to co-infection treatment. Therefore, when planning your antibacterial protocol for co-infections, it would be wise to also prepare to treat for Borrelia shortly following or even overlapping the co-infection treatment.

Principle #10: **The longer you treat for one particular problem, the more likely it is that other problems are cropping up and will require treatment soon.** This is why it is important to consider changing treatments as soon as possible after a plateau in progress is reached. This principle applies to not just infections, but non-infectious problems as well.

Principle #11: **Combining treatments, especially antibacterial treatments, has a synergistic effect.** This is one of the most important principles. Certain therapies are much more effective when combined with other therapies. This is especially true when it comes to pharmaceutical antibiotics. The whole can be much greater than the sum of the parts, so to speak. However, there are literally thousands of possible combinations of herbs, drugs, supplements, and supportive therapies, and addressing each possible combination would require hundreds of pages. That is why it is so important to be working with an experienced, Lyme-literate healthcare practitioner who understands various combinations of therapies. Without the help of such a practitioner, you can waste countless time and energy learning hard, unnecessary lessons. Do not reinvent the wheel at the expense of your time, money, and health.

Principle #12: **Resistance isn't the problem.** Bacterial resistance isn't the reason why antimicrobial treatments stop working. Instead, the problem is that the infections are protected by biofilm and by the complex, poly-microbial community structure. This is a critical distinction. It means the antibiotics and herbs you are using aren't ineffective; they are just not reaching the organisms they are supposed to target. It also means that after a given treatment stops working, it will likely again be effective later when the particular infection it targets again becomes the dominant, or top, layer of the infection. This means you have a renewable arsenal— the treatments you use to fight the infections, although they may lose effectiveness, will again be effective later. Similarly, we can conclude that increasing the dosage of any given treatment will likely not increase the value of that treatment if the treatment seems to be ineffective. Instead, the treatment is probably ineffective not because of the dose, but because the targeted microorganism is unreachable by the treatment. A more prudent course of action would be to rotate to a different treatment, instead of increasing the dosage of a treatment that isn't working. Here's a real life example of what we are talking about. This is an excerpt from an email conversation I had with an experienced Lyme doctor.

> *I talked with a Lyme patient who was taking a very high dose of tinidazole (in order to address Borrelia, see Chapter 11), but she was only seeing some very small improvement in her condition. Her doctor suggested she take even more tinidazole. She complied and doubled the dose, but the increased dose didn't provide any additional benefit. She changed doctors, and the new doctor put her on a course of Mepron to address Babesia; he also took her off the tinidazole. After she had taken Mepron for two weeks, the new doctor added the tinidazole back into her treatment protocol but at half the smaller dose she had previously taken. This time, now that her Babesia was being treated effectively, the tinidazole was incredibly effective for her and launched her forward in her recovery, with dramatic Herxheimer reactions and improvement. See the point here? The dose of the tinidazole wasn't the problem. A smaller dose was more effective, but only after Babesia treatment*

began. Any drug, regardless of the dose, will only be effective if the target infection is exposed and vulnerable to the treatment.

A similar example can be seen when you look at what happens by taking "systemic enzymes" (that is, an enzyme supplement such as Wobenzym taken on an empty stomach instead of with food) followed by using tinidazole (or some other antimicrobial therapy). The enzymes break down biofilm and pave the way for the antimicrobial to reach its target, and results can be dramatic.

(Of all the treatments I suggested in my past book, *The Top 10 Lyme Disease Treatments,* systemic enzyme therapy is among the most important. Even using systemic enzyme therapy alone—not in combination with other treatments—has yielded fantastic results for biofilms.)

Principle #13: **Pharmaceutical antibiotics hold a very important place in Lyme disease treatment, but overusing them can have serious drawbacks.** The right pharmaceutical at the right time can cause permanent and severe damage to the infective colonies, damage which justifies the side effects of the drugs. However, if this kind of extremely favorable cost-to-benefit ratio doesn't exist for a particular situation and antibiotics are used anyway—especially if they are used for a long period of time—then their side effects can outweigh their benefit. The key principle to realize here is that pharmaceutical antibiotics do not have a healing and strengthening effect on the body. Instead, they weaken the body and the immune system. If they are used in short bursts with maximum cost-to-benefit, then they can be very useful. But over the long-term, they can do a lot of harm. Yet, I still observe that many top Lyme doctors use them almost exclusively over long periods of time. For some people, that kind of treatment may yield good results, but for many others, it isn't a good trade-off. You will have to determine which camp you fall into and how pharmaceuticals should be integrated into your treatment program. Note that different pharmaceuticals can have different side effects. Some drugs are relatively mild and well-tolerated. Others can have profound and even permanent negative effects. And the side effects can vary from person to person, depending on the individual's unique biochemistry. To summarize: Pharmaceutical antibiotics themselves aren't good or bad. What makes them good or bad is how they are used.

Principle #14: **In most cases, the occurrence of Herxheimer reactions, or other kinds of healing reactions, is a good sign and should guide your selection of treatments.** So, if you are unsure which treatment to use next in your rotational protocol and you resort to trial and error, it is likely that the treatment which produces the most productive Herxheimer reaction (and subsequent improvement) is the correct treatment to use. Unfortunately, I can recount numerous stories of people I've talked with who used a treatment for months on end without any perceptible Herxheimer reaction or improvement, because "the treatment just seemed so important and the logic for its use made so much sense." Without Herxheimer reactions and improvement, it is quite likely that such seemingly ideal treatments are not providing continued benefit. Likewise, the experience of only Herxheimer reactions with no improvement whatsoever can be a warning sign: improvement should ensue at some point during the use of a treatment. So, in summary, there are two characteristics which mark successful treatments: Herxheimer reactions, and improvement in symptoms. If a treatment seems logical and popular but doesn't provide you with results, it may be that that particular treatment just isn't working for you, even if it seems to be working for everyone else.

Principle #15: **The recovery process may proceed in fits and starts (that is, it may proceed rapidly at some points and slowly at others).** You may experience periods of time in which almost everything you do doesn't help, and other periods of time in which everything seems to work very well. Knowing that this may happen can help you prepare for the recovery process. For example, if you happen to be in a period during which not much is working, you might decide to start dedicating a little bit more time to researching new treatments, so you can get your recovery back on track. And, during times when everything seems to be working, you might take advantage of this success by rapidly rotating the best available treatments to leverage whatever weaknesses you've been able to expose in the infections.

Principle #16: **Layers of the infection are protected by biofilm, which is a film-like shield that guards bacteria from environmental threats.** The realization of this fact allowed Lyme disease doctors and researchers to make leaps and bounds of progress in the treatment of Lyme and co-infections. When anti-biofilm treatments are utilized, the protective abilities of Lyme disease and co-infections diminish, and treatments become more effective. Information throughout this book will help you address biofilms. Anti-biofilm therapies should be used regularly within your rotational protocol to ensure that the other treatments you are using will have maximum effect. If biofilm is not addressed, treatments which would otherwise be highly effective can have little or no effect. Be warned, though: once you penetrate the biofilm, there may be no turning back as what's behind the biofilm is released and must be dealt with.

Principle #17: **Detoxification therapies are needed throughout the entire recovery process, regardless of which other treatments you are pursuing.** The specific detoxification treatments you use may vary over time depending on which problem you are primarily dealing with. Detoxification is so important that it is worthy of at least as much of your time and effort as the treatment of the actual infections. The right detoxification treatment at the right time can eliminate almost all of your symptoms fairly quickly and can render the whole recovery process much more comfortable and tolerable. This is especially true when you still have a high load of microorganisms and toxins in your body.

Principle #18: **Convincing yourself that it is time to rotate therapies or get more aggressive with your treatment may be difficult.** Human beings are incredibly adaptable. After having a chronic illness for any length of time, you may quickly adapt to a state of illness. A very well-known and well-respected Lyme doctor has made the observation that one of the symptoms of Lyme disease and co-infections is the inability to perceive, or have insight into, the extent of your own disability or illness. In other words, you're no longer able to actually determine how sick you really are. You don't feel the urgency which you should feel. Another very well-known Lyme doctor has said that "Lyme disease patients will never self-navigate out of their own disease." This is one of the reasons why people only begin to really understand their disability after they've made significant enough healing progress to allow their brains to function well enough to conduct an accurate and valid self-analysis. Sometimes, after a person has taken a significant leap forward in their healing progress, they can feel even more desperate and depressed, because, at their worst, they were not able to completely comprehend how sick they were. Typically, when they finally do get aggressive treatment, they have psychological breakthroughs in which they are often shocked—and even traumatized— by the realization that they have been so sick for so long. One of the results of this lack of insight is that very sick people sometimes do not have the wherewithal to commit themselves to an aggressive anti-Lyme protocol, or, if they do, they do not have the awareness necessary to determine if/when the protocol is no longer working. When you recognize this limitation, you will be able to more easily take an objective look at your situation and make appropriate decisions. Also, a good Lyme doctor is essential, because they can help nudge you along the correct path. Remember, the sickest people are sometimes the least able to make the kinds of aggressive and logical treatment decisions necessary to heal.

Principle #19: **Some of the treatments utilized in your rotational protocol will not be safe unless they are used along with specific supportive therapies or interventions.** It is important to recognize that certain treatments you may decide to employ are only safe and effective when combined with special supportive therapies. For example, the use of the drug Rifampin, which has been shown to be very effective against

Bartonella, should be accompanied by frequent liver function tests, as Rifampin is known to be very hard on the liver. Supportive liver supplements should be given when the drug is used (see Chapter 15). Furthermore, some people will be unable to use Rifampin in a rotational schedule because stopping and restarting that particular drug causes a "flu-like syndrome" side effect in some users. Rifampin is best used along with doxycycline because of their synergistic effects. And finally, Rifampin, like all antibiotics, can cause an imbalance in intestinal flora and should therefore be used alongside a good probiotic. This is not a complete list of Rifampin side effects and concerns, but it is a sampling of some of the customized considerations you'll need to face when using a given treatment. As you can see, it is very important to have adequate knowledge of the treatment you are considering in order to determine which supportive therapies may be required, and to decide whether or not the treatment will negatively interact with other items in your treatment protocol. This is one of the reasons why it is so important to have a knowledgeable doctor supervising your treatment. You can't just pick up a new treatment and use it; you really have to know what you are doing.

Principle #20: **The theory that numerous infections are like layers of an "onion" and that each infection takes its turn being the "top" layer of the onion is not science fiction. It is proven fact.** Modern science describes a method by which bacteria living together in a biofilm community are able to communicate with one another for mutual survival. This communication is known as quorum sensing (QS for short). Science tells us that quorum sensing allows the community of microorganisms to elect one species of microbe at a time, and the elected microbe takes the forefront on the battlefield for survival. If that particular species is defeated or suppressed—if you use appropriate antimicrobial therapies to target and remove it—then the community, which contains numerous kinds of microbes, will move on to elect a different species of microbe to take up the fight. Meanwhile, the previous species of microbe that was defeated is given time to recover and increase its numbers, so that it might be ready to take its position once again on the front lines, at a later date. This pathogen "merry-go-round," as some have described it, is the reason that the Antibiotic Rotation Protocol is needed. It is also the reason why carefully combined therapies may have profound benefit: ideally, if we could attack all the species at once with a carefully coordinated attack, we might be able to knock out the whole community without giving it time to recover. In practice, this is difficult to achieve, but combinations can still offer us synergistic benefits.

Principle #21: **Each new layer of the onion which you treat and remove will feel quite different to you and may respond differently to treatments you've used in the past.** This is one of the more difficult obstacles encountered during Lyme disease treatment, and failure to recognize this principle can result in extensive confusion, bad decisions, and halted progress. During certain times in the recovery process, a given antibiotic or herb may have a very powerful positive effect, and during other times, it may do little or nothing for you. For example, you may start taking artemisinin for Babesia and find that it is extremely helpful in alleviating your symptoms. You may then discontinue its use after you plateau. Later, you may try artemisinin again and find that it does nothing for you. You may therefore conclude that your Babesia is gone and artemisinin is useless to you, so you will throw away your artemisinin and check Babesia off the list of things to worry about in the future. "Well," you'll say, "I guess I conquered Babesia." The truth, however, may simply be that when you tried artemisinin for the second time, you simply happened to be working your way through a layer in which Babesia was not an active problem. In reality, had you held on to the bottle of artemisinin and used it again, let's say, two months down the road, you would have found that future layers of your infections actually did contain Babesia and that artemisinin may have been tremendously helpful for these future layers of infection. The key point to remember here is that a single experience with a given treatment is not enough to conclude that the treatment will or will not be useful in the future. The recovery process is full of roller-coaster like experiences, and you need to be prepared for these. This principle also applies to non-infection related issues such as detoxification:

during certain parts of the recovery process, your body may greatly need, for example, heavy metal detoxification support, and during other parts, heavy metal detoxification treatments may be more of a burden to the body than a help.

Principle #22: **There are various methods for deciding which treatment to use next in your rotational protocol.** It can be fairly simple to decide when it is time to stop a given treatment: treatments should be stopped after Herxheimer / healing reactions subside and after improvement in symptoms ceases. On the other hand, it can be much harder to figure out what to do next after a treatment is stopped. Methods for determining what to do next include, but are not limited to, energetic testing (also known as Autonomic Response Testing), your past experiences and knowledge of your body/disease, the guidance of your health care practitioner, the experiences and advice of other Lyme sufferers, and the study of new information available to the Lyme disease community. Of course, monitoring symptoms is also key; if you can tell which infection has taken the lead role in the "pathogen merry-go-round," you can address that infection with the proper therapies. After you've figured out which problem is the new dominant problem for you, one of the best kinds of treatment to use during your rotational protocol is a new treatment, that is, one which you've never used previously. A new, previously unused treatment can have dramatic beneficial effects because your body and your infections have not yet encountered it, and hence, neither your body nor the infections have adapted to the treatment. For example, if you've determined that the dominant problem you are facing is Babesia, using a Babesia antibiotic which you've never before taken can be very helpful. Of course, treatments you've used before can be helpful, too, but new treatments are especially helpful. It is for this reason that you should make it a high priority to stay up-to-date with the latest Lyme disease research, so you can always be adding new treatments to your arsenal. In the event that you are unable to find a new treatment, it is ideal to choose a treatment that you haven't used in a long time. The longer it has been since the last time you used a given treatment, the more likely it is that the current layer of the onion which you are dealing with will be susceptible to that treatment. You might even decide to put recently used supplement bottles in the back of your supplement shelf and allow them to move forward as other supplements move to the back of the line, in order to help you keep track of what you have recently used and what you haven't used for a long time. No, this methodology isn't a perfect science. It is just a tool to help you get organized. Use whichever organization strategy works for you.

Principle #23: **Especially during the last 10% of healing, treatments may need to be rotated or changed quite frequently.** The infections may change configuration, and new layers of the onion may be exposed very rapidly during the final phases of treatment. Early on, during illness, the same treatments may work for long periods of time. Later, however, rapid rotation of treatments may be necessary. It is important to adjust your plan to accommodate for this fact. While it is not conventional wisdom to adjust a treatment program on a frequent basis, it may be necessary for you to do just that—especially during the last 10% of healing. I will use a personal example to illustrate this point. At one point in my recovery process, rife machine therapy was doing very little for me; it was quite frustrating. However, I decided to take colloidal silver one day. Within 30 minutes after my first dose of colloidal silver, I had the urge to do a rife session (after you've used rife machines for years, like I had, you begin to recognize the signs and symptoms which indicate that rife therapy may be helpful). So, I reluctantly underwent a rife session and expected nothing to happen. To my surprise, this particular rife session resulted in a large Herxheimer reaction and marked improvement in my symptoms. This rapid sequence of treatments—first, colloidal silver, then, minutes later, rife therapy—was not the kind of thing that would have worked for me early on in the illness. Nevertheless, video is available showing spirochetes converting into dormant cyst forms in a matter of only minutes after being exposed to an antibiotic. If the infection can respond that quickly to a changing environment, we must also be willing to act quickly if we are to win the fight. One of my healing mentors, a very wise woman who lives in Asia and recovered from Lyme disease using mostly biophoton therapy (see Chapter 10), told me that during her last few months of treatment, she literally had to rotate treatments daily in order to keep up with the changing needs of her body. She primarily used energy testing to figure out what to do next. She told me that sometimes, Bartonella would be the dominant infection in the morning, and Borrelia would be the dominant infection in the afternoon! Conventional wisdom about how frequently treatment protocols should be changed cannot be our guiding compass. Instead, we must evaluate and respond to the unwelcome infections living within us, even if those infections disobey conventional wisdom. We must act on the truth, not on the system employed by doctors to ensure an efficient flow of patient visits.

Principle #24: **"Pulse Therapy" can be helpful in treating infections.** "Pulse therapy" is simply the term used to describe the intermittent use of antibacterial treatment. For example, a particular antibacterial treatment may be used for 10 days, followed by 10 days off, followed by use of another round of that antibacterial treatment. During the time off from the antibacterial treatment, the infection may drop its guard and again become susceptible to treatment. So, using the treatment intermittently may be more effective than using it continuously. And likewise, higher doses of medication can be used with fewer side effects, because pulsing allows the body to take a rest from the treatment and recover from its potentially toxic effects. The logic behind pulsing is, in fact, agreed upon by many well-respected Lyme-literate practitioners. For example, one of the best-selling Lyme disease books of all time documents the author's experience with pulsing for not only her own case of Lyme disease, but also for that of a very well-known doctor. Both she and the doctor beat their own Lyme disease via a pulsed antibiotic treatment schedule. According to her book, the break between pulses was long enough to allow a "relapse" to take place before the next pulse was initiated. Again, the concept is to trick the infections into thinking that the coast is clear. Then, the infections are hit hard with an antibiotic or antimicrobial treatment. Had the antibiotic simply been used continuously, the infections would have never relinquished their dormant, defensive, impenetrable configurations, so the treatment would have had diminishing effect. Personally, I believe that rife therapy can be integrated very effectively with pulsed antibiotic treatment—rife therapy works best during breaks from antibiotics, so it can be used when taking breaks from antibiotic pulses.

Principle #25: **A very well-known and experienced Lyme doctor advocates using less antibiotics, with lots of breaks taken between their use, to allow the immune system to learn to fight the infections.** This way of thinking is in alignment with how I believe that chronic Lyme disease should be treated. While many Lyme doctors use continuous, high doses of antibiotics, I advocate carefully targeted, brief courses of antibiotics—and lots of time when no pharmaceuticals are in use—to allow the body to rebuild its natural defenses.

Principle #26: **Whichever infection is on the top layer of the onion is the limiting factor in recovery.** You can't bypass this layer and work on other infections or issues. If you can't effectively treat the infection on the top layer of the onion, your progress will slow or halt. This is why it is so important to be under the care of an experienced doctor, someone who can recognize what is happening on the top layer of the onion and who understands which treatments work best for that particular problem. It is for this reason that co-infections like Babesia and Bartonella cannot be ignored if they are present, because the entire recovery process will halt if they are not addressed.

Principle #27: **When it comes to pharmaceutical antibiotics, and other toxic treatments, the longer the treatment is used, the less beneficial that treatment will become.** Furthermore, the longer the treatment is used, the more likely side effects will develop. Therefore, the initial period of use for most treatments is the most beneficial, and the cost-to-benefit ratio decreases steadily over time. After a long period of time, the treatment will cause lots of harm and be doing only a little bit of good.

Principle #28: **Some people need to rotate treatments more often than other people**. Some people need to rotate weekly, others monthly or even longer. Time frames can be different, but the measuring stick is always the same: when a plateau is reached—that is, when Herxheimer reactions and improvement cease—the treatment should be discontinued, and a different treatment should be initiated.

Final Words on Building Your Treatment Template

As we leave Part 1 and move on toward the rest of the book, let's reflect on where we've been and where we're going.

This chapter and the entirety of Part 1 have established some foundational guidelines to help you figure out when and for how long to use the various antimicrobial and supportive treatments that you'll encounter later in this book and in other resources. Part 1 wasn't written to provide information on any specific treatments, but instead to provide a strategy, or template, into which you can drag-and-drop specific treatments.

If you are disappointed that you never encountered a standardized, easy, complete treatment template in Part I, I can understand your feelings. Ultimately, though, success is found not by following a simple treatment recipe, but instead by gaining understanding so you become capable of developing your own, unique treatment template. Lyme disease affects people very differently, so there's no one-size-fits-all approach. Arming you with this understanding has been the purpose of Part 1. Now it's up to you to take what you've learned and apply it to the specific treatment options you'll find in Part 2 and Part 3. It is up to you to take the building blocks I've given you and weave them together to create your own treatment template (if the phrase "treatment template" is confusing, you can instead use "treatment plan," "treatment strategy," or "treatment philosophy").

As I've mentioned throughout the book, wisdom on how and when to use various treatments is, in my opinion, much scarcer than information describing the treatments themselves. In this way, Part 1 is much more important than Parts 2 and 3, because after you master the information in Part 1, you should be able to perform the research and analysis contained in Parts 2 and 3 without my help! You should be ready to evaluate and use lots of new treatments which are currently available and also those which haven't even been discovered yet. Part 1 is the most valuable because it has given you tools which will far outlive the relevance of the rest of this book. You've heard the saying: "Give a man a fish, and you've fed him for a day. Teach him how to fish, and you've fed him for life." I hope that Part 1 has taught you how to fish for new treatments and understand how to use them.

As you construct your treatment template, avoid becoming obsessed with the choices available to you, and resist becoming paralyzed with indecision. These can be easy traps to fall into, given the open-ended nature of the treatment strategy we've examined. Paralysis of analysis is harmful because trial and error will be a big part of your education. So, simply trying new treatments can be much more productive and helpful than spending endless time analyzing them (of course, if the treatments you are considering have possible side effects or interactions, make sure you do conduct adequate analysis before using them).

Investing time and thought into understanding what's taking place in your body is the key; the more energy you invest, the better results you will get. Surprisingly, many people don't make this investment. Many people just look to their doctors for all of the answers. While doctors have wisdom you can benefit from, it is you who are living inside your body; you are best equipped to figure out what your body needs. Yes, take your doctor's advice, but make sure that advice lines up with what you know to be true of your body and its needs.

Lastly, before moving on, I would encourage you to put a rough draft of your treatment template down on paper. Make a list of the current health challenges, infections, and co-infections you are dealing with. Document which layer of the onion you believe you are presently battling. Write down your medical history, and include notes on how past treatments have affected you. Ask yourself in what ways you are similar to other Lyme sufferers and in what ways your body appears to respond completely uniquely. Flesh out a tentative future plan which describes which health issues need to be addressed and how serious they are. Then, as you move through the rest of the book, you can decide how and when to use the treatments you read about; you can see where they will fit into your treatment template. Remember that your treatment template needs to remain flexible, since your situation can and will change. Don't be obsessed with your treatment plan; just develop a rough draft and be willing to change it as needed.

Now, let's move on to examine the new treatment protocols (Part 2) and the new individual treatments (Part 3) which can be used according to the treatment guidelines we've explored in Part 1.

PART 2

The New Treatment Protocols

In this section of the book, we will look at the new treatment protocols. Read *Information For The Reader* (located near the beginning of the book) to understand how the individual treatments described in Part 3 differ from the treatment protocols described here, in Part 2. The treatment protocols contained in Part 2 are separated from the Individual Treatments (Part 3) not because the protocols are more important than the individual treatments, but instead, because they are simply more involved and require more ink and paper to describe.

Part 2 of the book doesn't give guidelines on how to use the treatment protocols described here. Those guidelines are contained in Part 1 of the book, where you learned how to build a treatment template for your own unique situation.

Note that some of the treatment protocols described here, in Part 2, will not fit easily into the treatment template you built in Part 1 of the book; some of them, such as dietary recommendations, can be adopted as general lifestyle suggestions.

Each of these protocols will hold a different level of value for each different Lyme disease sufferer. Some of the protocols may be tremendously helpful for certain people but useless for others. Furthermore, how and when each protocol should be used will differ for each person.

Chapter 4
The Paleo Diet for Lyme Disease (and Other Nutrition Hacks)

NOTE: Dietary information for Lyme disease sufferers is covered in many available books and resources. The information in this chapter highlights dietary lessons and key information which I personally have found to be interesting and useful, but the chapter is not intended as a complete discussion, nor is it intended as a one-size-fits-all approach. The correct diet for you will vary depending on your individual needs. Please consult your physician prior to making any changes to your current diet.

Why the Paleo Diet?

During my Lyme disease recovery, I experimented with many different ways of eating and noticed that each diet had big pros and big cons. Ultimately, most of the diets were too extreme. For example, veganism makes a lot of sense since vegans eat a nutrient-rich, fiber-rich, alkalizing diet which has countless health benefits. However, the vegan diet lacks many essential macronutrients which aid in Lyme disease recovery, such as saturated fats, cholesterol, and readily available protein. (In this chapter, we will see why these nutrients are so important). Even vegetarianism, it turns out, is usually too extreme and doesn't provide the nutrients needed to power a recovery from chronic illness.

But let's not throw the baby out with the bathwater. Let's keep the benefits of eating a vegan diet without completely eliminating the other required macronutrients found in other diets. This logic is what guided my selection of an eating plan. I like to think that I've taken the best of many diets and combined them all into one. Only, I don't get to take credit for this kind of diet, as it wasn't really my idea. The diet is known as the Paleo Diet, and it's quite popular across America right now.

The fundamental premise of the Paleo Diet is that over the last 200 years, the human diet has changed more than it has in the previous 5,000 years due to the advent of agriculture and food processing technology. The Paleo Diet advocates eating a diet which predates these developments. Paleo proponents argue that our bodies aren't designed to handle these new modern food changes. While many people view the Paleo Diet as just another fad, it is far from that. In fact, it's one of the oldest diets on planet Earth (hence, it's name), as it advocates eating foods which are similar to what our ancestors consumed. The modern American diet, on the other hand, is composed of foods which are relatively new to humanity, including processed carbohydrates and excessive sugar. So, people need to be careful when talking about the Paleo Diet as a fad, as that is an inaccurate characterization.

There are different versions of the Paleo Diet, and I won't spend time explaining each one; instead, I'll talk about the modified version which I find to be most beneficial for Lyme disease sufferers. Paleo Diet experts may object to my description of the diet and tell me it isn't completely accurate; they would be correct. I don't advocate a strictly Paleo Diet, but instead, a version which makes sense for chronically ill people. Accordingly, my recommendations in this chapter will deviate somewhat from a strictly Paleo Diet.

Let's look at the Paleo Diet in more detail.

One of the basic rules to consider when understanding the Paleo Diet is to avoid foods which have a list of ingredients. Instead, the diet prefers whole, unprocessed foods. These are foods which are not modified from their original, natural state and which ancient humans could acquire and consume without the help of modern food processing technologies; hence, the name "paleo" as in "Paleolithic." So, a bag of almonds is a good choice—only one "ingredient;"a bag of potato chips is a bad choice—multiple ingredients which have been processed. Foods chosen for the Paleo Diet should be readily available in nature and easily gathered and prepared by a person using minimal farming and technology. Cooking is acceptable because cooking can be accomplished with very primitive means.

The Paleo Diet also attempts to avoid dairy as well as many types of carbohydrates, including grains, beans, and potatoes. Processed carbohydrates are especially undesirable, so paleo eaters stay away from breads, pastries, desserts, etc. Sugars and processed carbohydrates are highly inflammatory and lead to significant exacerbations in Lyme disease symptoms. Since fruit can be found in its whole, unaltered form in nature, without the need for processing or agricultural cultivation, fruit is allowed in the Paleo Diet, although it should be consumed in moderation. More on this later.

We've talked a lot about what not to eat. What should we eat? The foods most important in the Paleo Diet include animal meat, fruits and vegetables, and nuts and seeds. Some types of dairy may be permissible if tolerated—we will talk about dairy more in the coming paragraphs.

As I mentioned earlier, some of my dietary recommendations aren't strictly in line with those of the Paleo Diet. Lyme disease sufferers have some unique needs, so we'll talk about how the diet meets these needs and where it should be modified to account for Lyme-specific health challenges. For example, when the Paleo Diet is used for weight loss, which it often is, total daily carbohydrates are severely restricted. My version of the Paleo Diet for Lyme disease allows a higher level of carbohydrates to be consumed. As you formulate your own diet, remember this one, guiding principle: if a particular food makes you feel good, then eat it. Our bodies can offer us a lot of wisdom, and since each person's body is different, the best diet for you will be different than the best diet for me. The goal isn't to follow the diet in a rigid fashion, but instead, to use the parts of the diet which make sense for your individual biochemistry.

Also, I will focus on some of the more controversial aspects of the diet because these aspects are the ones which are most likely to confuse or divert potential adopters. If you keep up with what's going on in the modern study of nutrition, you'll know that there is a heated debate raging over much of what I discuss in this chapter. So, this chapter will explain my positions on these controversial topics and will provide the logic behind my positions.

And lastly, while weight loss isn't the primary goal of the information in this chapter, I do believe that obesity can be a huge obstacle in healing from any chronic illness, so the dietary objectives set forth here also take into consideration maintaining a healthy weight.

Fat and Protein: The Foundation of the Paleo Food Pyramid

While vegetables are a major part of the Paleo Diet foundation, most of the daily calories consumed will be derived from meat and healthy fats. More specifically, the foundation includes foods like poultry, eggs, butter, fish, coconut oil, and even red meat and bacon (in moderation). These items would make the bottom, or foundation, of the paleo food pyramid. You will notice that these foods are high in protein and fat, two nutrients which, despite popular opinion, provide tremendous benefits. For the general population, protein and fat serve as very satiating foods, which leads to less hunger and less of a propensity to overeat. Furthermore, these foods avoid insulin and blood sugar spikes, which result from carbohydrate intake and which are associated with a plethora of health problems such as obesity, diabetes, cancer, insulin resistance, inflammation, hypoglycemia, and depression, just to name a few.

Putting fat and protein at the bottom of the food pyramid is a huge shift away from the traditional belief that complex carbohydrates should comprise the majority of our calories. However, new research debunks the theory that carbohydrates should be our primary food source; this is a flawed assumption for chronic illness and the general public alike. If you still think that fat makes you fat, you need to do some reading. Fat actually helps prevent you from getting fat, because it satiates you more effectively and keeps your blood sugar in a lower range, thus decreasing the level of insulin circulating in your blood. The food that makes you fat, instead, is refined carbohydrates. A detailed discussion of the physiology behind this statement is beyond the scope of this book; however, this is a critical point which you should research on your own if it is a new concept for you. I highly recommend reading the excellent writings of Dr. Joseph Mercola (www.drmercola.com).

For Lyme disease sufferers, fat and protein have special, specific benefits. This was a lesson that took me a long time to learn. For years, I tried avoiding fatty and high protein foods thinking, instead, that vegetables were the key to good health. It turns out that vegetables shouldn't actually be in competition with fats and proteins: both classes of foods are critical and indispensable. You run into problems when you create a false dichotomy and force yourself to favor either one or the other. Sadly, I believe this is where many chronically ill people reside—in extremes. We'll be looking at how fat and protein can benefit Lyme disease sufferers in the coming sections.

The higher levels of the paleo food pyramid primarily include fruit, nuts, seeds, and dairy in moderation. You'll notice the very conspicuous absence of grains, corn, potatoes, beans, and rice from the above discussion. Since I'm not a fan of extremes, my version of the diet permits these foods, but in extreme moderation. For more information on the paleo food pyramid, I suggest doing a Google search for *Paleo Diet basics* or *paleo food pyramid.*

How Fat and Cholesterol Provide Specific Benefits to People Healing From Lyme Disease

One of the main ways in which fats and cholesterol help people with Lyme disease is to aid in the synthesis of hormones. Lyme disease wreaks havoc on the endocrine system, and the body has a great need for the basic building blocks of new hormones. Cholesterol is indispensable in hormone production; in fact, it is the nutrient from which pregnenolone—the mother of all hormones which is used to create nearly every other hormone—is synthesized.

"But wait," you say. "I thought cholesterol was bad for us?" I believed the same thing for many years, and for some people, excess cholesterol may be bad, but for those with Lyme disease, cholesterol is critical to the recovery process. This explains why many Lyme disease sufferers crave eggs[5] (specifically egg yolks), a food which ranks among the highest for cholesterol content. It also explains why many Lyme sufferers actually test low for cholesterol, not high.

Furthermore, saturated fats, both from animal products and also those found in foods like coconut oil, are critical to hormone synthesis. Again, this flies in the face of conventional wisdom which tells us that saturated fats are bad. In fact, it is the trans-, or hydrogenated fats, that

---

[5] Eggs are a fantastic food! The yolk is rich in dozens of critical nutrients including cholesterol, B vitamins, choline and inositol, DHA, minerals, and more. The whites provide high-quality protein. Eggs are also affordable.

are bad. Saturated fats actually provide a great deal of support as well as help repair body tissues during Lyme disease recovery.

If you are still reeling from the above statements—that cholesterol and saturated fats are actually healthy—I can relate. I was reeling, too. You should do some independent reading on modern studies, and you'll find that the thinking on this topic is changing in many research circles. Of course, when combined with a sedentary lifestyle and overconsumption, these nutrients can turn into poisons—and so can most other foods. It goes without saying that exercise, as well as moderation at the dinner table, are critical components of any healthy lifestyle.

One of the missing links which helped me to better understand the role of cholesterol and saturated fat in Lyme disease recovery was the discovery that adrenal fatigue plays a huge role in Lyme disease. There are separate chapters in this book to address adrenal fatigue, but for the purposes of our discussion here, the adrenal glands are responsible for producing many of the body's hormones, and when these organs get stressed, as occurs in Lyme disease, hormone production drops to unhealthy low levels. Since adrenal fatigue often accompanies Lyme disease, those suffering from it require extra support for hormone production, and consequently, more consumption of saturated fats and cholesterol than people who don't have Lyme disease. This is another reason why the Paleo Diet is so appropriate for Lyme disease sufferers. It also explains why the general population may not need the same levels of cholesterol and saturated fats as the Lyme disease population.

The simple reality is that people with Lyme disease will usually feel much better and heal more quickly if they include adequate intake of cholesterol and saturated fats in their diet. These nutrients do not, however, replace the need for other kinds of fats, such as the Omega fatty acids found in foods like fish and flax oil. Therefore, Lyme disease sufferers should also consume hearty servings of fish and/or flax oil. Fish can be tricky due to high mercury content; therefore, some people (such as myself) prefer to use flax oil instead of fish. While flax oil doesn't have the extremely beneficial DHA component, it does have the building blocks that allow the body to synthesize DHA. Fish-free DHA supplements are also available.

Another important benefit of fat is that it stimulates bile flow. Bile is, of course, your body's primary way to eliminate fat-soluble toxins which are abundant in Lyme disease. So, fat can aid in the detoxification process. *Note: Because the body naturally recycles upwards of 95% of the bile used for digestion by absorbing it in the intestinal tract toward the end of the digestive process, fat soluble toxins can also be absorbed, preventing their elimination. This creates a circular flow of toxins, as bile is first introduced into the gastrointestinal tract to aid in digestion and then absorbed out of the gastrointestinal tract later. Hence, there are various treatments and strategies available which help to prevent bile and fat-soluble toxins from being absorbed; these therapies may break the circular cycle so that toxins are excreted in the feces rather than being retained in the body. These treatments are known as "binders" and are discussed in various places throughout the book, especially Chapter 9.*

Protein

Now let's move on to the discussion of protein, the other macronutrient at the bottom of the paleo pyramid. During one of my stints as a vegan (it only lasted a few weeks!), I was feeling horrible and stayed up late to research dietary philosophies. I happened upon an article written by one of the top healers of our time. The article explained how the body's detoxification system relies heavily on amino acids (i.e., protein). Glutathione, the master detoxifying antioxidant, is synthesized from the amino acids L-cysteine, L-glutamic acid, and glycine. And guess what? Lyme disease sufferers burn through glutathione much faster than other people because our bodies have to work so hard to detoxify all of the toxins and dead organisms associated with Borrelia and co-infections. So, we need more, not less, amino acids than the general public.

Sure, vegetable-only diets will allow you to consume many types of vegetable protein, but only animal protein arrives in the form that your body can use right away. Most vegetable proteins require your body to work hard to synthesize them into more readily usable forms of protein, and when you are sick with a chronic disease, this work can be devastating and drain the body's resources even further. So, we see yet another reason to avoid vegetarianism and veganism: you simply aren't able to get enough protein, and the protein you get isn't the best kind for you.

In addition to detoxification processes, protein is important for so many other body functions, such as maintaining muscle mass, healing tissues, and balancing brain chemistry (most neurotransmitters are, in fact, amino acids). During chronic disease, protein is critically important for building new blood vessels and cells, strengthening the immune system, and keeping the body strong to fight infections.

Sure enough, after discovering the above information and discontinuing my vegan diet, I began to feel better immediately. My energy returned, and I was like a new person. I doubt there will ever be another time in my life when I attempt to give up animal protein. Are there some people in the world who may actually benefit from a vegan, or at least, a vegetarian diet? Probably. And you might even be one of them. But chances are, if you have Lyme disease, you will do much better to consume animal protein.

Some animal proteins are healthier than others. It's a good idea to minimize red meat consumption, not because of the fat content but because red meat is very acidic. Poultry, fish, and eggs, on the other hand, are better choices.

Before leaving the topic of protein, we must address one of the most important proteins available—whey protein. And that requires a discussion of dairy products.

Whey Protein & Dairy Products

Dairy products are the schizophrenics of nutrition. Are they good? Are they bad? It depends on whom you ask, and the fads seem to flip flop each year. There is actually good reason for the controversy, believe it or not. That's because dairy is both good and bad.

Most dairy products can be broken down into the following constituents. Once you learn about these constituents, it is easier to evaluate various dairy products.

1. **Milk protein**. There are two primary types of milk protein:

   a) **Casein**. This is the "bad" protein. It is linked with many degenerative health problems. It is found in milk, cheese, and related dairy products. While it is sometimes used for bodybuilding (especially as a night time meal due to its slow absorption), it is generally recognized as unhealthy. Most people who are intolerant of dairy products are intolerant of casein and lactose.

   b) **Whey**. This is the "good" protein. It is one of the most bio-available sources of amino acids and is a very useful dietary supplement. It contains little, if any, casein and lactose. If you are familiar with whey protein only as a body-building supplement, you need to take another look: it also has many properties which make it very useful for healing from chronic illness. Few people are allergic to whey protein, and it is generally well-tolerated. One of the greatest benefits of whey protein is that it contains a broad spectrum of amino acids which are easy to digest and absorb. It offers incredible benefits for Lyme sufferers.

2. **Milk fat**. Also called "cream," this is the dairy product that is used to make butter as well as heavy whipping cream products. It is high

in saturated fat. "Half & Half" is composed of half cream and half milk. Heavy whipping cream and butter have very little, if any, casein and lactose.

3. **Lactose**. Lactose is a disaccharide sugar. Many people are lactose-intolerant, and even people who can tolerate lactose are probably still slightly sensitive to it in ways they may not recognize.

Earlier in the chapter, we looked at the many benefits of protein, saturated fat, and cholesterol. **Therefore, when it comes to a diet for Lyme disease sufferers, most people will benefit from consuming whey protein and milk fat while staying away from lactose and casein**. Varying degrees of lactose and casein may be tolerated, and these amounts will be based on individual biochemistry and sensitivities. As a general rule, foods containing lactose and casein should be consumed in moderation or avoided. Hypersensitivity reactions including inflammation, stuffy nose, brain fog, and other allergies often result when a person is sensitive to, and consumes, lactose and casein.

I buy pure whey protein and make smoothies with it (more on that later). I also use heavy whipping cream in the smoothies. As mentioned, whey protein and heavy whipping cream contain only traces of lactose and casein. While my family doesn't consume much breakfast cereal, on the rare occasions that we do, we use 50% heavy whipping cream and 50% water as a milk substitute. As noted, most kinds of milk are loaded with lactose and casein, so we avoid milk.

Heavy whipping cream is preferred over Half & Half because it doesn't contain milk (Half & Half is ½ milk and ½ cream). We are using the whipping cream to get the fat content; therefore, any milk mixed in is superfluous and only gives us more of the bad elements of dairy. Note that butter and heavy whipping cream are very similar in composition, and liberal consumption of butter can provide important fat that helps with satiety and recovery from adrenal fatigue.

Yogurt is another dairy product which has many benefits (in moderation). We all know about the beneficial bacteria found in yogurt, but it is also a preferable form of dairy because it doesn't contain much lactose; the bacteria consume the lactose during fermentation. Yogurt can be consumed if you can tolerate it but watch for food allergy reactions.

Now that we've looked at a brief overview of dairy products, let's move on.

But What About the Vegetables?

We've talked about dairy products, protein, and fat. Does that mean that we don't need vegetables? Of course not! Vegetables are a critical part of any diet—the more, the better. Vegetables are nutrient-dense, high in fiber, and alkalizing. Remember, our preferred diet doesn't like extremes; we take the best of all the other diets and combine them. A vegetable smoothie is an amazing shortcut that allows much easier access to this food group, and I'll provide the recipe I use for this smoothie in a few pages.

I won't spend much time here singing the virtues of vegetables, since any information I provide will likely be obvious; you've heard it a thousand times. Instead, I'll spend more time talking about the more controversial, less known aspects of dietary decision-making. Suffice it to say, eating vegetables is good, and the more the better.

Fruit

Fruit should be consumed only in moderation. While fruit is fiber- and nutrient-dense, it is also high in fructose, a kind of sugar that can have many negative health consequences. One guiding principle to keep in mind when it comes to fruit is this: if you are reaching for a carbohydrate, favor fruit over other carbohydrate sources. The logic is as follows: we are going to be limiting carbohydrate intake to some degree, so you have to choose carefully, because you aren't allowed unlimited carbohydrates. Choosing fruit maximizes the benefit you get from your carbohydrate foods, because fruit is the most nutritious of all carbohydrate-rich choices, especially when compared to empty, nutrient-poor carbohydrate foods like potatoes and rice. It is also helpful to check the calorie and sugar content of various fruits. Different people will have different tolerances for fruit; some people will need more fruit to feel well, and other people will only feel worse when consuming lots of fruit.

Fruit also has a tendency to feed yeast and worsen candida problems, so this should be taken into consideration when deciding how much fruit to consume.

Berries like strawberries and blueberries are relatively low in sugar and calories, and high in fiber and nutrients, so they make good choices. Apples and bananas have more sugar and more calories but are great energizing foods for an active lifestyle. They are also nutrient-dense. I love raisins and dates, as they often satisfy sugar cravings and are great energizing snacks (consume them in moderation, though, as they are high in calories). An interesting study concluded that people who eat dates are less likely to be obese than people who eat the same amount of calories in the form of soda or processed carbohydrates!

Carbohydrates: Treating Them as Rocket Fuel

So, what's the story on carbohydrates? We've already seen that the majority of an ideal diet should be composed of fat, protein, vegetables, and fruits in moderation. Is there a guiding philosophy when it comes to carbohydrates? How much is enough, and how much is too much?

This is where we start to completely diverge from conventional dietary wisdom, and this is where the controversy becomes heated. In fact, in my opinion, this is the area where most Americans go wrong, as the mainstream food pyramid shows that carbohydrates should be the foundation of a healthy diet. If there's one thing in this chapter that should stand out as important, it is probably the following information on carbohydrates.

Our goal for carbohydrate intake should be to strike just the right balance. We want to consume enough carbohydrates to keep our energy up and to avoid a state of ketosis (although new research is demonstrating that ketosis may be a powerful tool to fight cancer) but not so much so as to cause weight gain, blood sugar and insulin spikes, and excessive inflammation. This level of carbohydrate consumption is very small in comparison with the typical American diet. Unfortunately, most Americans don't just consume too many carbohydrates, they consume *WAAAYYYYY* too many. Carbohydrate-rich foods are front and center in most grocery stores and are the go-to snacks and meals for many people. Breakfast cereals, breads, pastries, rice, potatoes, fruit, pasta, snack foods—these are just the beginning. Even whole grains, which are widely believed to be healthy, are consumed in huge, excessive quantities. Cutting back on the carbohydrates is certainly the most difficult suggestion that this chapter will throw at you. It literally requires a redesign of all three of the daily meals as well as your snack food choices. You have to go back to the drawing board for breakfast, lunch, and dinner, which isn't easy to do.

I like to think of carbohydrates as rocket fuel: a little bit goes a long way. When it comes to powering a rocket, you certainly do need fuel, but you definitely don't want too much of it, or you get a huge explosion! Similarly, you do need to consume carbohydrates, but you don't want to consume too much. The exception would be for people who are very athletic and burn a lot of energy on a daily basis. For these folks, high levels of carbohydrates are necessary and get quickly burned off. However, in all cases, the goal should be to consume just the right amount—no more, no less.

Chronically ill people must be even more careful than others when it comes to carbohydrates, because most chronically ill people don't have the energy for strenuous exercise, and therefore, are much more susceptible to obesity. Carbohydrates that enter the body during a state of reduced exercise/activity are immediately converted to fat. The higher level of activity you can tolerate, the more carbohydrates you can consume without gaining weight. If you are chronically ill, you really can't afford to be obese, as obesity further throws off your already battered hormone balance as well as introduces a plethora of health problems which you really don't want to be dealing with while you are recovering from Lyme disease. Furthermore, obesity increases the chances for connective tissue injury, which will, in turn, make you even more immobile; it's a vicious cycle. Obesity is often a struggle for those with chronic illness, but it should be addressed if at all possible.

So, for carbohydrates, how much is enough? Well, it is different for each person. The rule I use is basically this: I eat mostly fat, protein, and vegetables, until my body tells me it's time for some carbohydrates. Over time, you will learn what this feels like. The difference between the Atkins' Diet and the diet I'm advocating is that the Atkins' Diet doesn't allow any carbohydrates. My diet, in contrast, allows carbohydrates but only as much as I need and nothing more. Carbohydrates are eaten with awareness and intentionality; they aren't the first thing you grab when opening the cabinet. Also, whenever your body is stressed in any way, whether due to emotional factors, physical disease, Herxing, a common cold, or other causes, it will need more carbohydrates to function normally, so take this into account. During periods when you are feeling the strongest, you'll be able to consume the fewest carbohydrates.

It is true that a lack of dietary carbohydrates can cause lethargy, fatigue, malaise, and depression. So, another way to look at this eating plan is to make it your goal to squeeze the carbohydrates out of your diet as much as possible, without causing your energy levels to bottom out. If you have just eaten and are still hungry, eat more fat or protein, or more vegetables. Squeeze out the carbohydrates with other food choices. If you are really craving carbohydrates, and you can tell you need some rocket fuel, then by all means, eat some. Just be sure to stop after you've had enough.

Furthermore, be careful about the choices you make when choosing particular carbohydrate-rich foods. Stay away from processed, refined carbohydrates and from all types of refined sugars. Instead, choose fruits and whole grains like brown rice. Carbohydrate-rich foods high in fiber help to slow digestion and prevent the blood sugar and insulin spikes that result from eating refined carbohydrates. So, it's not just a question of how much to eat, but also, which carbohydrates to eat.

Ultimately, though, each person will need an individualized, custom level of carbohydrate intake. In my version of the Paleo Diet, I don't restrict carbohydrates to the point that my available energy is decreased, nor to the point that well-being is decreased. Bodybuilders and people who compete in physique competitions often deprive themselves of carbohydrates to the point that they feel fatigue, lethargy, brain fog, and lack of energy. I do not advocate this. People recovering from any chronic disease should eat enough carbohydrates to power their bodies and to energize them for daily activities. Again—and you'll hear me say this many times—the goal is to avoid extremes.

Lastly, I would like to offer some encouragement. I have personally found that the most difficult thing about changing my eating habits is the change itself. It is hard to change how you think about food, to pick new favorite foods, to change your shopping routine, and to re-stock your refrigerator and pantry shelves. These changes require discipline, thought, planning, and new knowledge. However, after you've made the changes, I can tell you from personal experience that it gets much, much easier.

Once new habits are formed, healthy eating will become the new norm, and you'll actually feel like you are going out of your way to eat any differently. It's all about developing healthy habits. I love the saying, "Habits are at first only as strong as cobwebs, but later as strong as cables."

Saying Goodbye to Grains and Gluten

I gave up gluten several years ago. After hearing for years that a gluten-free diet is critical for Lyme disease patients, I finally took the plunge and gave it a try. By this point in my recovery, I was already 95% well, so I wasn't expecting much to happen; boy was I wrong! Giving up gluten was one of the healthiest choices I've ever made. You don't really know how much damage gluten does until you give it up; only then can you see how much better you feel. The importance of a gluten-free diet is now widely accepted by most Lyme doctors and is gaining traction among the healthy population of the world, as well. Several recent books, including some New York Times bestselling books such as *Wheat Belly* and *Grain Brain* focus on the harm done by gluten. I won't spend much time talking about the dangers of gluten here, but if you make only one dietary change in this whole chapter, it should be to say goodbye to gluten. If you aren't willing to do this, you will be missing out on one of the most important, and easiest, ways to feel better. A Lyme diet that includes gluten is just a setup for failure.

My own journey away from grains didn't end with gluten; My family and I eventually reduced our consumption of most other kinds of grains, as well. Trust me—I know how hard that sounds. Before you close the book, throw it in the trash can, and proclaim how unrealistic I am, give me a chance to explain myself. You will see that my own experience has further reinforced the validity of the Paleo Diet for Lyme sufferers (the Paleo Diet advocates very low grain intake).

Here is how my story went. After my family gave up gluten, my wife replaced it with rice. We got rice everything—rice noodles, rice bread, rice pancake mix, rice tortillas. Our goal was to feel like we hadn't given up gluten; we wanted to keep eating the same foods we ate before. This worked for a while. We were happily able to eat the same foods that are normally made of gluten. We enjoyed gluten-free pizza, bread, breakfast foods, and more. However, as time went on, I started to realize that I just felt better when I left out the rice-based products. Over time, my wife agreed, and we slowly started to drop them from our diet. This transition was actually much more difficult than going gluten-free, because gluten-free eating didn't really change our meals much; we just used rice-based substitutes for the recipes that used to call for gluten.

Now, I want to be clear about something. We aren't completely grain-free. I will often make myself a sandwich using gluten-free bread. I'll take a few bites of brown rice from time to time. And when I'm in need of an energetic meal, I'll have a bowl of oatmeal. Remember, our ideal diet avoids extremes! The important thing is that I consume gluten-free grains in my diet as the exception, not the rule. And if I eat too much of them—even a little too much—I'll feel the effects. Grains and their high levels of carbohydrates rapidly turn into sugar once inside the body, and that spike in blood sugar and insulin causes all kinds of problems.

I will say that baby steps are important. Don't expect to radically change your diet overnight, or you'll be disappointed by failure. Take one baby step at a time.

Something interesting happened when we dropped most of the grains from our diet: I no longer had trouble keeping the weight off. I've never struggled with being overweight, but I have definitely gone up a belt loop or two, especially during the winter months. After dropping the grains, this is no longer an issue. While eating a mostly paleo-based diet, my physique began to resemble the body I used to have when I was a teenager. Muscle tone became much easier to achieve, and fat melted off. I wondered to myself: is the getting old process we all dread so much—punctuated by flab, weak muscles, and lack of energy—really caused by poor diet, and not just the aging of our bodies alone? I'm convinced it is. I've learned just how powerful nutrition can be.

A friend of mine who competes in amateur body-building contests once told me his secret: "Bryan," he said, "the secret to a good physique is that it is achieved 90% in the kitchen, and only 10% in the gym." Until my own eating transformation, I had always been skeptical of this claim. However, I now notice that with proper eating and moderate exercise, I've found it fairly easy to maintain the physique of my teenage self. Consuming a high-fat diet keeps me satiated and prevents overeating. The higher levels of protein in my diet allow me to build and maintain muscle much more easily, while the lower carbohydrate intake keeps me lean and trim and requires my body to burn fat as an energy source. A diet with the opposite composition—that is, high carbohydrates and low protein/fat—would have the opposite effect. Muscle mass would be compromised, and body fat would be gained.

What's even more interesting is the fact that I don't miss the grains at all. The foods I eat now are much more satisfying and tasty, and, most importantly, make me feel so much better than a grain-based diet. When I finally gave myself permission to eat the foods that have always made me feel good, and bucked the conventional wisdom about saturated fats, cholesterol, and protein, I began to feel satisfied after meals, my brain fog after eating went away, and I wasn't always struggling with a belt that felt tighter and tighter. For example, a breakfast of four eggs, a few slices of bacon, and an apple makes me feel so much better than oatmeal with a side of wheat toast. There's just no comparison in how I feel between these two choices—one makes me feel fantastic and energized, and the other makes me feel bloated and leaves me feeling hungry.

The biggest challenge to eating mostly grain-free isn't that it is hard, masochistic, or unpleasant. Instead, it is challenging because it is so far off the beaten path. The problem is the culture of carbohydrates that dominates our country. It can require hard work and intentionality to rebuild your diet from the ground up. Grains and refined carbohydrates are everywhere we look. Whole grains, which are admittedly healthier than refined choices, are still way too predominant in almost all food choices. Whether shopping at the grocery store or eating out with friends, it is nearly impossible to avoid coming face-to-face with huge loaves of bread, bowls of pasta, and other grain-based products. The hardest part of a low grain diet isn't giving up the grains, but instead, finding tasty substitutes which are accessible at home and when eating out. That is the real challenge, but once you find those substitutes, eating mostly grain-free becomes much easier. Once I discovered good replacement foods, I never looked back.

Putting It Into Practice: Meal and Snack Examples

Now, let's put it all together and take a look at some practical steps to implement the dietary guidelines in this chapter. Please note, though, that while I will give you some ideas here based on what we eat in my family, this is just a limited sampling of the many possible meals you can create using the Paleo Diet principles. Just do a Google search for *paleo recipes* and you'll find enough material to keep you busy for months!

Breakfast

Here are a few different meals you might consider for breakfast:

BREAKFAST IDEA #1: 4 whole eggs (including yolks) fried in coconut oil, served with a handful of baby carrots, a small bowl of plain yogurt (or Greek yogurt for twice the protein content), and a glass of V8 (or other vegetable) juice. Add an apple if you are planning an active day.

BREAKFAST IDEA #2: A few slices of bacon served with avocado, celery, and a chicken-apple sausage.

BREAKFAST IDEA #3: A paleo smoothie (described later).

BREAKFAST IDEA #4: A chicken breast served with a salad (consider adding a few handfuls of raisins or dates mixed with some whole, raw pecans, to the salad).

Lunch

LUNCH IDEA #1: A turkey sandwich made with gluten-free bread, avocado, lettuce, and tomato, along with a side of vegetables, and a few spoonfuls of peanut butter or coconut cream.

LUNCH IDEA #2: A baked chicken breast served with asparagus, and a cup of blueberries.

LUNCH IDEA #3: A filet of salmon served with quinoa, and a side of fresh sugar snap peas.

LUNCH IDEA #4: Homemade vegetable soup with a chicken broth base (chicken broth, especially homemade broth, is very healing to the adrenals).

LUNCH IDEA #5: A paleo smoothie (described later).

Dinner

DINNER IDEA #1: Shish kabobs cooked on the BBQ, including meat, vegetables, pineapple, and mushrooms, served with a salad made with ranch dressing or oil and vinegar dressing.

DINNER IDEA #2: Steak served with vegetables, a baked potato (allowed in moderation), a salad, and a handful of nuts.

DINNER IDEA #3: A paleo smoothie.

Again, these are just a small sampling of meal ideas to give you a general idea of how the diet can be implemented. Remember, flexibility is key. If you hold yourself to an impossibly rigid plan, you will likely fail. Experiment and find the foods you like, and extend extra grace to yourself while you are making the transition to healthier eating.

Snack Ideas

Snacks can be tricky, because we are so conditioned to reach for a bag of potato chips or pretzels. At snack time, I reach for some fruit instead. While I do advocate eating fruit in moderation, snacking on fruit can give you a little energy boost to help you make it until the next mealtime. Along with fruit, I recommend eating nuts at snack time (my favorites are pecans, almonds, and peanuts). The combination of carbohydrates in fruit, with fat and protein in nuts, can keep you satisfied and energized until the next meal. Dried fruit (my favorites are raisins and dates) as well as nuts are also very easy to pack for on-the-go snacks, and they don't require refrigeration or other special keeping. Of course, dozens of good snack options exist, including yogurt, vegetables, meat, and more. Snacking on meat, which may seem weird by our modern culture, can provide a high degree of satiety that will help you make it to the next mealtime. Remember the overarching guideline: pick snack foods that are whole and unprocessed and which don't have a list of ingredients.

The Marvelous Paleo Smoothie

We've mentioned this smoothie a few times in this chapter. Now let's take a look at what it is and why it is marvelous. The smoothie is designed to contain macronutrient ingredients which can power you through your day. The paleo smoothie literally changed my life in the kitchen—I have one almost every day and feel fantastic when I drink them. It is also an incredible meal substitute if you don't have time to make a nutritious meal. Instead of reaching for the bag of potato chips or a bowl of cereal, reach for the paleo smoothie. It offers the same brainless convenience but with a significantly better nutrition profile. We'll break the smoothie down into the various ingredient categories used to make it.

The Macronutrient Base

These are the ingredients which provide the calories, satiety, and macronutrients for the smoothie. When you start with these ingredients, you can build on them in many creative ways.

1. Whey protein: I generally use 1.5 scoops of whey protein isolate which contain about 27 grams of protein. Whey protein is low-calorie compared with other high-protein food sources, making it a good choice for smoothies. I prefer the Jarrow brand; it is listed as "Jarrow Formulas, Whey Protein, Ultrafiltered Powder, Unflavored, 32 oz" on Amazon.com and iHerb.com. You can also buy Jarrow's organic mix, but it is twice as expensive. Whatever you get, make sure your whey protein has only one ingredient—avoid any sweeteners, flavors, or additives. We will be flavoring and sweetening the smoothie with our own, healthy ingredients. I look for the lowest price and often find great discounts and free shipping when buying in bulk from iHerb.com. I also use Amazon Prime, an indispensable service which offers free 2-day shipping.

2. Heavy whipping cream: I will add a generous splash of heavy whipping cream which provides saturated fat for hormone production, satiety, and sustained energy. Remember, heavy whipping cream is preferred over Half & Half because it doesn't contain the unwanted milk component (see the earlier section on dairy products).

3. Ground flax seed: Add a large scoop of ground flax seed to enhance the nutrition of the smoothie with the critically important Omega fatty acids. Make sure you use ground, not whole, flax seed; whole flax seed does not get adequately digested. Flax seed is also relatively high in fiber and has potent anti-inflammatory qualities.

4. Add water to help with the blending process as well as ice to give it a cold, thick, refreshing texture.

The above macronutrients give you a high protein, high fat, low carbohydrate, nutrient-dense base which will power you through any challenge your day throws at you! Now let's see how we can doctor up the smoothie with creative flavors to make it taste great!

Creative Flavors and Additives for a Delicious Smoothie

After you have added the above macronutrient ingredients, you can experiment with other items to flavor and dress up the smoothie. A moderate portion of frozen berries along with half a banana create a delicious fruit smoothie. Sprinkle in some cinnamon and a dash of 100% pure, sugar-free vanilla extract, and you've got a recipe that will rival the taste of any McDonald's milkshake! Stevia extract is also available to sweeten up the drink (if you need a sugar-free, zero calorie sweetener, stevia is a decent choice; we use it in our kitchen). I shy away from using any type of sweetener, though. I find the moderate portion of berries or fruit is delicious and doesn't overpower the flavors of the other fantastic ingredients.

Another great flavor idea: get some organic, unsweetened, 100% pure cacao powder, and mix it into any smoothie recipe for a chocolaty flavor that is packed with more antioxidants than red wine and blueberries! Chocolate smoothies made from the macronutrient base ingredients along with organic cacao powder and stevia extract are among the most popular smoothies in my household.

There you have it—the paleo smoothie, one of my all-time favorites for a healthy snack or even a meal replacement. Please realize that the above recipe is very flexible. You can always drag-and-drop other items which you feel are a better fit for your preferences and lifestyle.

Paleo Hot Chocolate

Can you really consume hot chocolate and still be within the boundaries of the diet set forth in this chapter? It's your lucky day: you sure can! Simply mix some unsweetened cacao powder with heavy whipping cream, add a dash of stevia powder, mix with hot water, and you've got a yummy, healthy treat! For a more filling and satisfying hot chocolate, be generous with the heavy whipping cream and add a dash of whey protein.

Paleo Ice Cream

Paleo ice cream is one of my favorite things to make. It is just fantastic! It uses the same macronutrient base ingredients as the Marvelous Paleo Smoothie (and even the same flavoring add-ons). A date or two can be added to increase the sweetness of the resulting product.

You can control the consistency of the ice cream with the amount of ice and water you add. If you are in a hurry and want more of a milk shake, use less ice and more water for easy drinking. On the other hand, if you really want to take your time and enjoy it, add only a dash of water and a generous portion of ice; the result will have the texture of ice cream and can be eaten out of a bowl with a spoon. Eating foods that contain crushed ice is proven to be satiating and satisfying, offering a feeling of fullness, and the chewing that occurs when eating ice cream helps to give you the sensation of eating, which tells your brain to turn off hunger. Also, since ice cream is consumed more slowly than a smoothie, you are more likely to feel full by the time you are done eating. Yes, you are hearing me correctly: healthy ice cream can actually help you avoid the extra pounds as a result of these benefits!

The ice cream you make will taste so good that you will think you are cheating on your diet—but you aren't! You are powering your body with exactly what it needs and enjoying yourself at the same time. In fact, I've been known to eat paleo ice cream for lunch!

You can experiment with various ice cream recipes using the same macronutrient base ingredients. My wife prefers simple vanilla ice cream, which is made by mixing whey, heavy whipping cream, ground flax seed, 100% pure vanilla extract, a dash of stevia, half a dozen ice cubes, and about a tablespoon of water. Note that this recipe is carb-free, yet it tastes amazing. Go easy on the flax seeds or leave them out completely if the flax flavor seems overwhelming. The vanilla can be replaced with 100% pure cocoa powder (with no sugar added) to create chocolate ice cream instead.

The sky is the limit; you can be as creative as you want. The important thing is that the macronutrient base keeps the recipe nutritious, especially for the needs of Lyme disease sufferers. Next time you are looking for a snack or a healthy, easy meal, skip the unsatisfying, fattening, inflammation-causing refined carbohydrates and make yourself a smoothie or a bowl of ice cream instead!

There are many, many recipes like the ones mentioned in this book; you can find them in books and on the internet. A simple Google search for *paleo sugar-free recipes* will yield wonderful results. My wife also really likes the book, *Trim Healthy Mama*. You can find lots of great information in that book.

The Green Smoothie

What if you aren't hungry enough to justify eating all the macronutrients found in the Marvelous Paleo Smoothie or paleo ice cream, but instead, you want a healthy vegetable meal that is highly satisfying yet low in calories? I find that the biggest deterrent to eating vegetables is simply that they are so chewy, crunchy, and time-consuming to eat, especially the ones that are supposed to be really good for us. A big salad with a tasty dressing can solve this problem, but I have also discovered the green smoothie, and I love using it as an easy shortcut to getting vegetables down the hatch.

The green smoothie is where I get most of my dietary vegetables, and because of this, I make sure to pack it full of the most nutrient-dense, healthy vegetables I can find. I also use only raw vegetables, as these contain the most active enzymes and unadulterated vitamins and minerals. While it would be very difficult to consume raw asparagus, for example, it is easy when it is blended as part of the green smoothie. Likewise, broccoli is a chore to consume raw, but as part of a smoothie, it is easy. In fact, research shows that raw vegetables aren't even completely digested when chewed and swallowed, but when consumed as part of a smoothie, they are almost completely assimilated by the body because they enter the stomach as tiny blended particles which are much easier for the body to break down and digest.

I prefer smoothies over juicing because smoothies leave the whole vegetable, including the fiber, in the drink. I find this to be critical especially since the rest of the Paleo Diet is relatively low in fiber. However, juicing is, of course, a great option as well.

A typical green smoothie recipe in my household looks like this:

1. **Celery**
2. **Kale**
3. **Broccoli**
4. **Asparagus**
5. **Lettuce**
6. **Carrots**
7. **Beets**
8. **Cucumber**

Fruit, ginger, lemon, or even stevia can be added to improve the flavor (This recipe is not for the weak of heart. It tastes pretty intense!). My wife doesn't tolerate the taste very well and so adds a lot of fruit. I don't mind the taste, so I pretty much drink it with just the ingredients listed.

Adding plenty of water is important since all the fiber in these vegetables can make it difficult to drink. However, I find that with plenty of water, I can consume an entire day's worth of really healthy vegetables in about five minutes! It really is miraculous for me. Instead of laboring over a giant bowl of raw vegetables for hours, trying to choke them down by chewing and swallowing, I can simply slurp them down in a smoothie in just a few minutes.

Because these smoothies are so easy to drink in comparison with eating the actual raw vegetables, my wife and I find ourselves eating many more vegetables than we did before we started making the smoothies. We've noticed so many benefits of this, including weight loss, glowing skin, clear thinking, mood improvement, better memory, and other surprising results.

With regard to weight loss, I have been absolutely surprised by how filling green smoothies are. Every time I make one for myself, I think, "This can't possibly be as filling as a paleo smoothie without the macronutrient base ingredients." But, I always find that the green smoothie is even more filling than other types of smoothies. The high level of fiber accounts for this, as does the fact that green smoothies contain so many of the essential vitamins and minerals which the body requires to function. I really believe that my waistline would look a lot worse if I hadn't discovered the green smoothie.

The Right Smoothie at the Right Time

The green smoothie is very different from the paleo smoothie which provides macronutrients to fuel the body's many activities. While the green smoothie is very filling and satisfying, and contains essential vitamins, minerals, and phyto-chemicals, it lacks the building blocks for continued energy production and healing from chronic disease. Both smoothies contain nutrients that are essential for healing from Lyme disease, but they are each intended to be consumed under different circumstances.

The paleo smoothie is best as a meal replacement or for when you are substantially hungry. On the other hand, the green smoothie is great for when you know you didn't eat your vegetables for the day, yet you aren't super hungry, and you want to avoid a high calorie meal but still feel satisfied and full. I often find myself having a green smoothie for breakfast and then waiting until some real, substantial hunger sets in, at which time, I will have lunch or make a paleo smoothie. The green smoothie can sometimes hold me over to mid-afternoon, which is amazing considering it only contains a couple hundred calories.

This brings us to another important point. While the macronutrients fat and protein are essential to recovery, you should only consume them when you are substantially hungry. Consuming any food that contains a generous amount of calories when you aren't hungry will lead to weight gain. If you just want something to slurp down as a snack and you aren't really hungry, choose the green smoothie or a bag of baby carrots. Don't choose a high-fat or high-protein meal.

Tips for Success with Your Healthy Eating Plan

Now that we've seen some of my dietary suggestions and recommendations, let's move on to some of the general tips for success which can be applied to any eating plan.

The Poisonous Effects of Sugar

Because this book is intended for more of an advanced audience, I assume that you already know about the extreme dangers of consuming refined, processed sugar when you have Lyme disease. If you aren't aware of these dangers, you might want to do some research or read my previous books. A diet high in sugar will short circuit your recovery process and negate any other good dietary choices you make.

Don't be Afraid to Eat Things That Seem Socially or Culturally Weird

No dinner in the house? Don't worry. Just have a few carrots, a spoonful of peanut butter, and a spoonful of coconut oil, and you are all set! "No way," you say. "That's too weird!" Yes, it may be weird, but is weird a good reason not to do it? I notice that most people's eating habits are dictated more by culture and custom than by nutrition and science. And worse, many people fall to marketing hype and end up consuming processed foods produced by big corporations. Take a look around. Do the American people really exemplify the kind of health and lifestyle you want to emulate? Maybe, it is OK to be just a little bit weird, if it means you will be healthier than everyone around you. Sometimes, the healthiest food choices may seem to be the weirdest choices to the people you are hanging out with. But again, remember how Paleolithic people ate. A handful of nuts here, a banana there, a piece of meat a few hours later.

A bonus to following the Paleo Diet is that food choices are often very convenient and even as quick as fast food, with very little preparation, cleanup, or hassle. Remember, the Paleo Diet often prefers raw foods with only one ingredient. So the Paleo Diet is easy, not hard, for people on the go who don't have time to prepare healthy meals. A few handfuls of almonds is all it takes to replace a meal.

Plan Ahead—Especially When Traveling

This one doesn't need much explaining. Wherever you travel, chances are you won't find the kind of food you need to eat. Just make sure you are close to a grocery store when you get to your destination. Then you can get what you need instead of eating processed carbohydrate junk food. My wife and I sometimes joke that grocery stores are our restaurants, since restaurants typically don't have the broad food choices available which allow us to eat correctly.

Similarly, if you will be dining at a friend's house or restaurant, plan ahead. Know what's on the menu. If you can't or don't want to eat what is offered, simply eat a meal before you go and join in for the company and friendship, not the food. If you're invited to a close friend's for dinner, hopefully they will know you well enough to have a meal option for you.

While sometimes inconvenient, I've found that making good food choices instead of opting for the easier, culturally acceptable eating habits always makes me happier in the end.

Hunger is Your Friend, Food is Your Enemy

I love this saying. To most people, hunger is the enemy—an imposter intent on making you miserable—but the truth is, a little bit of hunger is your friend. It ensures you won't eat when you don't need refueling; it prevents obesity; and it develops in us an attitude of moderation when it comes to food. So remember, if you are a little bit hungry, don't open the refrigerator door right away—hunger is your friend.

On the other hand, for most people, food is the enemy—or at least, too much food is your enemy.

Fiber is Your Friend

Fiber has many important benefits for healthy people and chronically ill people. For Lyme disease sufferers, fiber is particularly important because it keeps the bowels moving, and the stool is the primary means for eliminating fat soluble toxins. Make sure you eat plenty of fiber.

Food Allergies

Avoid food allergens at all costs since food reactions can cause inflammation and reactivate old symptoms. Be especially aware of dairy products, which are very likely to cause problems in people with Lyme disease.

Paleo Desserts

Almost any dessert can be made with paleo ingredients and taste almost as good as the real thing. Do a Google search for paleo dessert recipes and you'll find results which allow you to keep eating many of your favorite dessert foods!

The Paleo Lifestyle Doesn't Stop With Food

The principles underpinning the Paleo Diet don't just apply to how we eat. They also apply to many other areas of our lifestyle. The next two chapters, Chapters 5 & 6 (especially Chapter 6), describe how these principles provide benefit to those healing from chronic disease.

Chapter 5
Adrenal Fatigue, Part I: Physical Symptoms and Physical Treatments

Note: Please be aware that the observations and opinions contained in this chapter and the following chapter are my own observations and opinions, and do not necessarily reflect the views of the various experts I reference throughout the chapters.

Adrenal Fatigue: A Condition That Affects Body, Mind, and Spirit

A drenal fatigue is a mystifying and fascinating condition. The more you learn about it, the more you see just how connected it is to almost every aspect of our well being: physical, mental, emotional, and spiritual. The condition of the adrenal glands will have an effect on you in every dimension of your life.

If you suffer from Lyme disease and related issues, it is a near certainty that you also suffer from adrenal fatigue, at least to some degree. The symptoms of adrenal fatigue can be very subtle, so you may not even know you are dealing with it. Be warned: if your symptoms are subtle now and you don't do something to heal your adrenal glands, your symptoms will surely progress and worsen as time goes on; the worse adrenal fatigue gets, the more difficult it is to reverse it. In fact, it becomes exponentially more dangerous the longer it is unrecognized and unresolved. The reason that adrenal fatigue is tricky to recognize is that some of the more common symptoms associated with adrenal fatigue (including emotional instability, fatigue, and other issues we will look at) are also associated with Lyme disease, making it difficult to identify which underlying issues a person has.

We will divide the topic of adrenal fatigue into two parts: the physical manifestations, and the non-physical manifestations. The current chapter will address the physical manifestations, and the following chapter (Chapter 6) will address the non-physical manifestations (which include mental, emotional, and spiritual aspects). The two chapters are inseparably connected and are intended to be an overview of the topic of adrenal fatigue. For more extensive, in-depth coverage, I will provide book and website recommendations at the end of this chapter, and I implore you to look at these additional resources. Adrenal fatigue is a very counter-intuitive, dangerous condition, and if you suffer from it, you really need to do some extensive reading on the topic if you hope to get well.

Introduction

The adrenal glands are endocrine glands that rest on top of the kidneys. When functioning properly, they produce many types of hormones, including stress hormones. These glands are critical to proper body functioning on numerous levels. Many problems, including thyroid imbalances, depression, chronic fatigue syndrome, panic disorders and agitation, mood imbalances, and a plethora of emotional symptoms may be due to adrenal fatigue.

Adrenal fatigue occurs when the adrenal glands cannot keep up with the quantity of hormones they are required to produce to maintain bodily functions. When this happens, the adrenals become drained, and the body experiences a growing net deficit of essential hormones. The result is that the body is no longer able to expend energy on physical, mental, and emotional activities. Since everything we do as humans is either physical, mental, or emotional (or a combination of the three), adrenal fatigue has an impact on each and every aspect of our lives. While there are many other features of adrenal fatigue, as we will see, the primary point to remember is that adrenal fatigue is a problem of energy inadequacy. When you have adrenal fatigue, you will get worse when you expend too much physical, mental, or emotional energy, and you will get better when you allow for sufficient physical, emotional, and mental rest.

Adrenal fatigue is a problem that leads to massive dysfunction throughout almost all body systems. In this way, adrenal fatigue is very unlike other kinds of health problems. For example, if you have chest congestion, you are likely to only experience a narrow set of symptoms limited to the lungs. Not so with adrenal fatigue. If you have adrenal fatigue, you'll experience dysfunction in nearly every other organ in the body, and you'll experience dozens of seemingly unrelated, yet severe, symptoms. Because of this, adrenal fatigue is a serious problem. People with severe adrenal fatigue are often confined to their beds for years at a time without enough energy to even walk down the stairs and eat breakfast. A long-time family friend is such a person, and I've watched her maintain this state for over two decades. It has been very sad to see.

Adrenal fatigue is typically caused by one or more of the following circumstances:

1. **Disease**—The adrenal glands are weakened and compromised by physical disease and are not able to operate at full capacity. In this case, the adrenals themselves are physically damaged by some disease process.

2. **Stress**—A person experiences extreme stress, worry, emotional distress, anxiety, or other feelings which trigger the fight or flight response for an extended period of time. In this case, the adrenals may not have been physically damaged by a disease, but they can still become depleted, drained and exhausted, if mental or emotional stress is prolonged or severe.

3. **Brain Dysfunction**—In circumstances when a person's stress level is normal and not excessive, the adrenal glands may still become fatigued if the brain is malfunctioning and sending over-stimulatory signals to the adrenal glands, telling them to produce excessive stress hormones. This situation typically results from some kind of dysfunction within the brain, not the adrenal glands.

There are other causes of adrenal fatigue, including dietary issues and other physical/emotional problems. However, the above three will be the ones we focus on. For Lyme disease sufferers, all three are typically in play. Lyme disease and co-infections (especially Bartonella) cause physical damage to the adrenal glands themselves, leading to #1 occurring. #3 happens when Lyme disease and co-infections cause physical damage to the brain, which disrupts signals sent from the brain to the adrenal glands, causing the adrenal glands to get false alarms and overreact to even the smallest stress stimulus. And #2 happens during the course of normal life events and stresses, but is exacerbated by #'s 1 and 3. While healthy people are susceptible to adrenal fatigue, they are typically only vulnerable to #2, and therefore, they can tolerate significantly more stress than can Lyme disease patients before their adrenals begin to fail. This discussion should illustrate that Lyme sufferers are much more susceptible to adrenal fatigue than the general population.

One last note before we move on: Adrenal fatigue is an issue that compounds as the adrenals become more exhausted. Exhausted adrenal glands become much more sensitive to stress. So, the experience of adrenal fatigue can be a downward spiral. When the adrenals are in bad shape, relaxation and de-stressing is desperately needed, yet finding relaxation and peace are much more difficult because the adrenals over-react to even the smallest stressful stimulus. This puts people with adrenal fatigue in a very precarious and dangerous position; a paradox of sorts. Moderate to severe adrenal fatigue is a very serious and life-threatening health problem which needs to be treated with the utmost caution and respect.

Symptoms of Adrenal Fatigue

The symptoms of adrenal fatigue can overlap tightly with the symptoms of Lyme disease. In many instances, this leads to poor recognition of adrenal fatigue as people mistakenly attribute all of their symptoms to Lyme disease. Some common symptoms of adrenal fatigue include exercise intolerance, sleep disturbances, lack of energy and fatigue, and feeling overwhelmed by the smallest of tasks. It is common to feel exhausted yet not be able to sleep. Since these are all potentially Lyme disease symptoms, too, it can be tricky to know what's really going on. One way to distinguish adrenal fatigue from the plethora of Lyme disease symptoms is to look for emotional instability, fatigue, sleep disturbances, and other symptoms which have their onset the day after exercise.

Also, while Lyme disease can cause fatigue and weakness, the fatigue and weakness that accompany adrenal fatigue are often much worse and much more debilitating. Lyme disease sufferers without adrenal fatigue may feel horrible hiking up several flights of stairs, but they can still do it. In contrast, those with severe adrenal fatigue may not be able to make it up the stairs at all, or if they do make it, they will experience a huge crash in the following days.

Another possible differentiating feature is that adrenal fatigue typically begins or worsens after a person experiences extremely stressful life events; for example, divorce, the death of a loved one, loss of a job, or other similar challenges. Numerous tests are available to measure the hormones produced by the adrenal glands to determine whether they are at normal levels. I am not convinced that these tests are significantly useful, but in the hands of the right doctor they may provide clues.

Shortness of breath, or rapid breathing, may also be present when the adrenals are exhausted, and there are several deep breathing techniques available to help reset the breathing patterns to normal. Of course, Babesia also causes shortness of breath, adding to the confusion. However, the shortness of breath that comes with adrenal fatigue is often accompanied by other adrenal fatigue symptoms, while the shortness of breath that comes with Babesia is often accompanied by other Babesia symptoms; therefore, you will have clues to help you determine what the root cause of your symptoms is.

The startle response can also be heightened when adrenal fatigue is present. The body may feel like it is always on high alert. Again, unfortunately, this symptom can also be caused by tick-borne infections when adrenal fatigue is not present, hence, the difficulty of determining which problems are caused by adrenal fatigue and which are caused by tick-borne infections.

For men, adrenal fatigue symptoms can be brought on or exacerbated by sex because the demand to create new hormones during and after sex drains the adrenal glands.

Adrenal fatigue symptoms are often experienced as "crashes." These crashes can include the sudden onset or worsening of symptoms. The initial crashes are often the worst, because they typically precede awareness of the problem, and are, hence, not addressed with the proper therapies and interventions. If the proper steps are taken and recovery begins, these crashes will be experienced with less frequency and severity over time, leading to a slow, uphill climb out of the depths of adrenal fatigue. However, if exercise or other taxing activities are resumed too soon during the recovery process, or if worry and stress overwhelm the adrenal glands, then backsliding can occur in the form of additional serious crashes. Adrenal fatigue experts, such as Dr. Lam, whose book is referenced at the end of this chapter, often use a graph to illustrate the "crash-recovery" cycle and the various phases of healing. Unfortunately, recovering from a severe adrenal crash can be a very prolonged process, often requiring six months to three years. The good news, as we will see in the following chapter, is that the lifestyle changes required to heal from adrenal fatigue are often very positive, healthy changes that can lead to a more satisfying and relaxed life.

Emotional Symptoms

We will address the emotional aspects of adrenal fatigue in the next chapter, but it is important to be introduced to these symptoms before we go any further.

The most debilitating symptoms of adrenal fatigue are the emotional symptoms. These symptoms aren't "all in your head." Weakened adrenals actually cause physical imbalances in the body and are the underlying physical cause for feelings of guilt, shame, insecurity, desperation, sadness, anger, and others. Remember, the brain is a physical organ, and how you feel is influenced by the chemical reactions taking place in your brain. Adrenal fatigue causes physical changes in many parts of the body, and these physical changes lead to brain imbalances that result in tremendous changes in how a person feels about him or herself, and how they feel about the rest of the world. It can be very easy to just write these symptoms off as normal emotional responses to being in a tough situation involving chronic illness or life trauma. However, research concludes the opposite: these symptoms are not a natural and normal response to being sick. Instead, they are physical in nature and a direct result of the damage that the infections are doing to your organs.

It is important to realize that the symptoms we are talking about here are the result of real, physical causes. This opens the door to treating them with real, physical treatments rather than limiting the treatment approach to therapies like counseling or meditation. While psychological approaches are helpful, and are indeed needed for adrenal fatigue recovery (as we'll see), they will never completely solve the problem as long as the problem includes unresolved physical dysfunction within the brain, organs, and adrenal glands.

The above paragraphs are not a complete list of the symptoms of adrenal fatigue; numerous other symptoms exist. At the end of this chapter, I will provide resources for other books and websites which can shed additional light on the symptoms of adrenal fatigue.

As I am fond of recommending, a therapeutic trial of treatment for adrenal fatigue may be helpful when you don't know whether or not you have the condition. If you respond positively to the therapeutic trial, it may help confirm the existence of adrenal fatigue. If you experience no response, then it may indicate that you are not suffering from adrenal fatigue. However, keep in mind that almost all victims of tick-borne infections have adrenal fatigue to some degree.

Treating Adrenal Fatigue

The treatment of adrenal fatigue is perhaps one of the most frustrating endeavors you will encounter during your recovery from Lyme disease but also one of the most potentially rewarding. As Americans, we are used to taking a pill to make our health problems disappear. In fact, not only do we want to take a pill, we want to be back on our feet as quickly as possible to participate in the busy lives that we lead. Even Lyme disease sufferers have this expectation: "Doctor, just give me my antibiotic prescription right away, and give me the highest dose possible!" And, in fact, Lyme sufferers do get better with aggressive treatment. Maybe antibiotic therapy alone isn't enough, but certainly other kinds of aggressive treatments can be helpful.

Adrenal fatigue turns this treatment paradigm on its head. When it comes to adrenal fatigue, we need to literally re-wire our thought processes and expectations for recovery.

In the beginning of this chapter, we talked about how the adrenal glands in people with Lyme disease are weakened by infections and are over-stimulated by haywire signals from a malfunctioning brain. This leaves those who suffer from Lyme disease destabilized and compromised, and even less capable of dealing with the stresses of normal life. There is no pill or supplement which can fix this problem. The only way to heal the adrenal glands is to give them a rest and remove the stressors which are keeping them down.

So, removing the infections which weaken the adrenal glands, as well as healing the brain so that it doesn't send haywire signals to them, is important. However, eliminating life stress is also critical and is not easily done. In fact, it may require a complete re-working of your lifestyle, priorities, vocation, and even relationships. This is hundreds of times more difficult than popping a few pills. When we talk about removing life stress, we aren't just talking about avoiding fights with your spouse or boss. We are talking about re-thinking your entire outlook on life, and making peace with the many internal and external factors that add anxiety and worry to your life. To heal from adrenal fatigue, you almost have to figure out how to become a whole new person. The treatment for adrenal fatigue isn't an easy pursuit, and unfortunately, some people are unwilling or unable to make the necessary changes.

The next chapter will address these kinds of lifestyle changes in more detail. The simple reality is that to heal from adrenal fatigue, we have to literally change what we do on a day-to-day basis and how we think about our lives. These changes, while difficult, can ultimately be very rewarding, as we attempt to live a more balanced and relaxed life.

There are, of course, various supplements, prescriptions, and therapies which claim to help with adrenal fatigue. For some people, such interventions may be useful, but for most Lyme disease sufferers, they will do nothing more than artificially stimulate the adrenal glands which will lead to greater adrenal weakness at some point in the future. Or, in the case of interventions which provide the body with external hormones, the adrenal glands will atrophy and shut down, causing a dependence on the interventions and a permanent weakening of the adrenal glands. In both cases, the end result is not healing and rehabilitation but further debilitation and damage. Again, the only true, lasting recovery comes from removing the physical and emotional stresses from the adrenal glands, which allows them to heal and rebuild. I can tell you from experience that many Lyme sufferers (including myself) are reluctant to accept this reality and will first run through the gamut of quick fix treatments before they come to terms with the truth about adrenal fatigue.

While supplements and nutrients cannot be a substitute for rest and the elimination of stressors, they can provide support during the recovery process. Let's examine some of the available supplements and treatments, and discuss their pros and cons. Let's start by looking at vitamins and food choices, because they stand apart from other supplement options in their ability to actually provide true, long-term healing.

B Vitamins, Vitamin C, and Food Choices

While most available supplements and interventions are mere bandaids, the vitamins and food choices we will look at here are among the few interventions which actually lead to healing and rebuilding, not just temporary progress or masking of symptoms. Why are these particular interventions helpful? Because even when lifestyle modifications are correctly implemented and stressors are removed, the adrenal glands must still be given the raw materials to heal and rebuild. These raw materials are found in the foods and vitamins discussed now. Without these special foods and vitamins, recovery can take a lot longer.

Vitamin C. Scientists have noticed that vitamin C is found in high concentrations in the adrenal glands. In fact, there is no other part of the body which hoards vitamin C like the adrenal glands. Vitamin C is critical for proper adrenal function and during adrenal exhaustion, vitamin C reserves are quickly used up. As a result, vitamin C supplementation—specifically, liphophilic vitamin C, also known as "Lipo C," which is highly absorbable and bioavailable to the adrenal glands (and other body systems)—is extremely important during recovery from adrenal fatigue. Various companies manufacture Lipo C, including Researched Nutritionals and LivOn Labs. Lipo C will be discussed in more detail in Chapter 17. Note: vitamin C increases the absorption of iron, so if you have unhealthy high iron levels, be careful not to take vitamin C near the time of consumption of high-iron meals.

B Vitamins. All of the B vitamins, but especially vitamin B5 (pantothenic acid, or pantethine in the more active form) are essential for adrenal function and are quickly drained during adrenal fatigue. Consequently, supplementation with a B complex as well as higher doses of pantothenic acid and/or pantethine is necessary during recovery from adrenal fatigue. My favorite B complex, "B Right," is made by Jarrow Formulas and is available from Amazon.com and iHerb.com. Note that toward the end of adrenal fatigue recovery, doses of these vitamins may have to be decreased as the adrenal glands learn to function on their own. Excessive doses can overwhelm the adrenal glands.

Multivitamin and Multimineral. While not as important as vitamin C and the B vitamins, a multivitamin and multimineral are still important during recovery from adrenal fatigue. The adrenal glands use many vitamins and minerals as cofactors during proper functioning.

Food Choices. Dietary habits are very important during recovery from adrenal fatigue. The chapter of this book on diet (Chapter 4) includes not just healthy foods, but healthy foods which are specifically compatible with adrenal fatigue recovery. Cholesterol and saturated fat are very important for adrenal hormone production and should be consumed regularly. Chicken broth, especially homemade from an organic chicken, is particularly healing to the adrenal glands. Animal sources of protein and fat should be chosen over vegetarian sources. Frequent, smaller meals throughout the day provide support during the early stages of adrenal fatigue recovery: these meals should include animal protein. When badly beat up, the adrenal glands will need simple carbohydrates eaten in small portions throughout the day to help provide basic energy. High salt foods are also important in the initial phases of healing. Amino acid supplements such as pea protein, whey protein, and similar products can help the adrenals to rebuild. For more on a diet that promotes adrenal healing, see Chapter 4.

The above food choices and vitamin/mineral supplements are critical to the healing process and are more important than any other supplements or herbs. They provide the adrenal glands the basic building blocks necessary to rebuild and recover. Now, let's move on to examine other adrenal fatigue therapies which have less value in the healing process.

Adaptogenic Herbs

Adaptogenic herbs such as Maca, Ashwagandha, and Rhodiola are said to help the body to better cope with stress. They may also have a direct effect on the adrenal glands by stimulating them or attempting to regulate them. While these herbs can be helpful for people with very mild adrenal fatigue, or when used for very short periods in people with more advanced adrenal fatigue, they still do not address the underlying causes of adrenal fatigue and life stress. Therefore, despite what some marketers may say, they hold only a small place in the treatment of advanced adrenal fatigue. Overusing them may, in fact, over-stimulate the adrenal glands leading to even further problems and adrenal weakness.

Hormone Supplementation and Glandulars

Adrenal fatigue results in inadequate production of adrenal hormones such as cortisol. As a result, some patients and practitioners choose to supplement with cortisol, cortisol precursors such as pregnenolone, or natural substances (like licorice) which may act like cortisol in the body.

All of these interventions can lead to feeling better quickly. The problem is that they may turn off the adrenal glands and cause adrenal gland atrophy. As the body gets used to receiving hormones from an external source, it turns off endogenous production. This can have dire long-term consequences as the adrenal glands may never recover their original functionality and activity. While some doctors advocate very small doses of cortisol, even these have been correlated with future problems. Proceed with extreme caution when it comes to any kind of treatment which introduces hormones into the body from an external source. These treatments may be useful as temporary rescue interventions but should only be used during the initial phase of recovery, while you are busy getting your lifestyle straightened out and removing other stressors from the adrenal glands. Make sure you are under the care of an experienced physician if you use any of these interventions.

Licorice is one herb that is used because it may cause the cortisol secreted by the adrenal glands to remain in the bloodstream for longer periods of time before being eliminated from the body. While licorice is probably a less dangerous intervention than hormone supplementation, it should still be used with caution.

Glandular supplements are simply supplements made out of the glands of other animals such as cows. Adrenal glandulars are available for sale under many brands and are typically made from dessicated (dried) cow adrenal glands. The philosophy behind consuming glandulars is that you aren't just getting one hormone, like you would with, say, cortisol supplementation. Instead, you are ingesting the entire adrenal gland of the animal, which contains dozens of hormones, tissues, and nutrients, all in the correct proportions and quantities. Glandulars are also available for other organ systems, such as the brain, liver, thymus, and others. Many healers believe that you can heal the liver by consuming liver glandular, and you can heal the brain by consuming brain glandular, and so forth.

While adrenal glandulars may cause the same problems as other kinds of hormone supplementation, namely, the inactivation and atrophy of the adrenal glands, in my opinion, glandulars are more gentle, beneficial, and healing than direct hormone supplementation. Using glandulars in moderation may provide the adrenal glands with a temporary rest and allow them to rebuild. This makes glandulars my favorite adrenal fatigue supplement, but they come with the warning that they are not capable of providing complete healing. They are only capable of providing a temporary rest. Complete healing, again, can only come from removing the underlying stressors burdening the adrenal glands. For a therapeutic trial to test whether one may be suffering from adrenal fatigue, glandulars may be a good choice. Lastly, even glandulars may lead to adrenal atrophy, so they should be used only temporarily. Only use them when you are ready to make all the other lifestyle changes described in the following chapter. If you use glandulars and are unwilling to provide other kinds of support for the adrenal glands, you will be wasting their effectiveness on a temporary boost, and you'll be left right back at square one when you discontinue taking them.

Wisdom governing the use of adrenal supplements can be summarized as follows: Always prefer rest, a low-stress lifestyle, and nutrition when healing from adrenal fatigue. Every other intervention is a crutch which might be beneficial for a short period, but which will only be a bandaid covering symptoms.

Tips for Recovery, with a Focus on Lyme Disease

Let's now take a look at some general, guiding principles for recovery from adrenal fatigue, with a specific focus on the unique challenges presented by Lyme disease.

Symptom Support

When the adrenals are not working properly, many body systems get thrown off. You may require sleep aid, thyroid support, digestive support, and other interventions while you are healing your adrenals. The books and websites listed at the end of this chapter provide details on this type of support. Remember, though, this support is a bandaid intended to help you get started on the real treatment; that is, long-term, comprehensive, stress reduction, and removal of the infections causing tissue damage within the adrenal glands.

Getting Better and Getting Worse

Do not take the task of recovering from adrenal fatigue lightly. If you have some degree of adrenal fatigue now and do not do something about it, it will continue to get worse and may debilitate you. The further the condition progresses, the more difficult it is to reverse.

To understand adrenal fatigue recovery, consider this over-arching principle: When the stressors placed on the adrenal glands are less than the capacity of the adrenal glands, recovery progresses. When the stressors are greater than the capacity of the adrenal glands, recovery regresses. So recovery requires extended periods during which rest exceeds stress. Exactly how much stress you can tolerate without backsliding depends on how messed up your adrenal glands are. This logic leads us to the conclusion that the longer you wait before you begin healing your adrenals, the less stress you'll be able to tolerate during the recovery process without back-sliding. If you think about it, this can become a very serious, precarious situation. The sicker you become, the harder it will be to get better.

Those with severe adrenal fatigue can get thrown into a tailspin after seemingly inconsequential exercise, like walking up a flight of stairs. These people require extreme lifestyle modification and near complete rest, if they are to recover. On the other hand, people with minor adrenal fatigue can jog a mile and only experience mild adrenal symptoms. But one thing holds true: mild adrenal fatigue will progress to serious adrenal fatigue if stress exceeds rest.

Worthy of note, particularly with Lyme disease, is the need to eliminate the infections in order for recovery to take place. Because the adrenals are weakened by Lyme disease and co-infections, treating these infections is a primary component to getting well. In addition, it is important to control lifestyle stress, take in the correct nutrients, and maintain an adrenal-friendly diet.

Adrenal Fatigue as a Layer of the Onion

Adrenal fatigue can actually be one of the layers of the onion—it can come on at a certain point in the recovery process, based on the order by which you are removing infections from the onion.

This is true because Bartonella in particular can cause the most damage to the adrenal glands and the communication pathway between the brain and the adrenal glands. So, if you are dealing with layers in which Bartonella is dormant, you may have less of a problem with adrenal fatigue. However, once you reach the layer of the onion where Bartonella is active, adrenal fatigue may rear its ugly head. Be careful: increased stress on, and inflammation within, the adrenal glands can mean that small life stressors are experienced as out-of-proportion disasters, leading to a great deal of drain on the reserve capacity of the adrenal glands. The severity of

Bartonella can wax and wane throughout the recovery process, so the same can be true of the severity of adrenal fatigue.

If you are dealing with a layer of the onion during which the adrenal glands are particularly taxed, employ extra caution in your life to ensure a low stress lifestyle, and begin consuming the foods and nutrients which provide optimal support to the adrenal glands. And, of course, attack and kill the infections causing the problems (be careful, though. Herxheimer reactions and inflammation can temporarily worsen adrenal fatigue, as we will see in the next section).

Treating Infections can Temporarily Worsen Adrenal Fatigue

Yes, I have been telling you that in order to eliminate adrenal fatigue, you have to address infections. However, since the infections can actually live inside your adrenal glands, treating them can increase inflammation within the adrenal glands and can temporarily wear them down. Accordingly, while anti-infective treatments are still necessary, they should be undertaken with caution. If the adrenals are particularly weak, gentler treatments should be used. Furthermore, anti-inflammatory eating and supplements may be used to calm the adrenal glands during treatment. And lastly, anticipating more rest and less activity during anti-infective therapy is important. In the end, the infections must be dealt with in order to get well.

Other Hormonal Imbalances in Lyme Disease

Adrenal fatigue is not the only hormonal issue noted in Lyme disease. In addition to adrenal fatigue issues, practitioners and patients are increasingly recognizing the importance of all kinds of hormonal imbalances in the symptom picture of Lyme disease. All of the organs and body systems which produce and regulate hormones get hit when a person is infected with Borrelia and co-infections. While I do not believe that treating hormonal problems will fix the cause of Lyme disease, I do believe that doing so can lead to dramatic improvement in symptoms, and an accelerated recovery. The topic of treating hormonal imbalances is very complex and controversial. I will not be addressing the topic in depth here, but instead, I simply want to make you aware that many of your symptoms may be the result of various hormone issues. This should not be ignored during the recovery process. It can be very valuable to consult a doctor who is versed in treating hormone issues in patients with Lyme disease since there are many natural and pharmaceutical interventions which can provide symptom relief.

Adrenal Fatigue Can Take a Very Long Time to Heal

Even if you are doing everything right, adrenal fatigue can take months or years to heal. Don't be discouraged. Look for small, positive changes. Don't ask the question, "am I completely healed today?" Instead, ask the question, "Am I better than I was 3 months ago?"

Additional Resources

Adrenal fatigue is a peculiar and counter-intuitive condition. Without a deep understanding of the recovery process, one can flounder in frustration for months and even years. Please do not ignore this fact: it is very difficult, if not impossible, to recover from adrenal fatigue without first gaining a complete understanding of this mystifying and unusual condition. This is not a condition where you can expect to succeed by "throwing spaghetti at the wall and seeing what sticks." You have to take careful, planned, precise steps in order to get well. It is for this reason that I strongly suggest that you pursue the resources I have listed below.

In my opinion, the two experts with the best grasp of adrenal fatigue are G. E. Poesnecker, DC, and Michael Lam, M.D., M.P.H., A.B.A.A.M. Each of these doctors has fantastic books on adrenal fatigue and has greatly influenced my understanding of this condition. Dr. Lam's book is entitled, *Adrenal Fatigue Syndrome*. Dr. Poesnecker's book is entitled, *Adrenal*

Syndrome. Unfortunately, at the time my book was written, Dr. Poesnecker's book was already out of print. Sometimes, used copies can be found on Amazon.com. I strongly suggest obtaining both of these books, if you can. While other experts claim to have a grasp on adrenal fatigue, it is these two doctors who have the most accurate information.

Dr. Lam also has a fantastic website with dozens of extensive, free articles on adrenal fatigue. I highly recommend visiting www.drlam.com. Do not attempt to recover from adrenal fatigue without first reading Dr. Lam's materials.

Another fantastic resource is the chapter on Adrenal Fatigue contained in Connie Strasheim's book, *Beyond Lyme Disease.* This chapter can be viewed online as a free sample chapter by visiting:

www.lymebook.com/adrenal-fatigue-hypothyroidism.

Again, I would like to emphasize that I *strongly* suggest doing some further reading on adrenal fatigue. It is a very complex condition, and the two chapters in my book which address this topic only scratch the surface. If you believe you may be suffering from this condition, you should go beyond what I offer here and avail yourself of the resources mentioned above.

Chapter 6
Adrenal Fatigue, Part II: A New Worldview—Asking Basic Questions about Life as a Human Being

Moving from the Physical to the Non-Physical

You may be wondering why we are still talking about adrenal fatigue when the book has already covered this topic in the prior chapter. The reason is simple: Adrenal fatigue has two primary components—the physical, and the non-physical. The previous chapter looked at the physical manifestations of, and treatments for, adrenal fatigue. This chapter will examine the non-physical aspects, including the emotional, spiritual, psychological, and mental implications. If you haven't read the prior chapter, read it first, before reading this one.

As we learned in the previous chapter, supplements, dietary changes, and other interventions are only the beginning when it comes to treating adrenal fatigue. Reducing stress in your life and changing your worldview is the next step, and also, the most difficult one. These changes require you to rethink your place in the world, how you fit into the culture that surrounds you, and what's important in life. While researching, buying, and starting a new supplement product require only a small amount of energy, redefining your identity and your worldview is a massive undertaking. Unfortunately, the lifestyle changes that are required are so difficult and counter-cultural that many people won't make the necessary changes, and they'll experience only partial improvement in their adrenal fatigue. Yes, it is true that Borrelia and co-infections can hasten the onset of adrenal fatigue. However, once you have adrenal fatigue, it is not enough to just address these infections.

What do I mean by "counter-cultural" lifestyle changes? Let's take a deeper look.

Modern Life and Human Psychology

For a long time, I was one of the people who didn't make the healthy lifestyle changes necessary to recover from adrenal fatigue. I didn't listen to my wakeup call until my adrenal fatigue had progressed and spun out of control. Looking back, I regret not heeding the warning signs earlier. My recovery from adrenal fatigue took longer than it should have, due to my denial. It is my hope that this book will save you from the same mistakes. While I was able to recover, it wasn't easy, and I wish I had known this information years ago.

Adrenal fatigue isn't just another bodily dysfunction, as is so common with Lyme disease. Instead, it's your body's way of revolting against, or rejecting, the unhealthy parts of your entire worldview and lifestyle. It's all-encompassing. Early on in adrenal fatigue, your body gives you the choice and gently invites you to make changes. Later, if you don't listen, the changes may become involuntary as your adrenal fatigue progresses far enough to become debilitating and preclude you from participating in the complexities of modern life.

What exactly are the problems I am referring to when I talk about modern life? We'll look at these in more detail, but in summary, they include: a hurried life punctuated by ever-increasing work stresses and demands; relational turmoil and stress; lack of contentment and an ever-increasing desire for more; separation from nature and the natural rhythms and cycles of nature; and, probably most importantly, worry and anxiety as a way of life. Let's look back through human history to find out how and why these patterns of unhealthy thinking and behavior have developed.

While human existence has never been easy, it's only in recent human history that life has become so busy and stressful. Note that I use the word "stressful," not "uncomfortable." Surely humans alive today are more comfortable than we've ever been throughout history; we have mastered climate control, food distribution and storage, and other creature comforts unavailable to generations past. Humans of the past suffered from more disease, faced more physical challenges, and certainly dealt with more miseries than we do now.

However, life in past generations was less stressful than it is today, not in all ways, but in many of the ways that are important in adrenal fatigue. Before telephones, the Internet, and other methods for rapid communication across large distances, life was confined to your immediate village, town, or area. This made things much simpler, as you tended to the people and things around you and didn't worry about world events beyond your city or town. Before cell phones and email, most businesses were closed by 5 pm so people could go home, relax, and recharge. Now, people are "wired in" at all times, often conducting business at all hours of the day and night, and employers are becoming increasingly demanding; they expect their employees to be available all the time and to deal with problems in real time. In recent generations, people in America have become less satisfied with humble housing, vehicles, and provisions. We've become discontent, and we're constantly striving for more... more of pretty much everything, including more money, more power, more recognition, more luxury. These pursuits have cost us dearly and left us drained, exhausted, and burned out.

The type of work we perform in modern life is also very different from what it was in older times. While pushing a plow in a field with one's own hands certainly isn't easy work, it is, in many ways, healthier work than what we do today. Studies have shown that outdoor physical work, under the sun, with the breeze blowing in one's face, is much healthier for the body (and the adrenal glands) than sedentary office work in front of a computer. Farm work used to entail rising with the sun, and living and working in harmony with the cycles of nature. This is the kind of life our bodies have had for thousands of years; it is only in very recent times that we've completely changed how and where we spend our days. Farm work and other occupations of old no doubt caused other physical issues, but it is unlikely that they contributed as heavily to adrenal fatigue as modern life does.

What's interesting is the speed with which life has changed on planet Earth. Most of these changes have occurred within the last 150 years, and the rate of change continues to be exponential. Our society and culture is changing faster than our ability to evaluate the negative impacts of these changes.

If, as you read my description of old-fashioned life, you are taking deep breaths, relaxing, and longing for liberation from your techno-saturated, high stress, high pressure life, it's likely that you have a case of adrenal fatigue, and it's likely that modern life isn't doing much to help you! Your body is longing for a different life, a life more in tune with how humans have lived for thousands of years. For me, the longing is palpable and intense, and undeniable. It has also led me to make significant changes to my lifestyle, especially in how I spend my days.

Some of the stress we face isn't a result of modern life and culture. It is simply a product of human psychology. A mentality of "keeping up with the Jones's" has driven many people to work themselves into the ground in order to pay for the luxuries and amenities traditionally reserved for the rich. A culture of consumerism has driven an attitude of entitlement and discontentment. Extra money is often used to upgrade homes and vehicles instead of paying down the mortgage, paying off debt, and making life simpler. While these kinds of behaviors aren't new, they have intensified and become more uncontrollable in recent times. Satisfaction, thankfulness, gratitude, and contentment are feelings not experienced by many. Yet it is these very feelings which are healing and soothing to the adrenal glands. Some people spend their entire lives without ever really feeling content or grateful for what they have.

Other harmful feelings which result from basic human psychology are worry and fear. These feelings can be tremendously difficult to turn off. Yet, worry and fear cause stress, and that stress triggers the adrenal glands to work overtime in fight or flight mode.

In summary, there are two primary sources of stress in modern life: Stress that is new and results from modern jobs, technology, and separation from nature; and stress that is not new, which results from worry, fear, discontentment, jealousy, and consumerism. Both of these sources of stress must be addressed in order to recover from adrenal fatigue. The first kind of stress can be addressed by making external life changes (e.g.— changing one's career, moving out of the city to get closer to nature, turning all technological devices off after 5 pm, and spending more time hiking, camping, or participating in other activities in nature). The second kind of stress must be addressed by making internal life changes (e.g.— learning to be content with what we have, learning to replace fear and anxiety with trust and faith, and learning to find satisfaction in experiences rather than expensive merchandise). In this way, adrenal fatigue requires both internal and external lifestyle changes.

183

My Own Journey Out of That Deep, Dark Hole

Adrenal fatigue progresses if it is not addressed, and the more it progresses, the harder it becomes to ignore. Such was my own experience. After a particularly difficult series of life events, my very mild case of adrenal fatigue (which I hadn't even recognized yet as adrenal fatigue) progressed into a full-blown adrenal crash. It is hard for me to share this part of my story with you because it was such a difficult time in my life, and even the memories associated with it are stressful to recount.

Fortunately, I became familiar with the books and websites mentioned at the end of the previous chapter, and I knew I was in for big trouble if I didn't make some changes. The changes weren't easy, and I certainly can't say I've arrived, but I've begun moving in the right direction. The internal and external changes I have had to make were much easier once I realized that I didn't have much choice in the matter: either I learned how to change, or my quality of life would be lost. Looking back, now, in retrospect, I can see that those dark days of adrenal fatigue were actually a blessing; my life is so much healthier and more fulfilling now. It saddens me to look at people and see how unhealthy and unhappy many of them are, even those who aren't stricken with a tick-borne illness.

When my adrenals were at their worst, I was simply in survival mode. Really worn down adrenals cause horribly unpleasant symptoms such as near-panic level anxiety, terrible insomnia, a sense of impending doom, inability to deal with even the smallest daily tasks, severe depression, and explosive relational interactions (more on that later), to name a few. In fact, while many things Lyme disease sufferers face are horrible, I must say that the symptoms associated with adrenal fatigue were among the worst things I've ever experienced during my time on planet Earth. Exercise intolerance was also very limiting and depressing for me, as I am a very active person and things like hiking and mountain biking are a part of who I am. Now, looking back on those horrible days, I am so grateful I can enjoy the activities I used to take for granted. A simple mountain bike ride now provides me with indescribable joy, because I know what it feels like for these activities to be out of reach.

My first few months of recovery involved taking lots of vitamin C and B vitamins, consuming plenty of animal fat and protein, sleeping a lot, resting a lot, and trusting that things were going to be OK. And more than anything, it was important for me to forgive myself for lost productivity, missed life opportunities, and other losses that were incurred during this time. A sense of guilt and inadequacy are extremely common symptoms during severe adrenal fatigue, so it is important to recognize these emotions as symptoms of the condition, not as a true reflection of one's own self-worth. Extending grace to one's self during recovery is so important.

The first few months of the recovery process were the hardest, because improvement wasn't easy to notice, and I just had to keep going forward on faith that things would work out. It wasn't until later that I could clearly see a pattern of improvement forming.

By now you can see how much this chapter differs from the prior chapter. Both chapters are on adrenal fatigue, but you probably never guessed just how deep the non-physical aspects of adrenal fatigue can be!

After my adrenal fatigue recovery stabilized and I got on a good track, I still had to be careful. If I overdid it (either with physical stress such as exercise or hiking, or emotional stress such as bickering and arguing with friends or co-workers), I would experience a setback and a temporary resurgence of the really nasty emotional symptoms mentioned in previous paragraphs. These mini-crashes, or setbacks, are wonderfully explained and illustrated in Dr. Lam's material (both in his book and on his website—see the end of the previous chapter for references). Understanding why and how they were occurring gave me an objective perspective which helped tremendously in providing the fortitude and perseverance needed to work through that phase of recovery. As time went on, the mini-crashes were less frequent and less severe. But the process took a couple of years. This is why it is so important to catch adrenal fatigue as soon as you can since doing so can significantly shorten the duration of recovery. This is also why it's so important to learn how to treat adrenal fatigue properly, as incorrect decisions and actions can prolong an already extensive recovery window.

Now I will share some of the lessons that I learned from adrenal fatigue. These insights were gained from personal experience as well as from reading the work of top adrenal experts and doctors. It is true that many life stresses cannot be avoided. However, many of them can be avoided, and here are the lessons I have learned about how to avoid them.

Choosing Good Role Models

You've heard the saying, "If you don't stand for something, you will fall for anything." I believe that this statement accounts for much of the stress people experience in their lives. Because we have not intentionally chosen a healthy lifestyle to model our lives after, we will instead follow the "lowest common denominator" examples in our society and culture. Usually, these examples end up being those which are intentionally put in our path by corporations and their marketing departments. The single and primary goal of corporations is to relentlessly convince us that we are inadequate, dissatisfied, un-whole people who will be fixed by the products they offer. If we listen to this message, we start to believe it. We start to think that we really don't have enough—enough money, friends, vacations, good looks, talents, or fill-in-the-blank attributes. This dissatisfaction creates a desperation to change our circumstances and gain more acceptance and approval from society at large, so we increase our work loads, spend less time relaxing and taking care of ourselves, and set off on the busy task of filling our lives with more—more of everything. This pattern of behavior is one of the primary triggers of adrenal fatigue. And, it just so happens that many people with adrenal fatigue are "Type A" personalities; so for us Type A's, it will require even more self control in order to turn off these unhealthy patterns of thinking and behaving.

While simply recognizing the above patterns, and attempting to avoid them, is helpful, I find it has been very valuable to pick out examples of people whom I want to emulate. A few years ago, my wife and I met some folks who are now among our best friends. They had decided to quit their high stress, high power, high paying jobs and live a simpler life. At first, their newly found lifestyle seemed crazy to us—almost irresponsible. That's because we were viewing it through the filter of modern society's lense: that is, the highest and best achievement for life should be a busy, productive, over-achieving lifestyle. Eventually we began to see the wisdom in our friends' simplification of their lives, and having them as an example in our own lives served to greatly weaken the default, culturally influenced belief that more of everything is always better.

If you don't stand for something, you'll fall for anything. So, pick someone who stands for something, and use them as an example, instead of the messages of corporate marketing.

People Pleasing, Perfectionism, and Taking Care of Yourself

People with adrenal fatigue are typically also perfectionists and people pleasers. These patterns of behavior tend to weaken the adrenal glands, because we experience anxiety and stress when those around us are displeased with us, or at least when we think they are. We also experience anxiety and stress when our expectations of perfection in people or situations are met with the reality that people and situations aren't perfect.

Weakened adrenal glands cause symptoms of emotional instability, which makes us even more susceptible to our perfectionist and people pleasing tendencies. So, you can see that it can become a vicious cycle.

Recognizing this pattern is very important. Since ultimate self-acceptance can never come from an external source, our anxiety and stress can never be quenched by other people. Likewise, people and things will never be perfect, so our anxiety and stress will never be quenched by discovering perfection in our lives. Therefore, we must extinguish the anxiety and stress with acceptance: Acceptance of ourselves, and acceptance of the imperfect people and things in our lives.

In addition to the unhealthy feelings involved in perfectionism and people pleasing, there is also an unhealthy level of work, energy expenditure, and effort. Perfectionism lacks a finish line, or end goal, to life's activities and interactions with others, so perfectionists never grant themselves rest. In other words, people pleasers and perfectionists never feel like work is done, settled, good enough, or acceptable enough. We always feel like more could be done, should be done, and must be done. Guilt, in particular, drains us like no other emotion. This constant unease equates to a slight draw on the adrenal glands over a long period of time. Not only will this strain lead to adrenal fatigue, it will also prevent a person from recovering from adrenal fatigue. We must adopt the wisdom in sayings like, "Do your best, then let it rest." We must set reasonable goals for ourselves, and after we've met those goals, rest and ignore that inner voice which tells us, "No! You haven't done enough! You should still be doing more!"

While we could get into the psychology of people pleasing and perfectionism, I will save that for a psychologist. I'm simply here to tell you that people who have adrenal fatigue, perfectionist tendencies, and people pleasing traits must work very diligently to change the way they think about the world. At the top of the list of changes is to tell yourself and learn to believe the following statement: "Doing my best is good enough.

After I do my best, I deserve rest, down time, and sleep. Taking care of myself is a worthy priority." Until you really believe this statement, you will be susceptible to continued drain on your adrenal glands. Like a slow leak in a tire, that drain will prevent you from making forward progress.

We must also diligently look for other areas of our lives which may be causing a slow leak, or drain, on our adrenal glands. Past events, even those that occurred decades ago may still be draining us emotionally. Unforgiveness, guilt, shame, regret, and other feelings might be causing low-grade anxiety and keeping our adrenals from recharging completely. It may even be possible that we've been living with these feelings for so long that we don't immediately recognize them when conducting an inventory of our state of mind. The point here is that any kind of emotional distress, even at a very low level, places a small drain on the adrenals and must be addressed and healed if the adrenals are to fully recover.

Managing Expectations

The friends I mentioned earlier (who drastically simplified their lives) shared a poem with me over dinner one night. The poem is entitled "If," by Rudyard Kipling. You can read the whole poem online by doing a Google search; it is a fantastic poem and I recommend that everyone read it. I will share a small portion of it here:

> *If you can meet with Triumph and Disaster*
> *And treat those two impostors just the same;*
> *[...] Yours is the Earth and everything that's in it,*
> *And—which is more—you'll be a Man, my son!*

Here's what I love about these lines. Our adrenal glands get drained when life doesn't go our way, because we end up worrying that we will be living a life which we don't feel is "right" or "best" for us. We all have an idea of how life "should" go. When it doesn't work out as expected, we get stressed out. The wisdom in the poem shows us that both triumph and disaster should be seen as imposters. In other words, we will be OK even when they occur. We can feel safe, secure, and right, just by being who we are and living our lives the best we can. When we strike the lottery and get rich (triumph) or when we lose our jobs and end up poor (disaster), these are but imposters to what we really value in life. When we adopt this perspective, triumph and tragedy will no longer control our emotions.

Whether rich or poor, I can still take a walk, have a conversation with a friend, love my family, and play a game of chess. I can still enjoy the simple things in life. Convincing yourself that triumph and disaster are but imposters, distracting you from what really matters in life, will go a long way to calming your adrenal glands, allowing you to be content in the present moment, and dispelling unrealistic life expectations.

It may be surprising that triumph is also considered an imposter. Yet, take a look at the celebrities and other super-rich. It is clear that money and success can be equally as draining as disaster, in many ways!

Here's the take-away lesson. The hardest part about designing a simple life isn't actually executing it. It is getting over the lies society has beat into our heads: that what makes us valuable, successful people, is how much money we make, what kind of car we drive, and how successful we are.

Once you accept life as it is instead of worrying about how your life isn't perfect, you will also learn to accept yourself how you are. You will be less inclined to accept stressful jobs or pursue unhealthy activities in order to force your life to meet expectations which were never healthy in the first place.

Choosing Financial Simplicity

While we all need money to survive, many Americans choose to heap additional stress onto their lives by attempting to "keep up with the Jones's," always trying to achieve the lifestyle just out of their reach. A blog that changed my life, and which I recommend to you now, was written by a man who was able to retire at age 30, not because he got rich, but because he chose simplicity. The blog is both inspiring and practical in its advice on financial simplicity. Instead of re-writing the wisdom he offers, I will simply refer you to his blog so you can read it for yourself: www.MrMoneyMustache.com. It is currently one of the most popular finance blogs in the country. As more and more people wake up from their brainwashing, they are turning to blogs like this to help them navigate out of the maze of a life controlled by corporate marketing and driven by feelings of dissatisfaction, greed, and envy.

When you choose financial simplicity, and really start to believe that the materialism which dominates most of the first world is destructive and unhealthy, you will release yourself from the pressure and stress that comes with discontentment. Of course, you may still experience stress in attempting to make a living—we all have to put food on the table—but once your basic needs are met, you can free yourself from the constant feeling that your life isn't good enough without bigger houses, cars, and material possessions. Go and read Mr. Money Mustache: his writing is fantastic and will give you a whole new perspective on your financial life.

Accepting Yourself

People recovering from Lyme disease and adrenal fatigue have limitations which other people aren't subject to. For me personally, these limitations aren't huge, but they are still there. For example, I don't do well consuming alcoholic beverages. I can get a good amount of sun exposure, but too much drags me down. I can participate in most vigorous activities, including mountain biking and running, but I need days in between these activities to rest and recharge. I can be active throughout long, busy days, but I need my sleep.

You can choose to accept your strengths and limitations or be bitter about them, but you can't choose to change them—at least not instantaneously. While you are working on your healing and shrinking your limitations, it is best to have an attitude of self-acceptance. This doesn't mean you give up on improving your health. It also doesn't mean that you give up on the good stuff in life. It just means that you find the good stuff which fits within your current set of capabilities. When I was recovering from adrenal fatigue and could not participate in my much-loved activities of mountain biking and hiking, I decided to take up camping. Instead of being bitter, I found something that I could do. Camping turned out to be incredibly satisfying and joyful. While my daytime activities during camping trips didn't include strenuous, all-day hikes, they did include such things as short walks, mild hikes, swimming, rafting, cooking, enjoying friends' company, relaxing by the campfire, and other similar pursuits. See the crossroads, here? I could have become bitter about not being able to go mountain biking and do all-day hikes, or I could have simply made the best of my situation with the tools I had to work with. I'm not saying I never had any bad days. Of course, I struggled, but I made it a point to try to keep a positive attitude. And I won't leave you hanging: there is a light at the end of the tunnel. While it took a long time, my adrenal fatigue is 95% gone now, and I am back to regularly enjoying hiking, mountain biking, and running!

People with adrenal fatigue are not alone in their need to accept their limitations. I have a friend, an avid athlete, who hurt his back terribly, needed surgery, and had to give up many of his favorite activities. He eventually found a positive attitude, bought a fishing boat, and loves taking his family and friends fishing. He still goes to the gym almost daily to stay in shape. He can only do certain exercises because of his back, but boy is he strong: he's the strongest one in the gym for the particular exercises he can do.

Everyone has limitations and everyone has the opportunity to participate in activities that match their capacities and strengths. Yes, you heard me right: *EVERYONE* has limitations! Our attitude towards those limitations, and not the limitations themselves, is what defines us. Recovery from adrenal fatigue will progress much more smoothly if you accept yourself, don't push yourself beyond what you are capable of doing, and find joy in the activities in life that match your strengths and capabilities. Healing of your adrenals is possible, but in the meantime, make the best of what you've got.

The Triangle of Emotional Distress

We will now look at what I call the triangle of emotional distress, which comprises three points: unresolved emotional conflict, physical brain damage, and adrenal fatigue. As we will see, Lyme sufferers often have all three of these problems, and when combined, they can be very serious and challenging.

Let's begin with unresolved emotional conflict.

Unresolved Emotional Conflict

Many top Lyme experts have now agreed that unresolved, past emotional conflict can delay recovery. It is a mysterious concept, and one which took me a long time to accept. Somehow, unresolved emotional conflict remains locked up inside the brain and creates a blockade that prevents not only spiritual and psychological healing but healing of the physical brain as well.

Lyme sufferers often end up having a hard time letting go of feelings they've internalized in the past, including such things as unhealthy beliefs, assumptions, past wounds, and other hurts. These pent up emotions become locked away in the brain. While this can take place in the healthy population as well, there's something about brain trauma which makes those with Lyme much more susceptible to this phenomenon.

Unresolved emotions can include many different types of trauma, such as that derived from past relationships, experiences, losses, regrets, insecurities, and more. Somehow, these emotions become encapsulated in the brain and even become intertwined with infections and toxins such as heavy metals. During the recovery process, you can hit blockades in healing wherein your recovery process is literally halted by some kind of emotional conflict you've been carrying around in your brain for years. As hard as you try, you just won't get any better until you deal with the conflict, release it, and move on. Sometimes, Lyme sufferers even experience strong flashbacks and emotional glimpses during the recovery process, especially during intense anti-infective or detox treatments. These flashbacks can cause emotional crises. If the emotional crises aren't dealt with, healing can come to a halt.

This may sound far-fetched, but trust me, the more you learn about Lyme disease, the more you'll realize that simple, Western, compartmentalized medicine is far too limited and unsophisticated to accurately describe Lyme disease. The sooner you accept the unconventional truths of Lyme disease, the sooner you'll be able to get on with your healing. We truly are beings composed of mind, body, and spirit, and these parts are not necessarily separate and unrelated.

One possible explanation for this phenomenon is that the physical damage done to the brain by Lyme disease spirochetes, co-infections, toxins, and other imbalances predisposes the brain to have a more difficult time clearing emotions which would, in an otherwise healthy brain, be discarded.

This brings us to the second point in the triangle of emotional distress: physical brain damage.

Physical Brain Damage

Physical brain damage is the second point in our triangle of emotional distress. Borrelia spirochetes can drill their way past the blood-brain-barrier and infect the brain. Their toxins and physical presence can damage the brain and be the primary cause of brain dysfunction. This dysfunction can manifest as everything from depression, anxiety, forgetfulness, and obsessive-compulsive behavior, to more serious problems including schizophrenia, aggressive behavior, and even suicidal thoughts or actions. As a result, many psychological symptoms experienced in Lyme disease are not character flaws or lack of self control, they are, in fact, organ damage.

We accept organ damage as a legitimate cause of disease in someone with, say, kidney disease. It's time that we also accept that the brain is a physical organ and is susceptible to the same kind of physical damage. It's time to stop stigmatizing mental disorders as if they are somehow caused by personality defects or the fault of the person suffering from them.

Adrenal Fatigue

Finally, adrenal fatigue is the third point in the triangle of emotional distress. The adrenal glands, which are already weakened by the damage done by Lyme disease, become increasingly stressed by the first two points in the triangle. These stressors are just too much for the them to handle, so the adrenals become drained and weak, causing symptoms strikingly similar to the symptoms experienced as a result of the first two points in the triangle. Emotional symptoms of adrenal fatigue include anxiety, worry, insecurity, and a feeling of hopelessness, just to name a few.

Other Factors in the Triangle of Emotional Distress

We've just seen that the three points in the triangle of emotional distress are unresolved emotional conflict, physical brain damage, and adrenal fatigue. When combined, these three points are capable of creating serious mental and emotional dysfunction. However, it should be noted that there are other factors, too, which contribute to the overall problems taking place in the brain of a Lyme sufferer.

For example, heavy metal poisoning which often accompanies Lyme can cause severe psychiatric symptoms. Likewise, hormonal imbalances and hypercoagulation can have devastating effects. Finally, brain inflammation can wreak havoc on mental and emotional functionality.

The End Result

The end result of these various dysfunctions is a soup, or mixture, of unpleasant emotions caused or contributed to by each of the three points on the triangle (and by the other factors mentioned). Yet, while each individual point on the triangle has helped to cause the problem, the resulting emotions are intertwined, interrelated, and very difficult to separate and associate with their respective cause(s). Furthermore, each point on the triangle is synergistic with the others, meaning that the whole of dysfunction is much greater than the sum of the parts.

It's hard to know which came first, the chicken or the egg. Was an already emotionally compromised person more susceptible to getting Lyme and adrenal fatigue, or does the physical damage caused by Lyme and related infections compromise the hormonal systems, organs, and chemicals that regulate emotions? Perhaps the physical damage done to the brain by the infections is behind the emotional dysfunction? In reality, it is probably a little of each, but one thing is clear: It can be difficult to sort it all out, and the depth of emotional and psychological imbalance created by this triangle in those with Lyme disease is profound. The triangle is also typically much more pronounced during the end stages of recovery when most of the larger, physical issues have been addressed. One Lyme practitioner has said that the emotional symptoms of Lyme are the last to go.

There is one thing in particular which makes the triangle very, very dangerous. Many people who are victim to the emotional triangle have no idea what is behind their suffering. Unfortunately, if they aren't educated about the physical causes of their brain dysfunction, Lyme disease sufferers may walk around with awful feelings including guilt, perfectionism, hypersensitivity, worry, anxiety, depression, suicidal thoughts, and more. Without understanding the physical causes, these people may feel like they are worthless and have lost their grounding in life. This is why it is so important to educate Lyme sufferers, practitioners, and caretakers about these topics. Once understanding takes place, it can be much easier to deal with the symptoms and say to one's self, "I'm not going to let these feelings dominate me, because I know they are just physical dysfunction—they aren't really who I am."

Unfortunately, accurate education is severely lacking. All too often, Lyme disease sufferers are expected to experience improvement in psychological symptoms when they are given common treatments for depression, treatments which work for the general population. But true healing in the Lyme disease population will not occur when interventions are limited to such things as counseling, anti-depressant medication, or meditation. Instead, healing can only occur when the Lyme disease sufferer recognizes that they have compromised adrenals, that their brain is physically damaged, and that their unhealthy emotions are bound tightly—and physically—inside their brain. These problems which are specific to Lyme disease require solutions specific to Lyme disease! Unfortunately, even among many of the top healers, the triangle of emotional distress is still unrecognized and untreated. Even the more advanced "natural" healers who forego Valium and anti-depressant drugs in favor of more "naturally healing" options like herbs, hypnotherapy, and acupuncture will still find success to be elusive if they don't understand the triangle of emotional distress.

I'm not saying these other therapies won't help at all; I'm saying that they must be only part of a complete healing program. The most important factor in healing is understanding. Once the causes of the problems are understood, appropriate treatment can be used.

The stakes become even higher when you realize that adrenal fatigue, as well as physical dysfunction in the brain itself, gets into EVERYTHING you think, say, do, and feel—your work, your attitude, your family life, your goals and dreams, your relationships, and your self-perception—EVERYTHING. Your overall happiness and ability to get through the day are impacted. These debilities are especially pesky when they are bad enough to compromise you emotionally but not bad enough to completely change your behavior or raise red flags to your friends and family. When severe, at least you can look yourself in the mirror and say "Wow! What is going on inside my head? This really isn't me. I need help." When subtle and moderate, you may just attribute these emotions to the blues, or life circumstances, or "just how you are wired," when in fact, they are actually symptoms of physical dysfunction inside your body. People experiencing such mild symptoms probably won't even make it as far as a conventional doctor's office or natural healer's clinic. They may instead stay within the confines of their home, alone, devastated and be-lieving that their dismal thinking truly is a part of their authentic self.

Don't let the preceding paragraphs bring you down, or discourage you. In fact, with proper education and treatment, Lyme disease sufferers can return to health, and thrive. It is proper education and treatment which are the keys to success. Let the preceding information equip you with knowledge of what's happening in your body and empower you to choose the healing modalities which will help you return to health.

Help for the Burdened

Among other things, solutions to the triangle of emotional distress include, but are not limited to, treating the infections in the brain and detoxifying the brain, healing and recharging the adrenals, and taking steps to release unhealthy, encapsulated emotions. Decreasing inflammation, balancing hormones, and taking other steps are important, too. Don't forget that untreated co-infections can also slow progress. I talked to one Lyme sufferer who had no healing in her triangle of emotional distress until she treated Babesia with Mepron. After that, she found anti-Lyme therapies and other interventions to propel her forward.

The most difficult of the necessary treatments may be dealing with unresolved emotional conflict, because this endeavor requires not just herbs and treatments but deep reflection and self-examination. When it comes to this kind of healing, I have found that journaling (the act of writing in a personal diary) can help a person identify internal conflicts and resolve them. There are also a number of therapies available which address stored emotional conflicts, including EFT (Emotional Freedom Technique, also known as "tapping"), counseling, and others. While some of these appear to be a bit outlandish and far-fetched at first, I can say that after years of research, most of them are legitimate and have numerous followers who regained their health through their use. As the Lyme community becomes more aware of unresolved emotional conflict as a cause for their sickness, we are seeing an abundance of resources and books on this topic. I recommend the books and work of Amy B. Scher, who is an expert in emotional healing.

Finally, spirituality can play a large role in healing. In particular, trusting in God can help to relieve feelings of worry and fear about the future. There are many bible verses which speak of God's acceptance of us and his unconditional love; such truths can help relieve us of the pressing feeling that we are not good enough. My favorite book of the bible is Ecclesiastes, and one of my favorite verses from this book is 4:6:

"Better one handful with tranquility than two handfuls with toil and chasing after the wind."

I just love how this verse gives us permission to live a peaceful, tranquil life instead of working ourselves to the bone in order to get rich and have cultural status and power.

I would like to close this chapter with a topic that I have personally found to be very helpful, and healing—camping.

Camping and the Outdoors: Medicine for the Soul

Note: Camping is dangerous in areas with high tick populations and Lyme disease incidence. Yes, I am aware that this includes most of the continent of North America and the rest of the world! While I am conscious of the risks of encountering ticks in the outdoors, I have personally decided that the benefits of camping outweigh the risks. I do not ask you to follow in my footsteps in this decision; each person must evaluate the risks and rewards of camping for him or herself. Where I live, in Northern California, we have access to camp sites where foliage and forest density is less than some other parts of the country. Again, I'm not saying camping is right for everyone, everywhere, but remember, too, that living a life indoors, without exposure to nature, also has many serious disadvantages. Please consult your doctor and/or local forestry experts before going camping.

In Chapter 4, which focuses on the dietary aspects of healing from Lyme disease, I mentioned that the paleo lifestyle extends beyond just a way of eating. Indeed, when it comes to healing from adrenal fatigue, returning to our ancestral roots can provide huge benefits. While most of us can't quit our jobs and live in a cave, we can take steps to disconnect from the stress of modern technology, and modern life, as much as possible. Often, we spend more time on our computers and smartphones than we really need to. It is compulsion and addiction that drives much of this behavior, not necessity. We need to make the conscious decision to spend more time in nature, or reading a book on the couch, or going for a walk outside. We need to build more space into our lives, more "margin," more free time. We need to allow ourselves to rest, rebuild and recharge.

While there are numerous ways to rest, rebuild, and reconnect with nature, I would like to share my experiences with camping. I would not go as far as to say that camping is right for everyone, but I believe the experience of camping can teach us some important lessons about disconnecting from our modern, wired, always-on lifestyles. Furthermore, as I've said several times now, I believe that there is something fundamentally healing about spending time in nature. Just as a glass of water can quench thirst, I believe time in nature can heal the body, both physically and psychologically. Science is quickly coming to agreement with this idea; more and more research is identifying measurable, physical properties of the outdoors which calm our psyches and revitalize our bodies.

Below, I'll share an essay—published on a friend's blog—that I wrote on camping. First, though, I'd like to point out some of the benefits of camping (or, if not camping, simply spending more time in nature):

1. Camping brings us back into alignment with the natural rhythms of the Earth; we rise with the sun, and rest with the darkness. We leave behind artificial lights, computer screens, and television shows.

2. Camping brings us close to the ground. Lying just inches from the dirt, our bodies are exposed to the electromagnetic energy of the Earth. When I am camping, I always wake up in the morning with an unusually high sense of wellbeing, and I feel more rested than when I'm sleeping in my house. This is true even when it is cold outside.

3. Camping takes us away from the harmful electromagnetic exposure we receive when indoors and surrounded by all of our electrically powered appliances, smartphones, TV screens, computers,

and especially WI-FI signals (by the way, in my home, we do not use WI-FI; instead, our computers are wired to the internet via actual ethernet cords).

4. Camping forces us to relax. Work is far away, house chores can't be done, and the TV can't be turned on. We have little choice but to really relax and enjoy the present moment. I've always felt that three days of camping feels like three weeks. Time seems to stand still, and the days meander on.

5. Camping reminds us of what's important: we are in close quarters with our family and friends, without distractions, so we can spend time building relationships and investing time getting to know each other.

6. All-in-all, camping is a healthy experience that encourages balance and relaxation. I've talked with many other Lyme sufferers who also find camping to be tremendously beneficial.

Essay: A Boring Camping Photo—More Than Meets the Eye?

This is an essay I wrote on a camping trip several years ago. The essay was written about a simple photo I took while we were camping in Big Sur, California. The black-and-white replication of the photo here may be difficult to interpret, so I'll tell you what is represented in it. The photo itself is a simple, uninteresting image I shot while lying down in my tent. I was looking up at the canvas of the tent, with an unzipped tent window through which you could see the canopy of trees above. I think the image was taken during an afternoon nap, perhaps. As you will see, the photo itself is not the interesting part of my essay. Keep reading.

CAMPING ESSAY

Is there more than meets the eye in this seemingly uninteresting, commonplace photo I shot while lying in my tent for an afternoon nap, looking up at the canopy of Eucalyptus trees surrounding our campsite in Big Sur, California?

Is this just my view from the tent, or is there more going on here?

Let me start by saying this: this is my favorite of more than 100 amazing photos from an awesome camping trip we took with our friends.

No, there isn't a hidden item you should be searching for in the photo—no scary spider, no rare bird in the trees above my tent, no, "Where's Waldo?" challenge in this photo. What you see in the photo is what I see too—nothing out of the ordinary or remarkable.

While the other photos I took on our camping trip to Big Sur display fabulous activities, relaxing time around the camp fire, and great fun had by all (especially our children), this particular photo is the most profound. Let me explain why.

Many of the activities you participate in while camping are just that: activities. They are fun, maybe even relaxing, and perhaps even out of the ordinary. Hiking, swimming, cooking, and lounging around the campfire late at night come to mind. These are great activities.

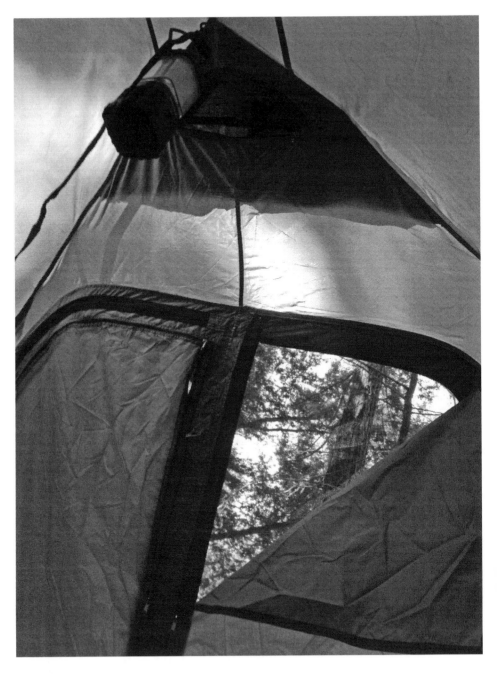

However, what I really love about camping and why it's my absolute favorite summer leisure activity is this: Camping completely turns your routine on its head. What do you do first thing in the morning when you are at home? What do you do before you go to bed? What do you do after lunch? If you are like most of us, you have a routine. And, I'll venture to guess that your routine is pretty intertwined with technology: I would risk assuming that you probably check your email first thing in the morning, and perhaps just before you go to bed.

You probably also have some unhealthy thinking patterns that go along with your routine. Maybe in the morning when you wake up and check your email, you worry about bills that you have to pay, or about your day's work ahead, or about the chores around the house that haven't been tackled. Or maybe, your unhealthy thinking is centered on some other, completely different topic. I can't know; I'm not inside your head. I can tell you that personally, my unhealthy thinking patterns are pretty much the same and predictable day-in and day-out: they have to do with work, productivity, and an inability to relax and see the big picture.

When I take a few hours off work and do something fun, it doesn't fundamentally change my routine, nor does it change my "stinking thinking" patterns. Why? Because most of a person's routine (mine included) happens not during the day, but around bed time, and in the morning. These are the times when you really set your compass for the day.

Now we're getting somewhere. Now you can understand why this seemingly boring photo is my favorite of dozens of camping photos. While I can relax and go swimming or go for a hike on any given day, the only days when I am really knocked out of my routine are the days when I'm in that tent, looking up through the windows, feeling the fresh air breezing in. At home, I'm always stuck in my routine because I'm always doing the same things before bed and when I wake up in the morning.

When you are camping, you leave everything behind—your computer, your routine, your chores, your worries, your thinking patterns. Camping is different enough from normal life that it sort of pushes the reset button in your brain. A hotel room doesn't do that for me; sure, hotel vacationing is awesome and relaxing, but you are still sleeping in a man-made structure, with your laptop sitting on a desk nearby, electricity just a plug away, and all the amenities, paperwork, parking, and other aspects of modern life within arm's length.

Camping is just about the only activity I've found that fully and completely pushes the reset button in my thinking. Three days of camping, and I'm refreshed completely. When I return home to my regular life, I have a new perspective on things. Does my new, clear thinking last forever? No, it usually deteriorates back to my normal thinking patterns within about a week or two. So that's when it's time to go camping again! Or at least, that's when it's time to reflect back to the camping experience, to remember what I learned and how I felt when the world wasn't barking at my doorstep, when my phone wasn't ringing constantly and when dozens of emails weren't pouring in at all hours of the day demanding my time.

The essence of camping isn't the activities you do during the day. It's the act of getting dislodged from your routine—of rising and sleeping with the cycles of nature, of leaving everything familiar behind for a few days. When you do this, you'll discover fun, relaxation, and intimate time with friends. But even more, you'll discover your soul. You'll find that your soul has been suffocating amid the modern demands of your busy, wired, technologically connected life; it has been pleading with you to give it some fresh air. You never heard your soul because you were too busy. What you were busy with differs among all of us, but I can say with certainty: you were too busy.

I'll end on a less philosophical note. Camping is cheap, so most people don't have a good excuse not to do it. If you loathe the work involved in planning and preparing, it means you are probably too entrenched in your routine—consider this a warning signal of impending burnout. Trust me, it's worth it. Put your computer down, gather (or buy) your camping gear, and plan a trip. Leave your life behind for a few days and discover a renewal that will refresh you, recharge you, and reset your thinking patterns like nothing else I've found on planet Earth.

Camping is my gift to you. Well actually, it's not my gift at all; it's God's gift to you. Accept the gift, and take some time to recharge your soul. And when you are lying in your tent, looking up through the open windows, you'll feel what I felt—the bliss of a break in your routine; a chance for your soul to drink in the natural environment it was intended to dwell in; and a rare opportunity to push the pause button on even the most consistent and normal aspects of your daily life.

Epilogue: The Word "Camping"

I really don't like the word "camping." It conjures up pictures of silly, superficial activities like eating s'mores, towing an RV, and lying on a sandy beach by a campsite. Really, the activity of "camping" is much more profound than that. Camping connects us with nature like no other activity: sleeping mere inches away from the dirty ground with no climate control and no walls. Camping pushes the rewind button on the world's calendar, and we get to live as if it were 1500 years ago, without the modern amenities and basics of modern life. These profound shifts in how we experience the world are deeply relaxing and inspirational—and even a bit philosophical. On my last trip, I was left alone to read while the family did a day trip hike. I sat by myself at the camp site for six hours. The heat, the bugs, the curvature of the Earth my chair was sitting on, the shadows moving across the ground as the hours passed—these were all experiences so different from my normal life that they inspired some pretty deep thoughts: "This is how people lived for thousands of years before modern times. Wow!" Such an experience made me think: Are we really better off in modern times with so much technology and connectedness? Are we healthier? Are we happier?

Your own philosophical questions might be different than mine, and your own experience will be yours alone, unique as you are—but one thing's for sure: camping is about a lot more than s'mores and RVs. It's a complete shift in the human experience and gives us insight into the experiences of our ancestors. Modern life with electricity, the Internet, and Espresso is but a blip on the radar of human existence. For most of history, we've lived a lot more like what we now call "camping." Most of us lack that perspective and just take daily life for granted. Yet that very perspective is the one thing which we may truly need in order to live a more balanced life.

So next time you hear the word "camping," remember that this is an activity with profound and deep implications and lessons about the human condition. In fact, because camping is so affordable, I'd make the argument that camping is one of the richest, most rewarding, interesting activities dollar-for-dollar of anything available on our planet.

Chapter 7
Parasites and Worms: The New Lyme Disease Co-Infection? (Don't Skip This Chapter!)

A New Frontier in Lyme Disease Treatment

L et's start with an important statement: Don't skip this chapter! This chapter contains essential secrets which can unlock new, unprecedented improvement for many Lyme disease sufferers.

Readers may be inclined to skip this chapter because they assume that parasite problems are limited in scope to the intestines, and while these people may have some minor intestinal symptoms, they feel that intestinal parasites are, at most, a small part of their problem. In fact, countless Lyme sufferers have done extensive parasite cleanses and experienced little improvement in their Lyme disease symptoms. These people may be thinking, "Okay, so parasites are probably a real problem, but they can't be a very big player in my body-wide symptoms like brain fog, depression, memory loss, irritability, fatigue, and others."

So then, why should we take a deeper look at parasite problems? There are several important reasons which we will examine over the next few pages. Don't jump to any conclusions until you've finished reading the entire chapter!

First, the anti-parasitic treatments included in most over-the-counter herbal cleanses are not typically powerful enough to accomplish the goals we are after; therefore, even if you've done parasite cleanses, you probably haven't addressed more extensive parasitic infestations.

But more importantly, while some parasitic infections are located in the gut, many are not restricted to the intestinal tract. If you've read my past book, *The Top 10 Lyme Disease Treatments,* you may recall this statement from the introductory chapter:

> *"Lyme disease is a bacterial infection caused by Borrelia burgdorferi, an elongated, spiral-shaped bacteria transmitted to humans through the bite of a tick. Known as spirochetes, these bacteria are unusual, not well studied, elusive and difficult to cultivate in the laboratory, and capable of advanced survival activities more commonly found in larger, more intelligent organisms."*

Pay attention to the last sentence. Years after I wrote that statement, it is now well-established that Borrelia organisms (and even the co-infections Babesia and Bartonella) are unlike many other kinds of micro-organisms in that they are highly advanced in their lifecycle activities, survival capabilities, and ability to respond to environmental threats.

However, there appears to be even more going on here. Many physicians and researchers now believe that there are also other, recently discovered community members living within the infectious colonies inside the body of an infected person. Modern science hasn't solved all the mysteries surrounding this discovery, but we are beginning to uncover some answers to important questions. For example, we know that these community members are larger than Borrelia, Bartonella and Babesia, and we know that they play an important role in the Lyme complex. They are likely worm, or worm-like organisms, or even a number of different species of worm-like organisms. It is also possible that these organisms may have merged with Borrelia, creating a type of hybrid organism with shared DNA.

Expanding the Definition of Co-Infections

Modern research tells us that the "co-infections" involved in Lyme disease may be much more numerous than we had previously thought. We need to be thinking about a diverse and thriving community of many different kinds of organisms. This community likely also includes parasites of various types, and maybe even worms or worm-like organisms. All of the different organisms protect one another, and some of them may even take up shelter *inside* larger organisms. Thus, when larger organisms are killed, smaller ones may emerge and begin to cause problems all over again. To think of Lyme disease as just Borrelia with a few buddies like Bartonella and Babesia is far too simplistic and limited: The disease includes these players *plus* other players which are even now just being identified. The ratio of different organisms in the community may change and vary over months and years, and may also change depending on which methods are used to attack the communities.

As it turns out, these larger worms or parasites have some surprising properties. First, they can live outside the gut and throughout the rest of the body. Historically, worms and worm-like parasites were believed to be mostly confined to the gut. These new worms or parasites can take up residence with Borrelia, Babesia and Bartonella, take shelter within biofilm communities, and become important partners in the survival of the infections. Over the last several years, different researchers have given these new organisms different names.

It now appears that many Lyme sufferers are infected with these newly acknowledged parasites, just like many Lyme sufferers carry co-infections. Furthermore, because of the symbiotic relationship between parasites and Lyme-related infections, without addressing parasites, overall progress in healing may be halted. Therefore, the topic of treating parasitic infections is a hugely important topic. Ignoring it could cause your entire healing process to come to a halt.

Additionally, evidence indicates that anti-parasitic treatments may, in fact, be able to target more than just these parasites; they may also target Borrelia, Bartonella, and Babesia. So, use of these treatments can have all kinds of important new benefits. Thinking of them only as "anti-parasite treatments" restricts their definition to a very limited scope and misses the important reality that they may have a larger impact on entire colonies containing numerous types of bacteria. Bacterial colonies cloaked in biofilm are complex communities, and we don't yet fully appreciate how various treatments are capable of weakening and compromising them.

But there's more. At least one top practitioner has discovered that worm DNA can be found in bacterial biofilm, meaning that larger and more complex organisms (worms) may be involved, to some degree, in the proliferation and survival of much smaller bacteria, such as Borrelia. In fact, it may be impossible to adequately treat Lyme disease biofilms without addressing this worm component. So, as you can see, the use of anti-parasite (and anti-worm) treatments may go a lot further than merely killing a few worms that may be living in the gut. Anti-worm therapies may have the capability to destabilize entire Lyme disease colonies located in deep tissue throughout the body, helping to destroy Lyme disease. Let's summarize:

1. Borrelia organisms and co-infections like Babesia and Bartonella may be susceptible to the advanced anti-parasite treatments listed later in this chapter, giving you a new weapon against these infections.

2. The protective biofilm surrounding Borrelia colonies may be degraded by anti-parasite treatments.

3. There may be worms or worm-like organisms living within bacterial colonies throughout the body, and these organisms may be susceptible to anti-parasite treatments.

4. Anti-parasite treatments may have a significant impact in weakening all of the infective colonies throughout the body.

5. If parasites are untreated, progress against the other infections, like Borrelia, Babesia and Bartonella, can come to a halt. In this way, treating parasites doesn't just provide the benefits discussed in this list, it also renders other co-infections more susceptible to treatment.

6. Finally, it's important to remember that the kinds of parasites we are talking about in this chapter don't just inhabit the gut; they can also inhabit many other parts of the body.

Profound Improvement Experienced with Parasite Treatment

These theories aren't just academic. In fact, many Lyme sufferers are noticing huge improvements when using various anti-worm protocols. But it is important to be very clear here: Most of the well-known and often-used anti-parasite cleanses and herbal preparations are not capable of eradicating the parasites involved in Lyme disease. Keep reading to discover new solutions which offer much greater efficacy.

When employing these new solutions, some people report gains that were previously impossible using any other treatment. Even cognitive symptoms such as depression, memory loss, irritability, anxiety, and others can respond rapidly to anti-parasitic treatments. It is for this reason that I believe this chapter has some of the most important information in the entire book. We aren't just talking about a theoretical breakthrough; we are talking about a new treatment methodology that has actually been making many people feel much, much better.

It makes sense that such significant healing is possible if prior Lyme disease treatment was only targeting Borrelia, Babesia, and Bartonella but missing an entire species of worm or parasite. My own battle with Lyme disease began shortly after I consumed contaminated snow on a hike, circa 2001. I had horrible intestinal symptoms for weeks after this incident, which gave way to full-blown Lyme disease. I believe that Borrelia, Bartonella, and Babesia were hiding out in my body prior to this but were fully activated by the presence of some new kind of parasites that were introduced on that hike. Is it possible that parasites I picked up from that snow somehow migrated out of my digestive system, joined forces with Borrelia and company, and began building infective colonies together? Could this be why my Lyme disease symptoms exploded after what should have been a parasitic episode limited to my gut? I believe this is exactly what happened. I think there is a lot more going on with this disease than we currently understand. I even believe it is possible that Borrelia and the intestinal parasites somehow morphed inside my body into one hybrid organism with customized DNA. In fact, I believe that many people infected with parasites and Lyme organisms may be harboring custom species inside their bodies, species which can be different from any other species in the world. Such DNA sharing has been recorded in the scientific literature, and these kinds of incidents could explain why everyone responds so differently to Lyme disease treatment. If we are all walking around with a slightly different variation of the disease, it makes sense that no two people will respond in the same way to the available treatments.

I'm not alone in my observations. Several top researchers have identified new organisms which appear in their Lyme disease patients. Some of these organisms are labeled as protozoan, some are labeled as bacteria, and some are actually thought to be hybrid organisms which display characteristics of more than one kind of microorganism. Anti-parasitic drugs are thought to be among the most useful treatments for these new organisms.

We may not currently have the medical technology and resources required to explain exactly why anti-parasitic drugs and treatments work to help Lyme disease patients, but we are certainly making progress in unraveling the mysteries. I believe the following point is key: If we wait for 100% understanding before we proceed with treatment, we may be waiting decades before feeling better. This approach is unacceptable in my opinion. If people are getting better now using anti-parasitic treatments, I believe we should consider these treatments, even while all of the facts are still being discovered. We may not know exactly what the treatments are hitting, but we know they are hitting something, and that people are getting better. Of course, I advocate using these therapies only to the extent which they are safe, and only under the care of a licensed physician.

Many top Lyme doctors agree with me and now prescribe anti-parasitic protocols to their patients. This chapter will examine some of these protocols, and will also provide my observations and opinions about them. Please remember that some of the information in this chapter is based on my own personal observations and experiences; do not assume that my perspective is the only accurate perspective.

The Subtleties of Synergism

While the direct effect of anti-parasitic treatments may in fact be substantial, the treatments also offer a more subtle benefit. To discover this benefit, let's consider what is happening in the bodies of people who have been sick with Lyme disease for a long period of time.

After the bacterial colonies (comprising Borrelia, co-infections, and parasitic components) have survived in the body for months or years and have been attacked by various treatments, they take on a much more entrenched, treatment-resistant configuration. In other words, if you have been sick with Lyme disease for a long time and have tried many things, your infected areas are a bit like battle-hardened military platoons. They are hunkered down, protected, and resistant to whatever you are trying to do to defeat them.

This means that anything you can do to destabilize these highly protected colonies will allow the other treatments you are using (or have used) to be more effective. If you can breach their defenses, then they will no longer be able to ward off the normal Lyme disease treatments you've been trying to use against them.

This principle does, in fact, undergird much of this entire book, and Chapter 3, which describes the Antibiotic Rotation Protocol, is largely based on it.

Because anti-parasitic treatments weaken biofilm and attack members of the protected community using mechanisms of action different from any antibiotic you've probably taken in the past, they provide a new method for destabilizing the infective colonies located throughout the body. Therefore, after having used anti-parasitic treatments, you will likely notice not only an improvement in your symptoms but also a general increase in the effectiveness of other anti-Lyme and co-infection therapies. This double-whammy—improvement experienced from anti-parasitic drugs alone as well as from renewed effectiveness of other treatments—is why it is so important for us to always introduce new treatments into our treatment programs.

When facing a stalemate against the infections for months or years, this destabilizing effect can provide huge benefits in the battle.

Herbal vs. Pharmaceutical Treatments

One of the most common statements I hear repeated is that people prefer to use natural, or non pharmaceutical treatments when combating Lyme disease. And of course, this goal can be a very beneficial pursuit as it spares the body the damage done by pharmaceutical treatments. Furthermore, because Lyme disease requires such extended treatment, pharmaceutical therapies can take an increasingly large toll on the body over time, and can lead to a serious breakdown of the immune system and other body systems.

Additionally, because the infectious organisms involved in Lyme disease are so treatment-resistant and often hide behind biofilm, many of the powerful pharmaceutical anti-infective therapies people use have negligible effects against the infections and don't even reach their targets. This can be especially true if you are using a drug which targets an infection that isn't currently the top layer of the onion.

Combine these factors, and you'll note that pharmaceutical treatments have a dismal risk-to-reward ratio: they can wreak havoc while providing only minor benefits.

> **Yoga vs. Drugs**
>
> The trend in modern alternative medicine is to demonize drugs, list all of their disadvantages, and strongly prefer natural therapies like Yoga. We juice, fast, exercise, eat organic, avoid pesticides, and protect our bodies from the chemical onslaught of our era. And of course, we should. But what if you found out that your true illness, the root cause of your illness, wasn't an invasion of chemicals into your food but a series of infections living in your tissues? And what if it were true that killing these infections would propel your health to new levels you never thought possible? Well, if you suffer from Lyme disease and co-infections, I'm here to tell you that this may, in fact, be the case. So, continue to buy your organic groceries and treat the aches and pains of life with natural remedies but don't pass over the "big gun" pharmaceuticals needed to eradicate the infections from your body. Medical experience has taught us that for the majority of cases, no amount of holistic living will lead to a full recovery from Lyme disease without the support of serious pharmaceutical treatments targeted toward wiping out the infections.

While this reality is unfortunately true in many cases, there are exceptions. A carefully targeted pharmaceutical attack, used for only the short duration before the infections become resistant, can provide unparalleled killing power with minimal side effects. This is true for all of the infections involved in Lyme disease, not just parasites. Such a strategy used in rotation with other effective strategies can provide huge leaps in progress. The key, of course, is to recognize the difference between extended, ineffective use of pharmaceuticals and precise, targeted, effective attacks.

Experience has shown that, while it is admirable to prefer natural treatments over pharmaceutical treatments, the healing and progress described in this chapter simply are not possible when pharmaceuticals are completely avoided. When used intelligently, the rewards of using pharmaceutical anti-parasitic drugs can outweigh the associated risks of side effects or negative effects on the body.

Now, we'll look at the most useful of the pharmaceutical options as well as a few of the powerful herbal remedies which have a proven track record.

The Anti-Parasite Protocols

IMPORTANT NOTE: *The protocols listed in this chapter draw from the research and wisdom of numerous Lyme disease doctors, researchers, and patients. However, these protocols also incorporate my own findings, based on my own research and experience. Therefore, as you read this information, please realize that it is not a "one-size-fits-all" approach to healing. Your own situation and needs may differ significantly from what is offered here. Please use this information only under the guidance of a licensed physician.*

Also, please note that some of these drugs are untested and unapproved by the FDA, and they may be potentially unsafe. In addition to the approval of a licensed physician, I suggest collaborating with other Lyme disease sufferers to share your experiences with the protocol and get feedback from others about how they use the protocol. I have found that peer-to-peer collaboration can be invaluable when using protocols that do not have a great deal of established methodology and "best practices."

Furthermore, before taking any of the below treatments, I suggest you extensively research them to understand their potential side effects, interactions, and issues. It is also helpful to be familiar with how extensively the drugs are absorbed, whether food increases or decreases their absorption, which organs are needed to metabolize and excrete them, what the drugs' half-lives are, and what kinds of infections they are most often used for. You will also want to know about any interactions. Should they be taken with food or on an empty stomach? And if with food, should they be taken with a fatty meal or a normal meal? It is my own personal policy to become as much of an expert as I *possibly can on new drugs prior to putting them into my body. Even my guiding physician doesn't know everything about every drug, and I believe it is critical for people to take responsibility for their own healing and health. If you are unwilling to study up on these drugs and collaborate with an experienced doctor on their use, then <u>I strongly suggest avoiding these treatments</u>.*

It is also important to start only one new drug or treatment at a time, so you can carefully interpret what that treatment is doing within your body without the confusion of multiple new treatments.

Finally, people who are working with experienced doctors are much more likely to succeed with Lyme disease treatment because these doctors may have had many, or dozens, of patients on these drugs, and therefore, they know what kind of things to watch for and which warnings to issue to their patients. Using these treatments without an experienced, supervising doctor greatly increases the risk of failed treatment and side effects. I very strongly recommend that you pursue pharmaceutical treatments <u>only</u> under the care of a licensed physician.

I will not be specific about drug dosing in this chapter as the recommendations vary among different health care practitioners. Some doctors advocate doses which I believe to be much too high. Therefore, I will leave it to you and your physician to customize the dosages.

The Basic Parasite Protocol

The following drugs are listed in the order in which they should be used. They are not used in combination; they are used separately and sequentially.

Biltricide—Use for 4 days.

Pyrantel pamoate—Use for 17 days.

Ivermectin—Use for 17 days.

Albendazole—Use for 17 days.

Alinia—Use for 17 days.

Notes on the Basic Parasite Protocol:

While the above recommendation for the number of days to use each drug can serve as a general guideline, I recommend that you tailor these recommendations based on the Antibiotic Rotation Protocol principles (see chapter 3). In other words, if you feel a drug is beneficial for longer than the prescribed period, then stay on it for additional time (assuming that the side effects are manageable and that you are under the care of a physician). Alternately, if your Herxheimer reactions and improvement dissipate before the end of the time period, consider stopping the drug early. No dosing schedule should be rigid. Some people benefit from much longer periods of use of the same drug, while other people do better on a more rapid rotation schedule.

Also, because parasites can reproduce rapidly and are difficult to eradicate from the body, it may be necessary to use the above sequence of drugs more than one time; in fact, it may need to be used many times over a period of years. Some people report that if they revisit this protocol once or twice a year, they experience renewed improvement and additional results. Interestingly, the subjective experience of using these drugs can be different with each subsequent rotation, indicating that the same drug may be hitting different layers of the onion each time it is used. For example, one year, Ivermectin may cause improvement in memory and mood, and the next year, it may lead to improvements in energy, muscle aches, and stamina.

Finally, because these anti-parasite drugs may uncover other infections or render them more vulnerable, combining this protocol with protocols targeted toward Borrelia, Babesia and Bartonella can be very helpful. For example, one Lyme patient reported that combining Alinia with Tinidazole caused rapid and unprecedented symptom improvement. However, please consult a physician before combining these or other pharmaceutical drugs, because some combinations may be toxic and dangerous.

My Comments on the Drugs in the Basic Parasite Protocol

These comments are based on my personal research and experience; they may not apply to everyone equally. As always, please consider the advice of your doctor to be more accurate than this book.

Biltricide: This is one of the weaker choices. It is taken first to eliminate some intestinal parasites and liver flukes. It has had limited benefit for some Lyme sufferers but may still be included as part of a complete treatment protocol.

Ivermectin: This is one of the big guns of parasite treatment. It is widely recognized as one of the most effective drugs for Lyme disease patients. It has a very broad spectrum of activity and is absorbed systemically. It is believed to target some of the mystery bugs which researchers are just beginning to identify and name, and which are now being recognized as commonly occurring Lyme disease co-infections. If you do a Google search for *Lyme disease ivermectin*, you will find a great deal of information as well as patient testimonials and write-ups. Some top physicians now believe that this drug can partially address Bartonella. Ivermectin is generally well tolerated, and although some physicians recommend very high dosages, I personally do not feel comfortable with those dosage levels.

Of interest is the finding that Ivermectin targets bacteria as well as parasitic organisms. This finding further reinforces my earlier statement that anti-parasitic drugs aren't just targeting new mystery organisms, but they may also be helping us fight Borrelia, Bartonella, and Babesia as well. Consider the following research from France:

> *Ivermectin is currently approved for treatment of both clinical and veterinary infections by nematodes (worms), including Onchocerca cervicalis in horses and Onchocerca volvulus in humans. However, ivermectin has not previously been*

221

shown to be effective against bacterial pathogens. Here we show that ivermectin also inhibits infection of epithelial cells by the bacterial pathogen, Chlamydia trachomatis, at doses that could be envisioned clinically for sexually-transmitted or ocular infections by Chlamydia.

-Source: University Paris Sud, France

This information is fascinating, indeed! Now we can start to see a clearer picture of why anti-parasite drugs can have multi-faceted benefits and be so useful in Lyme disease.

Pyrantel pamoate: Available over-the-counter. Can profoundly impact Lyme disease and co-infections. Generally well tolerated.

Albendazole: A cousin of the popular Mebendazole, Albendazole is much more powerful, has more significant side effects, and targets a broader range of organisms. Due to potentially serious side effects, close monitoring is necessary. Can have significant benefits.

Nitazoxanide: This drug is typically sold under brand name Alinia, but much more affordable brand names can be purchased from overseas pharmacies.

Nitazoxanide is considered to be very useful by a large number of practitioners and can target numerous kinds of protozoan, including Babesia. It is also useful for other types of parasites, and is considered to be a "cyst busting" drug by some researchers, so it can impact Borrelia, too. For these reasons, it is one of my favorite drugs in this chapter, and it has broad application for Lyme disease patients.

As if the above-mentioned benefits of nitazoxanide weren't enough, the drug also impacts biofilm formation. This was shown by research published in Oxford's *Journal of Antimicrobial Chemotherapy,* in a study entitled, "Nitazoxanide inhibits biofilm formation by Staphylococcus epidermidis by blocking accumulation on surfaces. " Several other studies also demonstrate nitazoxanide's inhibition of biofilm. And lastly, nitazoxanide has even been shown to inhibit numerous viruses, including hepatitis. Peer-reviewed studies have demonstrated this anti-viral effect.

So, yet again you can see the diverse and much-needed benefits of anti-parasitic drugs. To summarize, nitazoxanide is used to kill parasites, Babesia, Borrelia cysts, viruses, and to disrupt bacterial biofilm. It's no wonder that Lyme patients, who are often afflicted with most or all of these problems, can feel so much better as a result of using nitazoxanide. Nitazoxanide is one of the most multi-talented and broadly applicable drugs available to Lyme sufferers, and I consider it to be one of the most important new treatments presented in this book.

Nitazoxanide is generally well tolerated but physician monitoring is still advisable.

Other Useful Drugs

The Basic Parasite Protocol described above is the most established and tested parasite protocol recognized by various Lyme disease doctors, researchers, and patients. However, my own, independent research and experience has revealed a few other anti-parasitic drugs which I believe have the potential to augment and complement the existing protocol. Remember, most of these infections (including Borrelia, co-infections, and parasites) develop resistance to most treatments, so expanding the arsenal of available options can lead to dramatic improvement and destabilization of the infective colonies. So, it is beneficial to have as many choices available to us as possible.

Again, I want to remind you that these treatments are experimental; proceed with caution. I have personally used all of the drugs mentioned in this chapter, but I do not recommend nor endorse them for use by others.

A drug may be well tolerated by one person, but cause significant side effects for another.

Mebendazole: A weaker cousin of Albendazole, some people find this drug to be useful. It may also be useful for people who cannot tolerate the more extensive side effects profile of Albendazole.

Diethylcarbamazine: Sometimes referred to simply as DEC, this is a very interesting drug. It is unique because it operates by a mechanism of action different from any of the other parasite drugs. Therefore, it may be useful when resistance has developed to the other drugs.

Various sources also cite anti-inflammatory, hepatoprotective, immuno-modulatory, and other beneficial effects of the drug, making it an interesting option for people with weakened livers or extensive inflammation. In fact, this drug's immuno-modulatory effects are so profound that some researchers suspect its killing ability is related more to fine-tuning the immune system to see the pathogens than to the direct chemical effect of the drug against worms and micro-organisms.

My conclusion, based on research and experience, is that it accomplishes both objectives: it modulates the immune system for much more effective targeting of infections, and at the same time, kills worms and micro-organisms via direct, chemical activity.

Also, this drug has strong activity in the endothelial cells, which is exactly where Bartonella likes to live. So, Diethylcarbamazine may directly inhibit Bartonella or at least kill the parasites protecting Bartonella.

Diethylcarbamazine seems to be one of the anti-parasitic drugs which leads to the most immediate and pronounced reduction of Lyme disease symptoms (possibly because it isn't just targeting infections, but it's also modulating the immune system). This plethora of very useful actions makes Diethylcarbamazine one of my favorite anti-parasite drugs, if not my single favorite drug. It is difficult to locate DEC in the United States, but it can be purchased affordably from other countries.

DEC is typically well tolerated and has a mild side effects profile for many people. When I reflect on what I now know about DEC, I often find myself thinking, "I really wish someone would have told me about this drug years sooner in my Lyme disease battle!"

Moxidectin: This drug is a cousin of Ivermectin. It is more lipophilic than Ivermectin and has a much longer half-life. Due to the long half-life, extreme caution must be exercised with dosing: if too much is taken, the drug will remain in the body for a very long time, so overdoses can be serious medical emergencies. Information on use in humans is limited; however, at least a couple of studies demonstrate that it is safe for human consumption. As always, consult a physician before use.

Non-Pharmaceutical Options

As you may already know, dozens of herbs and natural preparations are touted to be useful for parasites. Honestly, based on my own experience and research, the majority of these have limited effect for most people, at least with the entrenched, systemic parasites we see in cases of Lyme disease. The two herbal preparations with the most convincing user testimonials for Lyme disease and co-infections are **Humaworm** (www.humaworm.com) and **Parastroy** (made by Nature's Secret, available from various retailers including www.iHerb.com). Due to their low price and relatively limited side effects, these preparations are worth a try, but for some people, the results will not be nearly as forthcoming as when pharmaceutical drugs are used.

On the other hand, there is one herbal preparation which may be as effective as the drugs, if not more: **Mimosa Pudica.** Although it has a very funny-sounding name, Mimosa Pudica is very powerful and has demonstrated a broad spectrum of activity against many of the parasites which accompany Lyme disease. Some research shows that this herb also targets Babesia. People who use it typically report dramatic results in many pesky and difficult symptom areas, including cognitive problems. You need to be careful of one thing, though: Product quality can vary vastly between different suppliers. Some versions of the products have been foul, unhelpful, and maybe even toxic, according to some of my sources. Purchasing it from a compounding pharmacy where quality is more closely regulated is a very good idea. Also, there are some data which indicate that Mimosa Pudica can have toxic side effects. Please use this (and all potentially dangerous treatments) only under the care of a licensed physician.

Various other herbs exist. Their exclusion here doesn't necessarily mean they aren't worth using, but the above listed options are the ones which I have found produce consistent results. Note: Several other herbs with anti-parasitic uses are listed as Individual Treatments in Part III of the book. Some of these, such as moringa oleifera, can be quite beneficial.

Tips for Success When Treating Parasites

Treatment Timing

Like most of the other treatments covered in this book, parasite treatments only work when the treatment being used matches the susceptible organisms located on the top layer of the infective onion we are trying to unpeel. If those particular organisms are in dormancy, covered by layers of other infections, protected by biofilm, or simply in non-susceptible phases of their life cycles, then the treatments will be worthless. Unfortunately, I am unfamiliar with a reliable way to ascertain which infections are susceptible to which treatments at any given time (except in instances where you can match up particular active symptoms with particular infections). Energetic testing can provide clues. Also, parasites are generally more active during the full moon phase, so increased symptoms during that time can indicate the presence of parasites. It can also be noted that the full moon phase is a very good time to target parasites, as they are more active and susceptible to treatment during this time

The moral of the story is that trial and error may be required to figure out which drugs and herbs should be used at various times throughout the recovery process. When I was working through my own recovery process, I found that at certain periods of time, anti-parasitic treatments were immensely useful, and during other periods, they did absolutely nothing.

Remember also that the treatments which were helpful for a time but then stopped working will almost certainly be useful again at some point in the future, when the right organisms have their turn as the top layer of the onion. In fact, treatments which you've already used in the past and which have become totally ineffective may yet be extremely effective again, if only they are used at the proper time. So, take those parasite drugs back off the shelf after you've rotated through the whole lot of them; they will, with certainty, be useful again at some point.

Mind Games

In December 2012, the New York Times reported that many kinds of parasites actually take control of their host's mind. As scary as it sounds, it is a reality. With Lyme disease, the most common manifestation of this phenomenon seems to be that parasites limit a person's drive, ambition, and motivation to get well. Somehow, people are convinced that they are not that sick, and that aggressive treatment is not required or desirable. This is one of the reasons why it is so important to be under the care of a good doctor who can prescribe the necessary treatments. Be aware that you may have been pacified by the parasites in your body, and you may need to work diligently to get well despite the feeling that your problem isn't urgent.

Source: http://www.nytimes.com/2012/12/11/science/parasites-use-sophisticated-biochemistry-to-take-over-their-hosts.html

Where to Purchase Anti-Parasitic (and Other) Drugs

Several of the drugs listed in this chapter are available from U.S. pharmacies at reasonable prices. Others may be available in the United States but are exorbitantly expensive. Finally, some may not be available in the U.S. and are only marketed in overseas countries.

Therefore, shopping for drugs from online, foreign pharmacies may be one option worth considering—either for the purpose of saving money or to find drugs which aren't available in the U.S.

I have personally found several overseas pharmacies which have demonstrated reliability, honesty, and dependability. I will not print their names here, because even though I've had good experiences with them, I am still not confident enough in their product quality and dependability to publically endorse them. However, I will give you some of the tips I have followed for finding and using good online pharmacies.

WARNING: Please research the legality of importing drugs into your country, state, and city. Do not order drugs from foreign pharmacies if doing so is illegal in your area.

Hints for Finding and Using Reliable Online Pharmacies

1. **Canadian Pharmacies.** There is a group of Canadian pharmacies which require a regular U.S. prescription and appear to be highly reliable. The downside to using them is that their pricing and availability tend to mirror that of U.S. pharmacies, but occasionally you can find a deal. To search this group of pharmacies for a particular drug, visit www.pharmacychecker.com. This website also has a general listing of the pharmacies as well as user reviews for those pharmacies. Do not use any pharmaceutical drugs without a valid prescription from a trusted physician. At the

time this book was written, a few of these pharmacies had brand name Mepron (atovaquone) for less than half the price of my local pharamacy.

2. **Non-Canadian Overseas Pharmacies.** The rest of the overseas pharmacies—i.e., those located outside of the United States and Canada—appear to be based in India, Europe, or more exotic locations. These are the pharmacies you need to be most careful of when it comes to their integrity and reliability since there have been multiple reports of un-received orders and stolen funds. Additionally, there is a risk of inauthentic or even dangerous and counterfeit drug shipments. One method for screening these pharmacies is to do a Google search for *online pharmacy reviews.* There are several sites which I've used and which are very helpful for ranking these pharmacies based on actual user reviews. I've ordered from several of these pharmacies and have had mostly good luck. Advantages of working with them include lower prices and a wider variety of products. In some cases, I've found products which are only one tenth the price of the same products available in the United States! Again, though, proceed with caution. While I have used these pharmacies personally, there are significant risks associated with purchasing from them, so I don't recommend that you make the same decisions I've made without first conducting significant research and consulting your physician. I would actually prefer to avoid these pharmacies all together, but in some instances, they carry drugs which can't be found anywhere in the USA or Canada.

3. **Research Specific Brand Names.** Most online pharmacies will display the manufacturer name of the drugs they sell. While these manufacturers are typically not names you would recognize, some of them are reputable Indian or European manufacturers. You can Google the manufacturer names and read their websites, or read other news articles about the manufacturers to verify that they are high-quality, legitimate brands. **WARNING**: Not all online

pharmacies ship legal, legitimate, safe, authentic drug brands. Please proceed with caution. Some are fraudulent and will steal your personal information and not ship your products. **DISCLAIMER**: I do not personally recommend that anyone shop from online pharmacies. Instead, I am simply sharing my personal experiences here.

4. **Ask The Lyme Community.** Many other Lyme sufferers are looking for the same drugs you are looking for, so there's no need to reinvent the wheel. Join large discussion forums such as www.lymenet.org and ask around for sources for the drugs you need. Many participants in these forums have used online pharmacies and can share their experiences.

5. **Check With Compounding Pharmacies First.** Some USA-based compounding pharmacies can source rare drugs. It is safer to purchase drugs from these compounding pharmacies than from overseas pharmacies. Therefore, check with the many compounding pharmacies in the United States before looking overseas.

6. **Double Check with Your Physician.** Make sure you check with your prescribing physician before using any drug. In all cases, your physician's advice should be considered more accurate than this book.

Lastly, please note that there may be many risks associated with ordering from foreign pharmacies, including the risk of receiving dangerous counterfeit drugs, having your financial information stolen, never receiving the product you ordered, etc. <u>I do not suggest that you place orders with foreign pharmacies. I am not advocating this course of action for any individual.</u>

Climbing the Mountain of Victory and the End of Adrenal Fatigue

In conclusion, I would like to share a personal story which took place several years ago and which illustrates how parasitic infections can play a profound role in the Lyme disease complex. This story touches on the topic of Adrenal Fatigue, which is addressed in Chapters 5 and 6.

The debate rages on. Is adrenal fatigue caused by infections that wreak havoc on the adrenals and brain, or do the stresses of life weaken the adrenal glands and open the door for infections to take root? Which came first—the chicken or the egg? On and on the debate goes; where it stops, no one knows.

Except we do know, or at least we have clues. I will share with you what I have learned, and the clues I've gathered.

It was a smoky afternoon in my hometown in Northern California (my city gets smoke sometimes from nearby fires which rage across the Sierra Nevada Mountain Range). It was mid-August and peak fire season, but otherwise, it was a beautiful day. My better judgment, however, told me not to go for a hike; smoke inhalation would be extreme, and visibility was only about two miles.

An even more convincing reason not to go was my adrenal fatigue. At this point my adrenals had recovered to about 90%, but intense cardio exercise still brought me down. I wondered when this would ever end. When would I be able to hike the high, 10,000+ foot peaks of my hometown, again? Several years ago, I experienced a very, very stressful life event combined with what appeared to be a Bartonella flare-up. The sum of these two stressors seemed to send my adrenals into a tailspin, and while I had recovered a great deal, I still wasn't able to embark on a big, epic Sierra hike.

Only today, something was different. I felt strong, much stronger than I had in a long time. Just a week prior, I had begun a course of the anti-parasitic drug **Diethylcarbamazine** (discussed earlier in this chapter). When I began taking it this time, I didn't expect much. I'd already done several rounds of it in the past several years, and it seemed unlikely that it would be useful yet again. The drug was hugely helpful when I first discovered it, but I was skeptical that further use would provide any benefit. Besides, I had already achieved a very happy 90% recovery from Lyme disease. How much more improvement could I gain? Intuition told me that the drug had already killed whatever it could kill. My past uses of the drug, ranging from about 1-3 weeks in duration, surely knocked out any susceptible bugs.

But in this particular case, I took my own advice and defied my intuition, instead acting upon tried-and-true principles which I knew to be accurate. I accepted the wisdom which states that these anti-bacterial and anti-parasitic treatments are almost always useful, time after time, if only they are used at the right point in the infectious organisms' lifecycles. I didn't know it was a good time to use Diethylcarbamazine, but I figured a little trial and error wouldn't hurt. I took a chance; I made a guess. I remembered giving the drug a try just six weeks prior with almost zero response. Maybe this time it would be different...

And it was different. For some reason, this time, the drug kicked some major butt. I had very little Herx reaction—almost exclusively improvement. Strangely, I felt a tingling in the area of my mid back, the place that is home to my adrenal glands. I also experienced strange dreams reminiscent of the very early days of my original Lyme disease infection, and I had a new-found appetite for food, reminiscent of my teenage years. It just seemed that things in my body were changing, and changing fast. This hadn't happened before. Interesting.

While I had also been taking all of the other advice this book offers to heal the adrenal glands (And it had been helping.), this round of

Diethylcarbamazine catapulted me into a new level of adrenal health in just about 10 days time. If you know anything about adrenal fatigue, you know that things just don't happen in 10 days. Interesting…again.

So as I stood at the bottom of a fairly good sized mountain on this smoky August day, I felt strength in my legs and reserves of energy I hadn't felt in a long time. I charged up that mountain solo, breathing in dense smoke. On the top of the mountain—sweating, heart pounding—I was subtly aware of the smoke headache that was coming on; I'd experienced this headache before many times while hiking during other summers of heavy smoke pollution. Surely breathing in this much smoke can't be healthy, I thought. The headache was a nuisance but only occupied a small part of my thoughts. Instead of the headache, I was distinctly focused on how I felt: just fine. Normally, during the worst of adrenal fatigue, I would have experienced symptoms which were activated almost immediately upon exercising—symptoms which are a hallmark of adrenal fatigue. They would include light-headedness, a dead-weight feeling in my legs, soreness in my mid-back, salt and sugar cravings, and then after getting home, a fatigue that had me collapsing into the nearest bed and falling straight to sleep regardless of ambient noise or distraction. The next few days would have brought fatigue, depression, and emotional volatility.

Not this time. I didn't feel perfect, but I felt good, much better than I had in a long time. The following day brought some normal, relaxing tiredness which I remember feeling before chronic illness. It was the kind of fatigue that reminds you of the hike you did yesterday, but doesn't slow your day down; a gentle, restful recovery mode commonly felt by athletes when they are recovering from exercise (I know the feeling well, as I used to race mountain bikes and road bikes in college). While I have always suspected that infections are one of the root causes of adrenal fatigue, my day of hiking in the smoky Sierra's provided confirmation. The difference in my body from before this round of Diethylcarbamazine to after was nothing short of astounding.

Sure, many factors contribute to adrenal fatigue, including the presence of a Type A personality, the occurrence of acute, life stress, and the predisposing genetic weaknesses which run in certain families, but I now believe that in most cases, these factors alone would not be enough to bring on adrenal fatigue without the help of infections to ruin the adrenal glands and mess up the brain signals which are sent to them. The lesson I have learned is to keep chasing after the infections long after you think you can't do anything else. Go back to those drugs or herbs that worked for you in years past and give them another chance. If they don't work, wait another couple of weeks or months and try them again. The right treatment at the right time to target the right infections is just what the doctor ordered for sustained, continual progress in healing from this horrible disease. Of course, don't neglect the non-infection treatments offered by this book or elsewhere, but keep your sights set on taking out all of the infections, over and over and over again, until you find yourself standing on top of the mountain, like I have found myself.

You just never know when some lingering bacteria or parasites may be hanging out in your adrenal glands (or other organs). You just never know when the right course of the right drug at the right time can wipe these organisms out for good and let your tissues do what they've been trying to do for years—heal themselves. I will go back to a quote I heard from Doug, my original Lyme disease mentor, inventor of the eponymous "Doug Machine" (or "Coil Machine"), and long-time friend. Doug said to me, "While other people went on to investigate other health problems, I just kept chasing the infections, and I got well." I appreciate your wisdom, Doug, and I have followed in your footsteps.

Chapter 8
A Brief Update on Rife Therapy & Electromedicine

Important Disclaimer: This chapter is based on my own observations and research. I don't claim to be infallible or 100% correct on this topic, and I am not a doctor. Please view this information as the research and subjective opinion of only one person. Also, please realize that rife therapy is not approved by the FDA and may cause dangerous and harmful side effects. Do not use rife therapy without first getting permission from your licensed physician. While I personally chose to experiment with rife therapy, I do not suggest that others make the same choice. Unproven and unapproved devices sold as "rife-type" devices may be dangerous and harmful. I do not endorse the use of any of these devices. The information I share in this chapter should not be seen as an endorsement for using rife-type devices, but instead, my own personal opinions and experiences.

I wrote the book, *Lyme Disease and Rife Machines,* in 2004. That is now a long time ago. Surprisingly, I still feel that most of the information in that book is accurate and useful, at least to the best of my knowledge. New information, in most cases, adds to rather than replaces what's in the book. In other words, the information in *Lyme Disease and Rife Machines* isn't obsolete; it's just incomplete. So, for now, I won't be re-writing the book or replacing it. Instead, I'll spend some time building on it in this chapter, and I still suggest its use as a resource for anyone interested in the topic of fighting Lyme disease with Rife machines.

Please note that the topic of Lyme disease and Rife machines is evolving daily, so the information in this chapter shouldn't be seen as the final word. In fact, since I published *Lyme Disease and Rife Machines,* hundreds of new researchers and Lyme sufferers have reported their results and continue to provide new information. In my opinion, some of these people are now just as knowledgeable as I am when it comes to this topic. You can join in the discussion and get informational updates on the several Lyme/Rife chat groups available online.

For the discussion in this chapter, I will assume you've read my past book. It would be impractical to reprint the entire book here, as it is over 200 pages long, so our discussion will build on what was explained in the book. This is not intended as a sales pitch; if you don't want to buy the book, you can get up to speed in many other ways, including the free chat groups mentioned in the prior paragraph. There are literally hundreds of people who participate in these groups, and there's no reason why someone can't learn all they need to learn without reading my book.

The Limitations of Rife Therapy

If you are one of the people who has experienced complete, 100% healing from Rife machine therapy, that's wonderful! This chapter is not here to nullify your story. Like you, others have reported positive outcomes using rife therapy. However, there are those who have been less successful and for whom other pieces of the puzzle need to be identified and addressed.

After several years of additional study since my Rife book was published, I have come to realize that we know even less about electromedicine as it is used for Lyme disease than I had previously thought. While I do believe that one of the primary reasons rife therapy works is still the original explanation Doug MacLean (and Rife himself) provided for us (simply that certain frequencies are capable of vibrating, or resonating, spirochetes to death), I now believe that there are many other factors which determine the kind of results people are able to attain with rife therapy. Rife therapy has inadequacies that we must examine, and some of these weaknesses have more to do with the infections than with the rife devices themselves. Some of this new information has only come to light over recent years, as we've gained much more knowledge about what it means to have Lyme disease.

So, our discussion will now take us briefly away from rife therapy, and toward the nature of Lyme disease itself. We must look at the complexities and diversity found within a colony of infectious Lyme disease bacteria.

Once the body has been infected with Lyme disease and co-infections, these microbes create colony-like structures which are protected from the immune system by biofilm membranes. Inside these colonies, there exists an advanced network of different kinds of bacteria, parasites, viruses, and other microorganisms, including Borrelia, Bartonella, Babesia, parasites, and more. The colonies also contain diseased human tissue, toxic waste, heavy metals, dead microorganisms, and other components. As a community, the microorganisms inside these colony structures are synergistically beneficial to one another, and even communicate with one another via mechanisms such as quorum sensing. When you begin to treat one particular species of microorganism with a given drug, herb, or electromedicine approach, other species quickly sense the weakening of the colony structure and respond by increasing their own growth and proliferation activities. A fellow researcher, and friend, has described this process as "filling the vacuum": once a vacuum is created by a loss of the presence of one kind of microorganism, that vacuum is quickly filled by another microorganism. He has also jokingly described this process as the "musical chairs," and the "merry go round" of treating Lyme disease; as soon as you get a handle on one infection, another quickly rises up to become dominant, and the colony structure remains intact.

We just aren't sure how many of these numerous ingredients inside each infective colony are susceptible to rife therapy. Or, if they are susceptible, we wonder, to which type of rife machine are they most susceptible? Does the frequency always matter, or are there other components of the treatment which also help, such as the electric or magnetic field? Which kind of device works best—a contact device or a radiant device? The answer is most likely that each type of machine has a time and a place when it is most useful. Still, the trouble remains. Electromedicine may in fact be great for some problems (like active, free-swimming spirochetes) but may not be nearly as effective for other problems (like biofilm, other organisms, toxins, and poor circulation to diseased tissue).

We aren't really saying that rife therapy is not useful for Lyme disease infections. Instead, we are saying that rife therapy may not be useful for all of the infections in Lyme disease, nor for some of the other, non-infectious health challenges commonly seen in association with Lyme disease. Rife therapy turns out to be one of the many tools in the toolbox. For many people, it is one of the most useful tools, but, nonetheless, it's still just a single tool.

A top Lyme Doctor has identified more than a dozen factors which may be a part of the complete Lyme disease picture, including such things as infections, allergies, endocrine abnormalities, liver dysfunction, immune dysfunction, inflammation, environmental toxins, and more. In my opinion, Rife therapy can't address all of these problems, and for that matter, no single therapy can. Connie Strasheim offers similar information in her book, *Beyond Lyme Disease*, where she lists many health problems which go beyond infections and which are often found in Lyme sufferers.

So, it is clear that infections aren't the only thing keeping people sick. **Accordingly, rife therapy isn't the only treatment needed to get well.** Even if you didn't have any non-infectious problems before Lyme disease, you probably have them now, because Lyme disease opens the door for them to enter your body. Lyme disease is often referred to as the gatekeeper because of its ability to open the door to many other health problems.

Since I wrote *Lyme Disease and Rife Machines,* new frequencies, devices, and treatment protocols have been developed. While these new modalities are helpful, it is clear that they are still not a silver bullet. In fact, due to the multifactorial nature of Lyme disease, we can confidently say that no such silver bullet exists. It is certainly possible that rife therapy may be further developed in the future and will have an increased application in the treatment of Lyme disease, but even then, it is unlikely that any improvements would have complete effectiveness for all areas of Lyme disease problems.

Don't give up on rife therapy yet, though! Treatment of the free-swimming, spirochete form of Borrelia appears to be one of the strengths of rife therapy. And, rife therapy, in its many forms with its many frequencies, may also be able to go beyond merely treating the spirochete form of the infection. These may seem like small accomplishments in the face of so many intertwined health problems which make up Lyme disease, but in fact, these are big feats. Defeating free-swimming spirochetes without causing them to convert to their dormant, entrenched forms is a tall task, and rife therapy is still, in my opinion, the only treatment in existence to accomplish this feat. That alone makes rife therapy incredibly valuable for preventing the spread of Borrelia in the body and for keeping the infectious colonies contained during the recovery process. Furthermore, I still believe that when the time and circumstances are correct during the recovery process, entire infectious colonies are very susceptible to rife therapy, perhaps because, for a short time period during their lifecycle, all of the Borrelia organisms take on spirochete form. While I don't know for sure if that is the explanation, it has now been observed many times that at several points during any given year, rife users can experience dramatic leaps and bounds of improvement following rife sessions.

During these special times, which often take place in Spring and Fall, I have observed rife therapy to be essential and have no ideal substitute. For example, a person might go weeks—or even months—with no perceptible Herx reaction or improvement resulting from rife therapy, and then, all of a sudden, without notice, a subsequent rife session can produce a dramatic Herx reaction and significant improvement. While many mysteries still surround this process, I believe that this particular benefit offered by rife therapy can keep the recovery process marching forward. Double-blind studies have never been conducted on these observations, but I would go so far as to say that perhaps those who aren't using rife therapy are missing out on one of the most important therapies available when it comes to moving the trajectory of the recovery process toward a successful outcome.

The Lyme disease complex involves many more factors, and many more infections, than simply the spirochete form of Borrelia, which explains why you'll see antibiotic use (both pharmaceutical and herbal) more favored in this book than my previous books. New information since my books were published has demonstrated the presence of these diverse infections, so the simple reality is that more tools are needed than rife therapy alone. Working out the exact balance between rife therapy and other therapies will be something each individual Lyme sufferer will need to do on their own, depending on their unique health challenges as well as the current layer of the onion they are dealing with.

240

Rife Therapy in the Later Phases of Recovery

Ironically, if you do accept and embrace an understanding of the limitations of rife therapy, you must still prepare yourself for the possibility that, later in your recovery process, you may encounter a new layer of infection which is again highly susceptible to rife therapy. This occurrence is quite common, actually. Personally, after rife therapy had long lost its profound effects, during the period of time in which I was about 90% well, it again became very useful for a period of about two months subsequent to my use of chlorine dioxide (see Chapter 12 for information on chlorine dioxide as well as some very important chlorine dioxide precautions and warnings). I believe the chlorine dioxide destroyed entrenched, protective biofilms which were shielding some remaining bacteria, and after the biofilms were removed, these bacteria became active and were easily eliminated with rife therapy. Similarly, after the use of certain antibiotics or antibiotic combinations, the bacterial colonies may be forced to change their configuration, and once-dormant or non-vulnerable bacteria may again be susceptible to—and indeed best targeted by—rife therapy. So, the take-away lesson of highest importance is that you need to remain flexible: you need to prepare for the eventuality that rife may stop working for a time, and you also need to prepare for the possibility that it will start working again, sometimes spontaneously. The worst thought pattern in Lyme disease recovery is rigid thinking—that is, observing your body's response to a given therapy and assuming that such a response will be seen every time you use the therapy. In reality, your responses to treatments will change often, and you need to be prepared to re-evaluate each treatment you use, each time you use it.

While rife is definitely useful later in the recovery process, it will almost certainly be useful less often. Stop and notice that I didn't say rife becomes less important! It is just as important as it's ever been, but this importance occurs less often. What do I mean by this? When rife happens to be the right treatment for the particular layer of the onion you are dealing with, rife is extremely important, and there are no good substitutes for it. I will repeat: when rife is the correct treatment, there are no good substitutes for it. But as you get closer to a complete recovery, you will notice that the instances when rife is important may happen less frequently. This can be the result of many factors, including what was described in the previous paragraph, but also the fact that earlier use of rife therapy may have knocked out many of the organisms which are susceptible to rife. The problems still making you sick are things that aren't susceptible to rife, such as immune system dysfunction, hormonal imbalance, adrenal fatigue, and other issues. Toward the end of recovery is when these other problems seem to be most pronounced and demand the most aggressive corrective actions.

In summary, rife works great at killing spirochetes and greatly slowing down the progress of the infections; it even reverses some of them. Rife is the treatment that initially gave me back my life and allowed me to re-enter society as a functioning, productive person. It allowed me to go back to work and participate in the activities I love. It even helped tremendously during the last 10% of healing. However, during the final phases of my recovery, other treatments were the work horses, as the peripheral problems involved in Lyme disease began to move to the forefront of my recovery process.

Which Infections Are Least Susceptible to Rife Therapy?

The answer to this question is not entirely clear, but it appears that rife therapy is least useful for cyst and L-form Borrelia as well as co-infections such as Babesia, Bartonella, and parasites (although it may have some effect against these other infections). Therefore, one should turn to pharmaceutical antibiotics and herbs (or other proven beneficial treatments) if rife therapy is not eradicating these infections. Some useful herbs and drugs for these infections can be found throughout this book.

Many top Lyme doctors have concluded that Borrelia itself becomes much more vulnerable to treatment after the co-infections are addressed. So, after using herbs or drugs for co-infections, you may find that rife therapy is again useful, as new layers of Borrelia become exposed and active. This shifting dynamic of which treatments are most useful becomes more and more common the closer you get to being well (it seems that the last 10% of healing involves much more rapid rotation between dominant infections), so make sure that you keep your treatment plan and thinking patterns flexible and adaptable. Things are likely to change a lot during the final phases of recovery.

A simple rule to apply if you are no longer responding positively to rife therapy is to treat co-infections with drugs or herbs for a period of time, and then return to rife therapy. You will likely find that rife therapy will again become useful after doing this. The same goes for non-infectious problems, such as heavy metals. Sometimes, after detoxing heavy metals, a person will notice that their Borrelia infection is much more vulnerable and susceptible to treatment.

How Many Different Devices Do You Need?

I would like to answer a question which underlies all discussion of rife treatment. That is, "Why would someone ever need more than one device?"

This is a very important question. The reason is that different types of devices provide a slightly (or in some cases, extremely) different type of treatment output. Some devices are contact devices; some are radiant. Some use plasma tubes; others use a coil of wire. Some have a magnetic field; others only have an electric field. Some are capable of high frequencies; others are not. And there are even some devices which introduce new variables as well.

Why does this matter? Current research indicates that each device (and hence, its unique treatment output) probably targets the infection(s) in a slightly different way. As we've seen, the infections have very diverse colony structures which include biofilm, spirochetes, cyst-form organisms, l-form/cell-wall-deficient organisms, co-infections, and others, and each colony is located in a different body tissue or body environment. Some colonies may be more densely populated than others. If you look at a picture of a Lyme disease bacterial colony, these differences will be obvious. Accordingly, informal research seems to indicate that each type of rife device targets the colonies in a slightly different way. The problem is that we do not always know the specific effects that a given device will have on the colonies. In a perfect world, one device would be designed to incorporate all of the beneficial effects of the numerous devices. Until that is done, however, we are left with a broad selection of different kinds of rife devices, each offering a slightly different, and somewhat unknown, mechanism of action against the infections.

I am aware that this is not the ideal situation, and I would fully support any research that determines the precise effects of each machine. However, until that research takes place, we are left with the wisdom that owning a diverse selection of devices may be the most logical conclusion. Obviously, finances become a restriction. Some people have formed groups of Lyme sufferers which share in the cost of purchasing multiple machines, and many of the available machines can be constructed relatively cheaply.

Lastly, while it may be beneficial to own multiple machines, it certainly isn't necessary to achieve good results. Many Lyme sufferers have received tremendous benefit from owning a single device.

If you intend to acquire or use one or more rife-type devices, please consult with your licensed physician prior to doing so. Advice from your physician should be, in all cases, considered more valid than the information found in this book.

An Important Revision to the Theory Presented in My Earlier Book

This is perhaps the most important rife-related update in this chapter.

In my book *Lyme Disease and Rife Machines*, I built my treatment strategies upon the major assumption that you shouldn't continually suppress Lyme disease bacteria with pharmaceutical or herbal treatments such as antibiotics, because this suppression causes the bacterial colonies to become further entrenched, more treatment resistant, and less susceptible to rife therapy. I then suggested that a good alternative to suppression is to simply wait for the bacterial layers to activate out of dormancy and kill them with rife therapy as that happens. Suppressive therapies were said to be useful at times, but at other times, breaks should be taken to allow the infection to come out of dormancy, become active, and become susceptible to rife treatment.

Although much of the above paragraph is still what I believe to be correct assumptions, I need to make some important revisions to this information. First, while Borrelia may behave this way, and while some infections may also behave this way and even hide under the protection of dormant Borrelia organisms, other kinds of co-infections and co-conditions may not behave this way and may need to be actively targeted instead of treated with the "waiting game." This is a very important statement, since my first books advocated the waiting game as the primary means of getting well. In some cases the waiting game may be appropriate, but if Borrelia has faded into the background and other problems are primary, then the waiting game may be the wrong course of action. For example, if you find yourself dealing with hormonal imbalances, clearly the waiting game is the wrong approach: you need to actively be taking steps to improve the hormonal problems.

And second, when it comes to Borrelia, it is still true that we want to allow dormant, suppressed, inactive layers to activate, and the waiting game is sometimes effective in accomplishing this. Since other toxicities and infections live in close quarters with Borrelia, activating layers of Borrelia can even help us reach layers of other types of problems. We know that active layers of Borrelia are much more susceptible to treatment, and dormant layers are almost impossible to kill by any means— rife or otherwise. So, we can see that activating dormant layers of infection is still an essential part of the healing process.

The problem is, the dormant layers of Borrelia sometimes activate much more slowly than I had previously thought, even when anti-microbial therapies are suspended and even when we are doing a great job at playing the waiting game. In fact, some of these dormant layers may take months or years to activate, and some may not activate at all, leaving a person in an ongoing, continual stalemate with Borrelia. While certain factors can increase the rate of activation of dormant layers (such as the avoidance of suppressive therapies like antibiotics and the natural changing of the seasons throughout the year), these factors may not be enough. And, since other infections and toxicities can dwell in close quarters with Borrelia, dormant and inaccessible Borrelia layers may also prevent you from treating the dormant and inaccessible neighbors of Borrelia. So the problem with the theory in my prior books isn't that seeking to activate dormant layers of the infection is an undesirable goal, but instead, that the waiting game itself may not be an adequate means for achieving that goal.

Therefore, as of the writing of this book, my current observation is that it can be very, very helpful to employ special treatments which may increase the rate of activation of dormant layers. In fact, doing this can be one of the most important aspects of a successful recovery. Forcing dormant layers to activate doesn't just increase the effectiveness of rife therapy, it may also increase the effectiveness of many other therapies targeted toward the other infections, and even non-infectious problems. The trouble is, treatments which can accomplish this are few and far between—90% of our available anti-infective therapies are either suppressive therapies, which prolong dormancy, or therapies that only work when dormant layers of infection have become active. Very few available treatments are actually useful for digging deep within dormant layers and causing their activation. There are several ways in which this goal can be accomplished, such as breaking up biofilm to release dormant infections (perhaps by using systemic enzyme therapy), disrupting colonies with various energetic devices (such as Medsonix, discussed in Part 3), and using herbs or drugs which force Borrelia into its active form. At the time this book was written, these kinds of therapies are still scarce, but we should all be on the lookout for more of them as time progresses.

One caveat, though (and you'll hear me repeat this because of its importance): When going about the task of activating dormant layers, watch out! A newly active layer means a dangerous layer, one that can make you feel sick and even potentially spread the infection to new areas of the body. It's a dangerous game. Activating layers is, I believe, necessary. But it should only be done when you are ready. If you are already overwhelmed with the symptoms of infections, activating new dormant layers may be a bad idea, not a good idea. The activation of dormant layers should only be a goal in the event that you are at a stalemate with the disease, and you are unable to elicit productive Herxheimer reactions (and subsequent improvement) from your treatments. Of course, we don't always get to choose when dormant layers activate; much of the time, they activate on their own schedule, so we need to be ready all of the time.

When a new layer activates, whether because of a treatment you used or on its own schedule, make sure you have your arsenal of appropriate treatments at hand to deal with and kill the newly activated infections. Newly activated layers can contain more than one type of infection, toxicity, or body dysfunction, so make sure to review which anti-infective and supportive therapies have been most helpful to you in the past, and be sure you have those on hand. Review treatment strategies. Stay alert, and be ready for rapid changes if dormant layers are being activated. Once you've succeeded in activating new layers, rife may be very useful, because rife is best suited to target active infections.

After dormant layers have been activated, you may find that they can become dormant again, at which time you'd need to reapply the treatments that cause activation if you want to continue to experience progress. This push-pull phenomenon, where layers are activated and then become dormant again, is still productive even though it may be frustrating. Each time the push-pull cycle occurs, the overall bacterial population is decreasing, and the integrity of the bacterial colony structure is also diminishing. By controlling the fight—when and how it happens—you are winning, and the infections are losing.

The activation/dormancy cycle, or push-pull cycle, and its repetition, has been documented by some top, well-respected LLMD's. In a phone conversation I had recently with a Lyme doctor and friend, he told me that his own recovery took place after he intermittently used intravenous antibiotics. He would use IV antibiotics for about 3 months, and then take a 3 month break, and then repeat. He did this several times before he got well. After each course of treatment, he waited to begin the next course until he experienced what he described as a "full relapse." While this doctor's theories may differ from mine with regard to exactly what's happening and which treatments are best, the overall theme is very similar.

To further drive home the necessity of activating dormant layers of infection, I'll quote a rife machine inventor who was among the first to use rife-like therapy for Lyme disease. This gentleman prefers his name to be withheld from the public spotlight, but he once told me, "My machine will take you as far as you can go." At the time, I wondered what he meant. I asked myself, "Well, how far can I go? Why can't I go all the way? What is the limiting factor? How can a machine work to kill some, but not all, of the infection?" Now the picture is clearer to me. The limiting factor is the activation of dormant layers of infection. "As far as I can go" is determined by the amount of dormant infection I can successfully reach and kill.

In fact, I hypothesize that the ability to activate dormant layers of the infection really is the most important bottleneck in the recovery process. In other words, the limiting factor in the rate of recovery is how quickly dormant layers can be activated. While it is true that you wouldn't want to activate them too quickly, the opposite problem is often seen; that is, they activate too slowly. Most of our powerful treatments, including rife therapy, just don't work on the dormant layers. There can be many reasons for this, including the fact that dormant layers are likely protected by biofilm and other impenetrable shields. It probably isn't going too far to hypothesize that the whole concept of "dormant layers" and "layers of the onion" is nothing more than our way of conceptualizing a singular phenomenon: biofilm. Maybe, biofilm is the whole problem. Perhaps, if biofilm didn't exist, Lyme could be wiped out quickly and easily. I personally believe that biofilm is a huge part of the problem, but that there are also other aspects which define dormant layers and which cause them to be out of reach of our treatments. The future likely holds promising, breakthrough research that can help us to figure this out and develop better ways of attacking these dormant layers.

In any case, the conclusion is clear: Treatments which can provide reliable activation of dormant layers and/or penetration through biofilm carry a tremendous importance and premium, are very rare, and should be sought, if at all possible. They should also be used with great caution and preparation.

Where We Go From Here

The devices I introduced in my book, *Lyme Disease and Rife Machines,* continue to be at the top of my list for usefulness and track record. However, I have also seen a few new devices which seem to hold promise.

Most of these devices, however, as a result of their newness, don't have much of a track record (or at least, a track record I am aware of—remember that I am not the final word on this topic!).

Therefore, I will not list any new devices in this book. I made this decision reluctantly, and after careful consideration. I know many people are eager to hear my evaluation of various new devices, so I can understand how this decision may come as a disappointment. Still, though, I simply do not have enough information on these new devices to render an educated opinion, and I would rather err on the side of providing less information, instead of incorrect information.

You can still find out about the various new machines. The Lyme disease community has largely replaced me as the rife therapy expert. It's hard to admit when one loses their status as expert, but in this case, I believe exactly that has happened, at least when it comes to the availability of new information since my book was published. The simple truth is that rife therapy has become very popular, and a large community of people has begun to discuss it, develop it, and refine it. This community momentum did not exist when I published my Rife book, and now, it far outweighs what one person can contribute to the conversation.

Therefore, I suggest you look for further information in the Lyme disease community, and specifically, amongst the online chat groups which focus on using rife therapy for Lyme disease. There are several such Yahoo! Groups, with members totaling over 3,000, and there is also lively discussion of rife therapy on www.lymenet.org (in the "Flash Discussion" section of this website, there is a rife thread which is over 100 pages long). Another great resource with many hundreds of participants is www.rifeforum.com. These are all great resources, available free of charge, where you can conduct further research.

An important note regarding online discussion forums: I'm not suggesting that casual community discussion of rife therapy is better than scientifically designed clinical studies. However, until such studies are conducted, it is my personal opinion that discussion amongst the Lyme disease community can be very informative and useful. Personally, I wouldn't be as healthy as I am today had I not utilized rife therapy even in the absence of clinical studies. Still, please remember that rife therapy is not FDA-approved and has never been formally studied, so it should only be used under the care and supervision of a licensed physician.

Rife User Report by Jon Sterngold, MD

I would like to conclude this chapter with a user report from Jon Sterngold, M.D. I have communicated with Dr. Sterngold over the years and I've always found his story to be fascinating; I hope you learn as much as I did from reading it.

About Jon Sterngold, MD: Dr. Sterngold was a board certified emergency medicine physician with 25 years experience as an emergency medicine doctor. He now practices preventative medicine as well as counseling/therapy/life coaching. He has been a licensed MD for 40 years, and he diagnosed the first reported case of Lyme ECM rash in Northern California in 1983.

———

I didn't know if I'd ever get better. Intellectually, I could imagine getting my health back—leaving such intense, moment-to-moment suffering behind, but viscerally, it felt as far away as a visit to the moon. I could barely remember what it was like to be 'normal'—to not have to cope with every microsecond of every day, but I surely knew that I used to be exceptionally healthy and happy. I was a very high functioning guy. As a board certified emergency medicine doctor, I was chief of our hospital's emergency department. A health freak all my adult life, I was running a hundred miles a month and hitting the gym for weight training regularly. I played rock guitar in a band, and did the best I could as a father and husband. Mostly, I felt good. Sometimes incredibly good. And then, things changed.

I was taking a Tai Chi class in an effort to age a bit more gracefully than hard running and weight lifting might permit. Standing nearly still, moving ever so slowly, a gnawing ache in my upper back muscles gradually made these postures unbearable. I tried to go on, but was so miserable, I dropped out and just power walked for exercise. But that didn't free me from this new monster attached to my thoracic back. I'd have to stop and bend over to try to stretch out my ever-tightening muscles that had forgotten how to work properly. And then both feet started to hurt. But that was only the beginning.

Within a few months, my low back started to ache. Ache turned into severe pain and it was impossible to stand in the mornings without holding on to a stick. It took me several hours of stretching and walking on my treadmill to be able to stand up straight. By evening, all I wanted to do was to relax on my couch. But then when trying to get off the couch, I could barely move. I'd never experienced such stiffness before. About to turn age 60, I thought, 'aging really sucks'.

A colleague suggested that this was not aging but was a real disease. He thought I might have Lyme disease. I hadn't given Lyme much thought after diagnosing the first reported case of the Lyme ECM rash in northern California in 1983. It just wasn't on my radar. My standard lab tests were totally negative, but a specialized lab test was floridly positive. I began to search the Internet for information about how to treat Lyme disease and found an avalanche of recommendations from antibiotics, herbals, salt/C, Rife machines, the protocol using Benicar and low dose pulsed antibiotics, homeopathy, diets, heat, silver, allicin, hyperbaric oxygen, ozone, and myriad detoxification approaches. As a scientist and seasoned clinician, what could I make of this? The more accounts of Lyme journeys I found on the bulletin boards, the more chaos I saw. I decided that whatever all those folks were going through, this was not my life and I would simply get well when I chose the correct antibiotic.

Armed with almost no understanding of what I was up against and having a fool for a doctor, I decided to put myself on high dose oral amoxicillin, which at the time meant about 3 grams a day. I had read about 'Herx' reactions and wondered what that would be like. On the morning of day 4, I lost my Herx virginity. While sitting at my desktop, I suddenly felt a woozy, buzzing, stoned sensation not unlike the onset of 'bad acid', complete with what I later termed 'visual tinnitus' and within 20 minutes or so, a very unpleasant deeply intoxicated state in which all I could do was to lay back in a recliner and 'go out' for a few hours. But I remained profoundly affected until the next day, when I felt better, though still with my typical pains.

I had two more Herx reactions on day 8 and day 15 but by the end of the month, I was not only pain free, but felt like I'd been reborn. I hadn't felt this good in years. Subtle symptoms I'd attributed to a life of sleep deprivation as an ER doc were just gone. I was ecstatic. But who in their right mind would want to stay on 'all these antibiotics', I thought? I decided I'd pursue alternative treatments to continue my path to wellness and maybe to get rid of the tinnitus I'd been plagued with for the prior 6 years.

I tried many things, including silver, allicin, the protocol using Benicar and low dose pulsed antibiotics, followed by low dose antibiotics without Benicar, various herbs, and various extreme diets. My ecstatic rebirth morphed into a fall from grace as I got sicker and sicker. Not only did nothing help, but some made me much worse. Not only did pain return, but the curse of 'brain fog' set in. I was beyond miserable, with no idea of what was in store.

At almost 2 years in to this misadventure, I found myself a real 'Lyme doc'. He was the guy! With a broad foundation in both allopathic and herbal/alt medicine, I surrendered myself to his care and recommendations. He thought my case was a bit odd and doubted that my symptoms were from Lyme itself, but more probably one of the co-infections. I didn't agree based on my initial benefit from amoxicillin, but trusted his experience and judgment. At this point, I was taking low dose antibiotics left over from my miserable time using Benicar plus antibiotics. (It might help some folks, but the Benicar made me quite ill, causing severe muscle weakness and profound symptomatic and frankly dangerous hypotension, all of which resolved within 3 days of stopping it). My Lyme doc advised me to stop all antibiotics, take some naturopathic meds, and 'let's see what happens'. Okay.

About 2 months off antibiotics, I went from the frying pan to the fire. What had been a nuisance disease transformed into a horrid state of near constant torment with severe insomnia, a continuous body buzzing sensation that was everywhere—on my skin where I could barely distinguish hot from cold, to my insides where I felt as if bottle brushes were being run through every blood vessel of my body. I felt woozy and that 'toxic intoxication' I had in my early Herx reactions. Two tormenting symptoms with this were a physical sensation of anxiety (without any actual anxious thoughts or issues) and a falling sensation from my mid waist to my legs—a tingly, edgy feeling that screamed for resolution. My only relief would come at night when high dose Ambien and other benzodiazepines induced sleep. The next day was like the day before and after months of this, it was all I could do to not put a bullet in my head. But I would not do that to my beloved wife and kids. I would stay on the cross to keep them from suffering. Plus, it's my nature to want to know how this whole thing would turn out. I needed to stick around for that.

My Lyme doc had me try one herbal concoction after another, with no benefit. I sent blood to another specialized lab for a comprehensive Lyme panel (the prior one was done at a public health lab). The results were stunning. In contrast to no positive bands on my initial Western Blot screen, I had multiple positive bands for both IgM and IgG. I showed this to my Lyme doc and he said, 'oh, I guess you do have Lyme disease', or something to that effect.

I took antibiotics for the next three months and was miserable with near constant Herx reactions for about 10 weeks. By the end of those three months, the brain and other neurologic symptoms had cleared and I was happy. Lyme doc said, 'good, now let's stop that and mop up with a few months of intravenous antibiotics'. I wondered if I should stop what was working, but I felt so good, I was game to do some final bug killing, despite what I'd learned about Borrelia developing resistant forms under the influence of the cell wall antibiotics he advised me to use. But I trusted.

I relapsed a few weeks in to the course of IV antibiotics and spent the next five years trying to get my life back with multiple high dose oral antibiotics. I pulled my PICC line after four months and moved on. At that point I knew that my Lyme doc was guessing at what was wrong and had guessed wrong at nearly every juncture so I decided that I'd save some money and do my own guessing. By this time, I was plugged in to a Lyme network of professionals that was an incredibly valuable resource for information, my own education about the nature of the beast, and a connection to some of the top Lyme docs in the world.

With their guidance and an unwavering trust in the power of antibiotics against an infectious disease, I consumed enough antibiotics, often 4 at a time, to sterilize a small third world country. Or, so I thought. I did improve, some. But in the last year of that journey, then 7 years since the beginning, I got worse than I'd been in years. I did some testing that revealed a C4a level of 25,000! Having dedicated my life to never becoming as sick as my patients, I was now morbidly ill.

Prolonged disability depleted our savings and we were facing economic disaster. At this point I met up with my colleague and friend who had initially suggested that I had Lyme disease years before. He has Lyme and after the failure of prolonged courses of antibiotics, he got well using a Rife machine. He said he got 80% better in the first year, then up to 90% by the second year and went from total disability to gainful self-employment. He invited me to his home to try his machine. I was on antibiotics at that time but 10 minutes in to the session, I felt a Herx reaction coming on. The unmistakable (for me) wooziness, brain buzz/fuzz, and a sensation that my perception registered fewer 'frames per second' happened. That was my Eureka moment. That was the day I took my last antibiotic dose—now 19 months ago.

I bought a Rife machine and became connected with my 'Rife coach' who helped me with programming, creation of custom channels, and general guidance in the use of the device. I had one Herx reaction after another and was just miserable most of the time. But I'd become a believer and though I'm otherwise a faithless sort of guy, I did believe that I would get better with enough time.

Our finances looking more grim by the day, after four months using the machine, I decided to leave no stone unturned and acquired an even more powerful machine. Bryan Rosner's Rife book described this particular machine as the most potent of the Rife machines for Lyme disease and I felt that I needed all the efficacy I could get. I took delivery of the new machine at the end of January, 2013. My first session was 15 seconds at 432hz, a common starting point, and it induced a massive, nearly immediate, Herx reaction. I smiled in my misery and knew, or trusted, that this would eventually get me well. I had to embrace this belief as I was otherwise 'out of bullets'.

Four months after beginning my Rife treatments, I repeated my C4a level and it was down to 7,700.

By early May, seven months in, I began to turn the corner. I was less brain toxic and was sleeping better, needing less Ambien. By the end of that month, I had stopped using sleep meds altogether, and started to query my own medicine network for future employment. Though I hadn't formally worked in medicine for a long time, I spend much of my time reading current medical literature—staying up to date. During the whole time I was ill, I did maintain a small niche practice helping other folks with their Lyme and other challenging diseases. With all my brain symptoms, fortunately I hadn't suffered any impact to my intellect. It was just a sensory nightmare. But now, the nightmare was fading. I was awakening from a very long and very bad dream.

By mid-summer, I had lined up two jobs. At one location, I'd do counseling/life coaching and medical admissions and management at a facility that helped people leave unhealthful diet patterns to resolve diseases of 'western diets'. At another practice, I'd do functional and integrative medicine focusing on men's health issues. By August, we moved from our hometown of the past 3 ½ decades to a more populated area with a lot of resources that weren't available in the small town we left.

I was happy! And healthy—most of the time. I wasn't symptom free, but the horrid brain stuff was gone, unless I was Herxing from a Rife session, but that usually resolved by the next day. I had my brain back and was/am ecstatic to be out of the hell state that had destroyed my life for 7 years. I was happy to see patients and found myself able to tolerate long workdays without problems.

And now, nine months after our move and 19 months into my Rife treatment, I continue to thrive. I will use Rife machines for the rest of my life as we have no evidence that Borrelia can be completely eliminated from our bodies. I still have Herx reactions with most treatments, so I know I have a ways to go before going to a less frequent treatment schedule, but these reactions are much less intense than in the past. I haven't taken sleep medication other than some melatonin for over a year. I have my life back and my gratitude for those who helped me get here is unfathomable.

Chapter 9
The KPU Protocol and Heavy Metal Detoxification

IMPORTANT NOTE: This chapter is not intended to be complete instructions for undertaking the KPU protocol; instead, it is intended to be an examination of some of the parts of the protocol which I believe to be the most important and the least understood. Therefore, to actually use the protocol, you will need other, more detailed instructions. I am focusing this chapter on the nuances of the protocol instead of the basic instructions for use, because I believe information on the former is much more difficult to come by, while information on the latter is commonplace on many discussion forums, books, and websites. My goal in writing this book has been to provide important, scarce information which can't easily be found online, instead of simply repeating information which is readily available on the internet.

Also, some of the information in this chapter is subjective and based on my own personal experiences with the KPU protocol. This information should not be seen as the final word. Your doctor's advice should be considered more accurate than this book.

Dosages will not be provided for the substances described in this chapter, as dosages must be personalized for each individual by a licensed physician.

Due to heavy metal release and circulation in the body as a result of the KPU protocol, this protocol can be dangerous. Use the KPU protocol only under the supervision of a physician who is familiar with heavy metal detox.

KPU treatment can be intense and extreme for some people and may not be appropriate for everyone.

A Primer on Heavy Metals

B efore looking at the KPU protocol, it is important to understand that many, or most, Lyme disease sufferers have some degree of heavy metal poisoning. The most common culprits are mercury and lead. These heavy metals find their way into the innermost parts of Lyme disease bacterial colonies, and the microorganisms use the heavy metals to aid in their survival. As a result, Lyme disease recovery will not progress if heavy metal toxicity isn't addressed. Furthermore, heavy metal detox is typically required throughout the entire length of the recovery process—it is not a therapy which can be quickly accomplished and then forgotten about.

The KPU protocol is one protocol which helps to address heavy metal toxicity. However, understanding that heavy metal toxicity is a significant aspect of the Lyme disease complex is of critical importance, and heavy metals should be addressed one way or another, even if a person decides not to use the KPU protocol.

What Is the KPU Protocol?

Kryptopyrroluria, also known as KPU, is a condition in which the body becomes severely deficient in several nutrients, the most important of which are zinc and vitamin B6. Other nutrients which are sometimes helpful for treating KPU and which may be deficient include biotin, manganese, chromium, molybdenum, boron, arachidonic acid, and magnesium. Accordingly, the "KPU protocol" simply involves the supplementation of these nutrients. Sounds easy enough, right?

Although the KPU protocol is fairly simple, before you run out the door to buy all these supplements and start taking them, be aware that there's a lot more to this protocol than taking a few supplements. Zinc, in particular, can cause heavy metal toxins in the body to be released, and you have to be ready for this eventuality if you are to succeed with the KPU protocol. Throughout this chapter, we will focus on the necessary precautions which must be taken when using the KPU protocol. Let's take a closer look.

Heavy Metal Toxicity and the KPU Protocol

Many aspects of Lyme disease treatment can be accomplished by multiple and diverse means while still resulting in improvement and healing. The most obvious example of this is the killing of bacteria. Bacteria can be targeted via pharmaceutical antibiotics, herbal antibiotics, electromagnetic therapy, oxidative therapies, and other types of approaches. Combining and rotating these therapies can have the most beneficial results, but each individual therapy can have a significant impact as well.

On the other hand, certain parts of Lyme disease recovery do not respond to multiple modalities, but instead, to only one singular modality. In these cases, if you fail to employ the necessary treatment, you get zero improvement in the problem area.

One such case, in which there is only one correct treatment, is mineral deficiency (and many other types of nutrient deficiencies, for that matter). Replenishing missing nutrients is one of the goals of the KPU protocol. While the body can synthesize or recycle some kinds of nutrients (e.g., alpha lipoic acid can recycle vitamin C), minerals can only be present in optimal quantities in the body if they are added to the body through supplementation, diet, or environmental exposure. If you do not add minerals to the body, then it is impossible for them to exist in the body. This is what makes mineral monitoring and supplementation so important: not only do minerals play a critical role in the body, but the body has absolutely no way of getting them other than as a result of direct actions you take (knowingly or unknowingly) to get them inside the body. Some minerals, like mercury, are undesirable and get inside the body via inadvertent exposure. Other minerals, like zinc, magnesium and iodine, are desirable but may not be present in the body in adequate quantities, because you are not eating enough of them, you are not exposed to them through the environment, or your body cannot hold onto them once they are inside the body.

So, the KPU protocol plays a role in Lyme recovery which cannot be played by any other treatment or protocol, because it helps to restore mineral levels.

Zinc and the "Mother of All Detox Reactions"

According to various leading physicians, research demonstrates that zinc deficiency plays an important role in chronically ill patients, especially those with heavy metal toxicity. People typically think of heavy metal toxicity as too much of something, but it is also not enough of something—essential minerals like zinc. Zinc shares a similar structure to many toxic heavy metals, so when it gets displaced from its binding sites throughout the body, toxic heavy metals move in to take its place, making a person more toxic with these undesirable heavy metals (such as cadmium, aluminum, mercury and lead). As the heavy metals flood the system, the zinc is kicked out. One physician has referred to zinc as the "gas pedal for heavy metal detoxification"—as zinc is supplemented during the healing process, it will compete with toxic heavy metals and reclaim the binding sites that were intended for it, hence, accelerating the process by which toxic heavy metals are removed from the system. The competition between zinc and toxic heavy metals for binding sites throughout the body is also what causes very significant detoxification reactions when zinc supplementation is initiated. While vitamin B6 is also deficient in patients with KPU issues, zinc is the main cause of the heavy metal detoxification acceleration that occurs during KPU treatment.

Furthermore, while heavy metals can occupy many parts of the body, the heavy metals which occupy zinc binding sites are the ones that do the most damage since zinc plays so many important roles in the body. Consequently, if zinc is replaced by heavy metals, then those heavy metals are, by definition, impairing all of the processes that zinc should be allowing. On the other hand, heavy metals which are located in fat stores or other non-critical places throughout the body are not nearly as harmful. For these reasons, replacing zinc is an obvious important step in the recovery process for many people. In fact, this is one of the things that makes the KPU protocol such an ideal heavy metal detoxification regimen: you are targeting and eliminating precisely the heavy metals which are doing the most damage and occupying the most sensitive parts of the body, and you're immediately providing the body with the healthy replacement minerals that it needs to function normally.

This is what sets the KPU protocol apart from other detoxification protocols. However, this is also what makes it a potentially grueling treatment. Let's take a deeper look into why the treatment can be so grueling but also so rewarding.

A top doctor who works with autistic patients has noticed that many of his autistic children are severely zinc deficient, yet zinc supplementation seemed to make these children dramatically worse. This doctor recounts that for many years, this paradox was mystifying to him, and he was unsure about what to do with the whole zinc problem.

That is, until he viewed the problem of zinc deficiency in the context of KPU. He then found that aggressively supplementing zinc in his autistic children lead to severe and sometimes debilitating detoxification reactions. If the patient was properly supported and detoxed, and if they pushed through the reaction, then they would emerge on the other side with dramatic improvements in symptoms and functioning. Many supportive modalities were required to achieve these improvements, and if they weren't in place, zinc supplementation was often unsuccessful and could even lead to severe worsening of symptoms. Over time, it became evident that many people who suffer from autism also suffer from KPU.

The breakthrough for Lyme patients came when this doctor and others discovered that a large percentage of Lyme patients also had the condition, and that they, too, benefited from addressing KPU issues. In fact, it has been observed that Lyme disease and co-infections have a much more difficult time surviving in a body that has optimal levels of zinc. Remember that mineral deficiency cannot be addressed by anything other than adding back the deficient minerals into the body, and that zinc plays dozens of important roles within the body. Combine these two factors, and you can see why returning the body's zinc stores to optimal levels can have such an important impact on the recovery process.

Again, before you run out and buy zinc and vitamin B6 supplements, keep reading to become educated about some important considerations when addressing KPU.

Considerations in Heavy Metal Detox While Undergoing KPU Treatment

The heavy metal detoxification and release that occurs during treatment for KPU (due to zinc reclaiming the binding sites throughout the body and the heavy metals which used to occupy those sites being liberated) is profound, dramatic and intense. In fact, many seasoned Lyme patients and practitioners have observed that the KPU protocol is the hardest protocol they've ever undertaken or supervised. When supplemental zinc displaces toxic heavy metals from their binding sites, a flood of toxic metal material is released into the blood stream and can easily overwhelm the body's innate detoxification pathways and mechanisms.

Therefore, a discussion of supportive treatments for the KPU protocol is, essentially, a discussion of heavy metal detoxification strategies. In order for one to succeed with KPU treatment, one must be able to succeed with heavy metal detoxification therapy. A detoxification support program comprising various supplements and protocols is not only recommended when undergoing KPU treatment; it is mandatory. If there is one point in this chapter that you remember, this is it.

Unfortunately, heavy metal detoxification, regardless of how or why the metals are displaced and released, is highly controversial and complex. Even the top experts in the field disagree on how to properly usher metals out of the body and on which supplements and substances are safe to use as proper chelators. If these metals aren't safely ushered out of the body, they can be redistributed in body tissues and wreak havoc.

In this controversial environment, one of the most important aspects of detoxification support is to know your own body and be willing to adjust your detoxification program based upon your individual response, regardless of the one-size-fits-all program your practitioner may be recommending. In the same vein, it is also crucial to work with an experienced health care practitioner who is not only aware of KPU and its various complexities, but is also willing and able to adapt your treatment program to your individual needs, tolerances and biological uniqueness. Keep in mind that many people have been severely and possibly permanently injured by improper heavy metal detoxification techniques due to redistribution of heavy metals.

The following discussion of how to support your detoxification pathways during KPU treatment and zinc supplementation will only scratch the surface of this complex and controversial topic. In order to safely use the KPU protocol, the reader should really have a much broader and more extensive education on heavy metal detoxification (especially the use of chelating substances) than what is offered in this book. The authority who I trust most and whose book I recommend is Andrew Cutler, PhD. His book, *Amalgam Illness: Diagnosis and Treatment,* contains essential concepts and protocols for heavy metal detoxification and should be read by anyone who undertakes KPU treatment. In my opinion, Andrew Cutler's methods are the most gentle and predictable, so for ultra-sensitive people, I would urge caution when it comes to heavy metal chelation, and I would read Andrew Cutler's book and its warnings about various improper methods of chelation. Basically, the more toxic you are, the more careful you will have to be, and the more likely it is that you will end up hurting yourself if you aren't making good decisions about heavy metal detoxification.

Furthermore, heavy metal toxicity creates unique challenges in Lyme patients, and these should be understood by anyone pursuing KPU treatment (see my previous books on Lyme disease for basic information about these challenges). People with Lyme disease are particularly susceptible to heavy metal toxicity, and Lyme disease and co-infections utilize heavy metals as a protective strategy in their lifecycles. So, be aware of what you are dealing with before you begin any kind of heavy metal program.

In summary, the important points to keep in mind are that detoxification reactions from the KPU protocol can be severe and dangerous, that each detoxification support program for use alongside zinc supplementation should be individualized based on your own unique biology, and that the following sections should not be seen as the final word, but instead as an introductory discussion.

Lastly, due to the intensity of the KPU program and heavy metal detox in general, I think it is possible that certain people shouldn't even undertake this treatment protocol. Whether you are one of these people is up to you and your doctor to determine.

Cleaning Up the Body Prior to KPU Treatment

Before someone even begins supplementing with KPU nutrients and minerals (like zinc and vitamin B6), it is recommended that they implement a heavy metal detoxification support program (including the use of systemic chelators and gut binders, which will be discussed later). This should be done long before supplementing with KPU nutrients. All accessible toxic heavy metal stores should be cleansed as thoroughly as possible prior to releasing more of them from zinc binding sites. The logic for this is simple: the supplements and chelators, which are supposed to help you deal with the heavy metals that zinc releases, will not be of much assistance if they are busy shuttling out the toxic heavy metals that have not been detoxed prior to initiation of the KPU protocol (heavy metal chelators have a limited capacity for removing metals from the body).

Heavy metal chelation all by itself can be very intense and uncomfortable, even in the absence of KPU treatment. Only after a person gets enough metals out of their body that they are relatively comfortable during chelation should they begin treatment for KPU.

I personally have the most faith in and have read about the most positive outcomes with the chelation protocol described by Andrew Cutler, Ph.D. If a person decides to undergo this method of chelation before embarking upon KPU treatment, the chelators Andrew Cutler recommends (including DMPS or DMSA along with alpha lipoic acid) should be well tolerated before zinc supplementation is initiated.

Why the Body Needs Help Detoxing Heavy Metals

The logic for supplementing zinc and other KPU nutrients, such as vitamin B6, makes sense. These nutrients are clearly important and natural substances that belong in the body.

But we are still left with questions. Why is heavy metal detox support even necessary during the KPU protocol, or before the protocol, for that matter? Why can't a person simply take zinc (along with the other KPU nutrients) and let the body naturally detoxify and remove the heavy metals that are released? After all, the body does have its own amazing and complex mechanisms for removing heavy metals. Some of the heavy metal detox supplements, substances and protocols we will look at are not natural or native to the body, so why use them? Some are even synthetic chemicals—like DMSA and DMPS—so, won't these add to the toxic burden in the body?

These are very important questions to answer if you are to muster the needed motivation to undertake an extensive and complex detoxification regimen. The simple answer to these questions is that, due to our industrialized society, coupled with the weakening of our detoxification organs which occurs in chronic Lyme disease, our bodies accumulate much more toxic debris than our elimination organs can handle. We pick up heavy metals from our environment, our foods, the materials used in constructing our homes, and other sources. The body knows that it is being overwhelmed by toxins it can't remove, so, in a defensive action, the body stores these heavy metals in body tissues to get them out of active circulation. For people who don't have Lyme disease or those who only have a small amount of stored toxins, the body's wisdom may be correct and may, in fact, not require additional support. Some people may live their entire lifetime with these toxic metals stored safely away in non-critical body tissue, like body fat.

However, the scenario is different for Lyme sufferers. In order to experience complete healing from Lyme disease, we have to eliminate all of these stored toxins, or they just continue to build up as a result of the weaknesses caused by Lyme disease. We must basically tell the body that we know better than it does. We force our will in this regard by taking heavy metal chelators that force the body to release these toxic heavy metals back into active circulation. However, when we make the body dump large quantities of toxic heavy metals into circulation, we are asking the body to do something that it cannot handle—we already know it can't eliminate these toxins on its own, which is why it stored them in body tissues in the first place. So, here are the answers to our original questions: we must provide extensive and complete detoxification support if we expect to come out the other side without being made much sicker and without having the heavy metals redistributed from the storage sites chosen by the body to much more sensitive organs like the brain and liver.

There are a few other factors which make Lyme sufferers different from the rest of the population. For example, the presence of infections in your body adds to the toxic burden, as these infections release their own biotoxins. If the net toxic burden is to decrease, then you must remove the biotoxins at a rate faster than the rate at which the infectious organisms in your body are growing, multiplying, and producing new biotoxins. Next, as if things weren't bad enough already, these infections can utilize the toxic metals in your body to create biofilm and other protective niches. Studies show that bacterial biofilms are composed of heavy metals, among other substances, and it is now believed and even proven, in some cases, that these toxic heavy metals are a vital tool that infections use to survive within the body. So, Lyme sufferers have more urgency than the general population to remove these heavy metals from the body. Although it should be noted that even people without Lyme disease have a higher risk of neurological diseases such as Alzheimer's and Parkinson's if they are harboring large quantities of toxic heavy metals.

Now you can see just how serious this topic is, and why it may be necessary for Lyme sufferers to take the plunge and undertake heavy metal detox. You can also see why I strongly suggest pursuing KPU treatment and heavy metal detox only while under the care of an experienced physician.

Ultimately, due to the peril involved, pursuing heavy metal detox may be just too dangerous for some people. Those who are extremely toxic or who don't have the required support to succeed in heavy metal chelation may be better off avoiding heavy metal detoxification and the KPU protocol entirely. While failing to remove heavy metals has serious risks, as we've just seen, removing them improperly and without adequate support may have even more severe risks. In this way, the problem of heavy metal detoxification is really a difficult challenge: perils and risks are inherent in all of the available directions you can choose, whether you choose to detox heavy metals or not.

To provide some encouragement, many Lyme sufferers eventually do get most of the metals out and all the good KPU nutrients in. Personally, after a grueling battle with heavy metals, I am now able to consume all of the chelators and KPU nutrients described in this book without experiencing any detrimental effects or healing reactions. It did take a long time, though, to get to this place, and it took careful, skilled help from many resources and health care practitioners.

Binders vs. Systemic Chelators

Now we will begin to look at some of the specific treatments used for heavy metal detoxification.

The topic of supporting the body's detoxification pathways during and before KPU treatment starts with a look at the difference between systemic chelating substances and gut-only substances known within the Lyme community as "binders." Understanding the differences between these types of detoxifying agents is critical if you are to successfully usher out the heavy metals which are released during chelation and/or zinc supplementation.

We will first provide general definitions of gut binders and systemic chelators, and then we will look at the specific supplements which fall into these categories as well as how they can be used.

Binders

Heavy metals can and do accumulate in all major body organ systems and tissues. Systemic chelators (which we will examine next) are usually given orally and sometimes intravenously. They enter systemic circulation in the bloodstream and cause heavy metals to dislodge from their binding sites throughout the body. After the metals have been dislodged and enter circulation in the bloodstream, the liver attempts to process the metals and remove them. The liver uses bile as a dumping ground for many toxic materials in the body, including heavy metals, which end up being excreted into the bile after they are caused to enter circulation by systemic chelators.

This is where "binders" come in. "Binders," sometimes referred to as "gut binders," are substances taken orally that do not enter systemic circulation (or are absorbed very poorly) and simply pass through the intestinal tract and into the feces without being circulated in the bloodstream. In the context of heavy metal detoxification, binders are capable of absorbing, or "mopping up," various kinds of toxins that are located in the intestinal tract—in this case, heavy metals contained in the bile. Many binders actually absorb and inactivate the bile itself. Some types of binders do not have an effect on bile but instead have highly absorptive properties and can absorb many kinds of toxins and impurities from the intestinal tract (some binders also absorb beneficial nutrients, so careful consideration must be given to the schedules by which binders are administered in relation to meals). Of note here is that binders may also be useful for detoxing after Herx reactions resulting from the killing of infectious microorganisms.

The use of binders is critical because a large portion of the bile that is secreted by the liver and gallbladder into the digestive tract is absorbed and reused by the body. This recycling is very efficient and allows the body to conserve resources by producing less bile. However, the toxins contained within the bile also get absorbed when bile is absorbed. When undergoing the KPU protocol, a person is already extremely toxic and can barely stay ahead of the rush of toxins that are being released during zinc supplementation, so absorption of toxin-rich bile is unacceptable and can greatly increase misery and delay the process of getting well. Since most of the heavy metals in circulation end up in high concentrations in the bile, gut binders can be very helpful in efficiently binding to the bile and its toxins, and ushering them out of the body. When using binders extensively, it can be helpful to consume foods which are known to help the body make bile, since some bile will be eliminated from the body rather than absorbed.

Binders are not only beneficial because they sequester and usher toxins out of the body. They also facilitate the process of bringing deeper toxins stored throughout body tissues into the gut for elimination. As bile is prevented from being absorbed back into the body by sequestration in gut binders, the body is forced to make new bile. This production of new bile then provides additional capacity for toxin storage, and according to many experts, causes the body to actually stimulate detoxification processes. One well-recognized pioneer in the field of Lyme-related biotoxins describes this process as "removing a plug from a bathtub and allowing the water [toxins] to drain out." In other words, sequestering and removing bile from the body essentially prompts the body to create more bile, fill it with toxins, and get rid of it, so the use of gut binders has the secondary benefit of accelerating the body's detoxification processes.

Lifestyle choices can augment or diminish the benefit achieved by using gut binders. A healthy diet, and especially consumption of fiber, will ensure that the bowels continue to move. Fiber is also one kind of gut binder due to its absorbent properties. Drinking lots of fluid is also important to avoid constipation, which is one of the most dangerous enemies of detoxification because it stifles the elimination of toxins from the body.

So, systemic chelators are Step 1 in the detox process. They dislodge heavy metals from their storage sites throughout the body and allow the liver to process them and add them to the bile. Gut binders are Step 2 in the detox process. They grab onto the heavy metals in the bile and sequester them to ensure that they don't get absorbed on their journey through the intestinal tract, but instead, are removed via the feces.

Between systemic chelators and gut binders, gut binders are, by far, the safer substances because they do not come with the risk of dislodging metals from deep within body tissues, which could potentially result in their redistribution throughout the body. A complete discussion of how to avoid redistribution dangers can be found in Andrew Cutler's aforementioned book.

Now let's take a more in-depth look at systemic chelators.

Systemic Chelators

Some would argue that zinc itself is a systemic chelator because it enters the bloodstream and causes heavy metals to be released from their binding sites into circulation. The problem with zinc is that it only dislodges the toxic metals; it does not safely pacify and inactivate them, which is the other characteristic of a systemic chelator. Zinc gets the detoxification process going by knocking the metals loose, but once the metals enter circulation, they are free to be redistributed and bind to other highly sensitive body sites such as the brain, liver, kidneys, and other critical tissues. Therefore, while zinc is absolutely necessary—the body has no ideal substitute for it—it can also instigate a storm of circulating toxins that wreak havoc on the body. It is precisely this storm that makes the KPU treatment process so uncomfortable.

Enter systemic chelators. In some cases, zinc may do a better job of actually forcing heavy metals out of binding sites, but systemic chelators do a better job of safely inactivating the heavy metals once they are released into the bloodstream, rendering them less toxic to human tissues, hence, making it easier for the liver to remove them without being damaged by them. This makes zinc and systemic chelators a great team: as zinc reclaims binding sites throughout the body and kicks out the toxic heavy metals, systemic chelators are waiting in the wings to bind with the toxic heavy metals and more easily usher them out of the body.

Once heavy metals are safely bound to systemic chelators, the metals are much less dangerous. Some systemic chelators are lipophilic and are useful for detoxing the brain, and some are hydrophilic and are useful for detoxing other parts of the body. Each type of systemic chelator has a different biochemical profile and different affinities for the various heavy metals. Some are better for removing mercury, while others are better for removing lead. The complexity of this scenario mandates that anyone using the KPU protocol should not only be under the care of a well-trained physician, but should also educate themselves on this topic and have first-hand knowledge of the process.

Even the most powerful and useful systemic chelators are only partially effective. Systemic chelators are only capable of creating mild to moderately strong bonds with toxic heavy metals, and while using systemic chelators, a significant quantity of heavy metals is still undesirably redistributed throughout the body. This is why heavy metal detoxification is so difficult and controversial. At the heart of the controversy is the question of which chelators create the strongest bonds to heavy metals, what doses of these chelators should be used, and how often the doses should be administered. You'll get different answers to these questions from nearly every expert with whom you consult. The goal of removing as many toxic heavy metals as possible while doing the least amount of damage is the delicate balance that people who undertake chelation must face.

As we've seen, systemic chelators can work in harmony with gut binders. Systemic chelators travel throughout the body and mobilize toxic heavy metals (or bind to toxic heavy metals which are already in circulation). The liver then processes these heavy metals for elimination in the bile. Gut binders are then waiting in the gut to absorb and inactivate bile and/or toxins.

Optimal heavy metal detoxification programs should use both systemic chelators and gut binders. In addition to systemic chelators and gut binders, there are many other supplements, protocols and treatments that aid the body in detoxifying heavy metals. Some of these substances should be used continuously throughout the entire KPU protocol, while others can be used intermittently. The help of a trained physician is essential in developing a good detox protocol.

NOTE: Heavy metals share many common attributes with the biotoxins produced by the infectious organisms involved in Lyme disease and co-infections. Both are fat-soluble, tend to accumulate in the brain with devastating neurological consequences, are difficult to remove from the body, and can cause debilitating symptoms. Both can also be addressed by similar substances and techniques. Therefore, the detoxification strategies (and even some of the substances and supplements) found in this chapter will also be useful for detoxification purposes during anti-infective treatment and Herxheimer reactions.

Examples of Gut Binders

Now that we've defined gut binders and systemic chelators, let's take a look at some examples of specific supplements. Many kinds of gut binders exist. A complete list of these substances is beyond the scope of this book, but here, I will list a few gut binders that have been used by the Lyme disease community and those who are pursuing heavy metal detox. If you want to use any of these, I suggest researching the substance first, as each one has different pros and cons, and different side effects.

1. Apple pectin, and other kinds of pectins.
2. Activated charcoal
3. Fiber supplements
4. Cholestyramine
5. Clays

Examples of Systemic Chelation Agents

IMPORTANT NOTE: All of these agents are potentially dangerous and have the ability to cause severe and permanent redistribution of heavy metals into sensitive body tissues. These substances should only be used under the close supervision of a licensed physician. Furthermore, the agent chosen isn't the only important factor; dosage and dosage schedules can also render these agents safe or dangerous.

1. Alpha Lipoic Acid (ALA)
2. 2,3-Dimercapto-1-propanesulfonic acid (DMPS)
3. Dimercaptosuccinic acid (DMSA)
4. Ethylenediaminetetraacetic acid (EDTA)
5. Some forms of silica
6. Some forms of humic acid
7. Chlorella
8. Cilantro
9. Some forms of zeolite

Different individuals will have differing responses to these substances. Also, different kinds of heavy metals will be more or less responsive to each substance.

Be especially careful with item #'s 4-9, as these are less proven and less safe than item #'s 1-3. Still, even item #'s 1-3 can cause serious damage if used inappropriately. Remember, chelators are typically not what cause damage; it is instead their improper use that is the problem. Any chelator used improperly will do harm instead of help.

Other Supportive Supplements and Treatments

In addition to gut binders and systemic chelators, there are many other supportive therapies which can be used during KPU treatment as well as during detox of other toxins, including Lyme biotoxins. Here we will take a look at a few of them.

- <u>Homeopathic drainage remedies.</u> These substances can be very helpful during detox, as they catalyze the body's own detox processes. There are many of them, but my favorites are Lymphomyosot by Heel, ITIRES by Pekana, apo-HEPAT by Pekana, RENELIX by Pekana, Ubichinon compositum by Heel, Hepar compositum by Heel, and Solidago compositum by Heel.

- <u>Amino acids</u>. Amino acids are used heavily by the body during detoxification. See Chapter 4 for information on how to increase your amino acid intake. Consuming animal protein as well as whey protein isolate is a great place to start.

- <u>Increased fat consumption</u>. Various types of dietary fat help the body remove toxins and rebuild damaged tissue. See Chapter 4 for more information.

- <u>Sauna therapy</u>. Many people benefit from sauna therapy during detoxification, as it can help remove toxins via the skin.

- <u>Herbs with detoxification properties</u>. Many herbs are available which help the body detoxify.

- <u>Vitamins and minerals</u>. The body uses up vitamins and minerals faster during detox, so supplementing with these is important.

- <u>Liver support</u>. The liver is heavily taxed during detox, so liver support is crucial (See Chapter 15).

- <u>Drinking lots of water</u>. Water is essential to keep everything moving and ensure that toxins and detox supplements are moving out of the body.

Two Phases of Symptomology During KPU Treatment

Many people have noticed two distinct phases of symptomology during use of the KPU Protocol. It is helpful to know about these phases before you begin the protocol, so you can prepare for them and develop strategies to deal with them.

Symptomology Phase #1: Heavy Metal Release

This phase has already been discussed throughout this chapter. Typically, a person will experience symptoms of heavy metal circulation shortly after beginning KPU treatment. During this phase, zinc supplementation can be a Catch-22. As the body begins to receive much-needed zinc to replace the toxic heavy metals which occupy the zinc binding sites throughout the body, you may find that you feel much better.

The Catch-22 happens because the more zinc you take, the more heavy metals get released. So, while your body may be craving additional zinc, taking more zinc may actually end up making you feel more toxic from heavy metal circulation. For this reason, it is advisable to start slow with zinc supplementation and work up the dose over time.

Symptomology Phase #2: Immunological Activation

After you have been using the KPU protocol for some time (this time frame varies greatly between one month and six months, or even longer), the heavy metal dumping will slow down, and finally end. This is a victory, and it feels very good to be able to give your body the zinc it needs without making yourself miserable with the symptoms of heavy metal circulation. It is quite a milestone to get to this point.

Somewhere around this time, or possibly sooner, your body will begin to use the zinc that it has never had enough of to turn on body functions which were not previously occurring normally. Because zinc is involved in literally dozens of critical bodily processes, you may experience various changes in how your body feels.

The most notable area of change is usually new immunological reactions. Some people describe this phase of the recovery process as "getting cold after cold," or "flu after flu." Others may experience it as an increase in allergies, nasal congestion, or even inflammation. Zinc is a critical component of the immune system (you may be aware that many zinc supplements are actually marketed as aids for the common cold), so as your zinc levels are normalized and the immune system turns on, you may feel the effect of this increase in immune function. Some researchers believe that chronically ill people have a backlog of viral and bacterial infections that the immune system hasn't been able to deal with, and that zinc supplementation may finally give the body the tools it needs to go after these infections. This could explain the experience of having "cold after cold," or "virus after virus."

In my personal experience with the KPU protocol, I did indeed travel through this phase. While I did have the perception of getting numerous minor head colds, fortunately, none of them were quite as severe or annoying as regular head colds. I did, however, experience one challenge during this phase. At one point, I suffered from nasal congestion so severe that I wound up with a raging sinus infection. Up until this point in my life, I had never had a sinus infection—not even one. This particular sinus infection was so severe that I almost went to the emergency room. My entire head was in unrelenting agony, and despite trying antibiotics, nasal rinses, a Neti pot, and a number of other interventions, it just wouldn't go away. Two treatments finally killed the sinus infection: First, I used oral oregano oil supplementation; and second, I laid on my bed with my head dangling backwards off the side of the bed and inserted salt water into my nostrils, allowing the salt water to drain deep into my sinus cavities as my head was upside down (I believe the Neti pot was ineffective because the rinse water was not able to penetrate deep enough into my sinuses; gravity was the only force which allowed the salt water to get where it needed to go).

Eventually, zinc supplementation no longer caused me to experience heavy metal detoxification symptoms or immunological activation symptoms. When you reach this point in the process (which can happen as soon as three months into the KPU protocol or as late as a year into it), most practitioners recommend that you continue to utilize a maintenance dose of the KPU nutrients for life, since the underlying causes of KPU are believed to be life-long problems, and the condition may return if the supplements are not continued.

Which Binders, Chelators, and Detox Supplements Should Be Used?

Although beyond the scope of this book, you should develop the skills necessary to determine which detoxifying agents are most needed by your body. The agents that are most helpful will change over time, sometimes as rapidly as every few days. You will find that substance "A" is very helpful to you one day, and the next day, does nothing for you. Different people have different ways of knowing which detox supplements are most helpful at any given time. Many people in the Lyme disease community rely on "energetic testing" to determine which therapies are most helpful at any given time. Energetic testing is also sometimes referred to as "muscle testing," "Autonomic Response Testing," and other names. Basically, energetic testing is a system for learning what substance your body needs by placing that substance (for example, a bottle of homeopathic medicine) within the energy field of your body (sometimes, the substance is held close to the chest, near the solar plexus) and then asking your body if it needs that substance. Asking the body can be accomplished by holding out an arm and having a practitioner push down on your arm (the stronger the arm, the more your body needs the substance), for example. Some people can simply feel that their body either needs or does not need the substance when it is held close or near to the body. Various energetic testing devices and mechanisms are also available for helping a patient or practitioner determine whether a given substance is something that the body currently needs.

While energetic testing may seem like quackery, it is actually employed by some of the most well-respected and experienced alternative healthcare practitioners. One of my mentors, a woman who is completely recovered from Lyme disease and co-infections, has said that energetic testing was the only thing that facilitated a complete recovery for her. She feels that people who do not utilize energetic testing may get well, but it will likely take them much longer because they are wasting so much time experimenting and using trial and error to find out what their bodies need. I have to say, after years as a skeptic, I am now a firm believer in energetic testing, because I have seen it work so consistently and reliably in my own healing journey.

The KPU Nutrients: Should They Be Taken Together or Separately?

Note: This question is in reference to the minerals, vitamins, and nutrients used in the KPU Protocol, such as zinc, vitamin B6, manganese, etc. It is not in reference to the detoxification agents, such as apple pectin, charcoal, gut binders, or systemic chelators.

While various products are available which combine all of the recommended KPU nutrients, I personally believe that supplementing each of the individual nutrients separately is the most prudent course of action. Individual supplementation provides many benefits, including the ability for you to identify adverse reactions to each ingredient, the ability to customize the dosage of each individual ingredient, and the ability to experiment with different product brands for each ingredient. As you will learn, dosage levels for the various ingredients can be controversial and vary depending on individual tolerance, so using separate products for each individual ingredient can provide you with the necessary flexibility to adjust your protocol as needed. Also, please note that while some of the KPU nutrients are relatively safe and non-toxic (such as biotin), other nutrients included in the KPU program (such as vitamin B6) have known toxicity at higher dosages. Please conduct your own, independent research on each ingredient prior to use, and please use these nutrients only under the careful supervision of a licensed health care practitioner.

Copper Supplementation During the KPU Protocol

Zinc and copper compete for absorption in the intestinal tract. Since supplementation with zinc can lead to copper deficiency, copper supplementation may be required at some point during KPU treatment. Keep in mind, however, that copper toxicity is also very common in people with chronic disease. Be careful when supplementing with copper. The right amount can prevent copper deficiency, but too much can create other problems.

In the worst cases, copper deficiency can be irreversible and cause permanent neurological damage. It is for these reasons that caution and common sense should be employed during use of the KPU protocol. It should not be used unless it is supervised by a licensed health care practitioner. Zinc dosages should be carefully monitored, and zinc should not be taken in large, unsafe doses, as these can lead to copper deficiency.

Side Effects of Arachidonic Acid

Arachidonic acid is a type of Omega-6 fatty acid and one of the recommended supplements in the KPU Protocol. Users of the protocol should be aware that some people cannot tolerate Arachidonic acid, because it has, in some studies, been associated with heart attacks, thrombotic stroke, arrhythmia, arthritis, osteoporosis, inflammation, mood disorders, obesity, and cancer. It can often be detrimental to people who have chronic inflammatory conditions. For me personally, Arachidonic acid was not beneficial and did indeed increase inflammation. At first, I felt that this may have been a healing reaction or detox reaction. However, after continued use, it became obvious to me that this substance was negatively impacting my health. This is something to consider before using Arachidonic acid as a part of the KPU protocol. This type of problem is another reason why supplementing with the KPU nutrients individually, instead of within a supplement that contains all of them, may be a more cautious approach.

Do All Lyme Sufferers Have KPU Issues?

If you begin the KPU protocol and do not notice any detox reactions or symptom improvement from zinc supplementation or from supplementation with the other KPU nutrients, it may be possible that you do not have KPU issues and that you do not need to use this treatment.

Various tests are available to determine whether a person requires KPU treatment. While I'm not convinced of the accuracy of these tests, they may be helpful in deciding whether or not to pursue KPU treatment.

Conclusion

This chapter has certainly not provided exhaustive, extensive guidelines for using the KPU protocol. Instead, the chapter was intended to provide you with information on some of the nuances of the protocol as well as some of the misunderstood aspects of heavy metal detox. You can find more specific instructions for using the protocol in many locations, including other Lyme-related books, and by searching Google for *KPU protocol for Lyme disease.*

I also recommend reading Andrew Cutler's book, *Amalgam Illness*, to gain a foundation of understanding for heavy metal detox.

Chapter 10
Biophotons

The Powerful Immune System: Your Best Weapon in the Battle Against Lyme Disease?

B efore talking about biophoton therapy, I want to share a story, to set the stage. In the summer of 2011, I had the flu. It was one of those terrible flus, when you are gagging and on the toilet all night. A few times, I thought I may be dying and considered taking myself to the ER. I was running a fever of 102 for most of the course of the illness.

After two full days in bed, barely able to climb the stairs in my home, I finally started getting better. It happened quickly. Within a day or two, I was feeling like my old self again. As I reclaimed my body, I marveled at the amazing ability that the human body has to heal itself.

Our immune systems are astoundingly powerful. You need only look at what happens when the immune system isn't working to see how powerful it actually is. HIV patients sometimes can't recover from simple illnesses because their immune systems are not intact. My dear friend with cancer was told that he should report to the ER any time he had even a minor cold or flu, due to the fact that the chemotherapy he was taking crippled his immune system, a fact which could potentially render everyday colds and flus debilitating, even fatal.

Yet, here my body was, healing itself from this intense flu—and in only two days!

People with Lyme disease do not die from common colds, typically. The problem does not seem to be that our immune systems are not strong and healthy enough to hunt down and kill Lyme disease and co-infections. Instead, as I've described in my other books, and as the medical literature alludes to countless times, the problem seems to be that chronic tick-borne infections are capable of cloaking themselves, of hiding from our immune systems and tricking our bodies into living in harmony with them. The immune system is still powerful; it just isn't able to find the enemy.

This is why biophotonic treatment is so fascinating and promising. The fundamental premise behind biophoton therapy is the act of teaching the immune system to recognize invading, yet stealthy, chronic pathogens. Since the immune system is undoubtedly the most powerful weapon we possess, the ability to train and strengthen the immune system may be the most powerful treatment we possess. Personally, I believe that biophoton therapy is one of the most difficult treatments to master, but if mastered, it could be one of the most promising therapies in existence for Lyme disease and other chronic infections. Assigning the immune system the job of killing the infections, and equipping it with what it needs to do so, is simply an unbeatable strategy for healing from Lyme disease.

This chapter will give you an introduction to biophoton therapy and provide you with some additional resources where you can learn the specifics.

What Is Biophoton Therapy?

The treatment involves using homeopathic nosodes in combination with a device that emits light from LEDs. Homeopathic nosodes are solutions which contain diluted infective microorganism material, similar to other types of homeopathic remedies. In normal homeopathy, the remedies are consumed orally. With biophoton therapy, the small glass vials containing the homeopathically diluted material are held in front of the body, touching an area near the solar plexus, and at the same time, light from the LED device is directed to various parts of the body, including areas on the head, torso, wrists, and legs. No homeopathic material is consumed orally or otherwise; the entire treatment is done with the homeopathic material outside of the body.

If you are skeptical, I do not blame you. The treatment is so unusual that I would not expect anyone to accept it without having experienced it firsthand. There are various theories as to how and why it works. Personally, I believe that the most convincing theory is that the nosode, when placed close to the body, alerts the immune system to the presence of the invaders inside the body. Then, the biophotonic light emitted from the LED device energizes the immune system and identifies the infections. After the treatment is complete, the immune system goes to work killing the infections. Some people experience significant Herxheimer reactions following the treatment, demonstrating the real power of biophoton therapy.

One of the pioneers of biophoton therapy for Lyme disease is Ingo D. E. Woitzel, M.D., of Pforzheim, Germany. Many people from the United States have made the trip to be treated by Dr. Woitzel, and some are able to hand-carry a biophoton device back from Germany, as the German devices aren't currently sold in the United States. At over $5,000 USD, they aren't cheap devices to purchase. And when you add in the cost of travel to Germany and the fees of seeing Dr. Woitzel, the whole event can be quite cost prohibitive.

Fortunately, there is a much more affordable biophoton device sold in the United States, and many people have had success with that device. The best way to obtain information about both devices is to visit http://www.lymenet.org and ask around on the discussion forums. For various reasons, including my desire to remain separated from the commercial side of this Lyme disease treatment, I have chosen not to provide the device information here.

To learn more about Dr. Woitzel's treatment of Lyme disease, I suggest reading Connie Strasheim's book, *Insights Into Lyme Disease Treatment* (also published by BioMed Publishing Group). The chapter of the book focusing on biophoton therapy is available online, as a free book excerpt:

www.lymebook.com/bionic-880-photon-woitzel-germany-pe1

In my opinion, one of the most important advantages of biophoton therapy is that it awakens the native immune system to fight the infections. Many other Lyme disease treatments, such as pharmaceutical antibiotics, suppress the immune system.

Is Biophoton Therapy Really a Legitimate Lyme Disease Treatment?

If I hadn't experienced biophoton therapy for myself, I would adamantly question its legitimacy. This therapy is one of the most mystifying Lyme disease therapies I've ever encountered. Yet, it helps to remember that I'm an American, and in America, energetic medicine isn't well-accepted. In Europe, on the other hand, it is much more widely accepted and used, even by medical professionals. In fact, some of the biophoton machines with the best track records are manufactured in Europe, and even regulated by the European government as legitimate medical devices. Recently, I received this email from a Lyme disease patient:

> *When I was in Toronto at the conference this year, I picked up a brochure that had a quote from the Medical and Executive Director of the Borrelia Clinic of Augsburg (BCA), in Germany. Dr. N is an MD and a PhD. The BCA has recently begun to incorporate biophoton therapy into their treatment of Lyme. He says, "According to our experience, Photon Therapy can significantly support the anti-infective treatment of Lyme Disease."*

A good friend of mine, who is a trained engineer and holds a high position in an engineering firm, says something similar. He avoided trying biophoton therapy for years, but finally did, and he can't believe how well it works. He was very skeptical.

The list of Lyme sufferers who have benefited greatly from biophoton therapy is long. Many of them participate in the discussion forums located at www.lymenet.org, so you can join that group to talk to users of the therapy.

One Lyme sufferer maintains a blog in which she has detailed her success with biophoton therapy: http://sixgoofykids.blogspot.com. Her blog posts have a great deal of good information on the topic. You can find another interesting story at: http://betterhealthguy.blogspot.com.

There are numerous reasons why Lyme sufferers often pass up this therapy and never give it a try. Even if you can accept the legitimacy of the treatment, its use still requires a significant amount of education. Unfortunately, teachers and mentors who know how to properly use the treatment are much harder to find than mentors for more common therapies. But remember, our goal in this book is to evaluate therapies based on their effectiveness, not their popularity.

All I can tell you is to investigate the therapy for yourself. Keep an open mind. American, Westernized medicine isn't the only legitimate form of medicine in the world, and we have a lot to learn from other medical disciplines. This humility is so important that without it, we might arrogantly pass up many promising healing modalities.

What's Next for Biophoton Therapy?

This book will not provide detailed instructions on using biophoton therapy. Instead, this chapter was intended as an introduction to this treatment. You can learn a great deal by doing a Google search for *biophoton therapy Lyme disease.*

Also, at some point in the future, I am expecting to see publication of a book on this topic. Such a book would be fantastic, and helpful to many people. An expert living in Europe who is, in my opinion, the world's leading expert on this topic, has plans to finish a book which provides very detailed instructions on using biophoton therapy. If, and when, that book becomes available, I will notify those who are subscribed to my newsletter. If you would like to subscribe to my newsletter, please visit: www.lymebook.com/newsletter.

Chapter 11
Tinidazole: New Research on an Old Drug

T inidazole has been widely discussed and written about in the Lyme disease community for years. Here, I'd like to provide an update and some new information.

Based on all of the studies I've read, tinidazole is simply the best, most effective drug for attacking Borrelia in all of its three forms. If you are taking tinidazole and you aren't experiencing improvement or Herxheimer reactions, it probably means that your Borrelia is eradicated already, or more likely, hidden under other layers of the onion, or perhaps protected by biofilm. Whenever Borrelia gets exposed and becomes the top layer of the onion, tinidazole offers significant benefits and can really help you make progress. Another benefit of tinidazole is that it is generally considered to have a milder side effect profile in comparison with its cousin, Flagyl (metronidazole).

In my previous Lyme disease books, I dedicated a significant number of pages to discussing the major differences between various classes and categories of antibiotics. Each different type of antibiotic has a significantly different effect on Lyme disease and co-infections. Certain antibiotics are highly active against Borrelia but do very little in the way of targeting co-infections like Babesia and Bartonella. Other antibiotics, for example, target Bartonella effectively but do not eliminate Borrelia or Babesia. It has even been observed that some kinds of antibiotics may target one form of a specific infection but not another form (for example, some antibiotics target the cyst form of Borrelia but not the spirochete form). And the list of differences goes on from there.

Furthermore, some antibiotics have been shown to actually delay recovery and cause symptom worsening by activating what I refer to as "the Lyme disease defense mechanism," which can be summarized as an array of different biological activities the bacteria undertake to survive in a hostile environment.

Understanding different categories and classes of antibiotics and their effects on Lyme disease and co-infections is critically necessary in order to recover. Incorrect choices can cause lost months or years in the recovery process. This is one of the reasons why it is so important to work with a Lyme-literate medical doctor who is not only trained on this topic but who has also had years of experience working with Lyme disease patients and has been able to observe, in a clinical setting, the outcome of various antibiotics and antibiotic combinations. Additionally, it is important to understand how the treatment of co-infections can render Borrelia more vulnerable to antibiotic treatment, as is discussed elsewhere in this book. Finally, it is important to understand how biofilm and the colony structure of Borrelia and co-infections can protect the bacteria from treatment.

Although new research is emerging as Lyme disease is being recognized as an international epidemic, there is still a shortage of actual research on which antibiotics are most effective for the various infections.

That is why the new research I will present in this chapter is so exciting: it is one of only a handful of studies that provides us with insight into which antibiotics may be most useful to treat Lyme disease and co-infections. The information in the following study will also provide clarity and additional insight into the antibiotic treatment strategies discussed throughout this book.

Note: While I will cite various research studies in this chapter, please be aware that the interpretation of that research, and the conclusions drawn from it, are not the opinions of the cited researchers but are solely my own (Bryan Rosner's) interpretations, applications and conclusions. The researchers mentioned in this chapter have not read or agreed with my writings.

Recent Study Sheds New Light on Tinidazole

A study published in the *Journal of Infection and Drug Resistance* (Dove Press)[6] provided us with profound new insights into the importance of tinidazole (a 5-nitroimidazole antibiotic) in the treatment of Lyme disease and co-infections, specifically, tinidazole's effects on the different morphological forms of Borrelia. Two of the study leaders, Eva Sapi and Raphael B. Stricker, are known for their important and influential work in the field of Lyme disease research.

It has long been thought that tinidazole is helpful in targeting Lyme disease cysts, which are low metabolically active forms of Borrelia that are not easily killed. Borrelia spirochetes can convert to cysts in a hostile environment, and due to their resistance and low metabolic activity, cysts are thought to be one of the reasons why Borrelia can persist in Lyme disease patients who were previously treated with antibiotic therapy.

---

[6] "Evaluation of in-vitro antibiotic susceptibility of different morphological forms of Borrelia burgdorferi", by Eva Sapi, Navroop Kaur, Samuel Anyanwu, David F. Luecke, Akshita Datar, Seema Patel, Michael Rossi, Raphael B. Stricker; published in association with the Lyme Disease Research Group, Department of Biology and Environmental Sciences, University of New Haven, New Haven, CT, USA, and the International Lyme and Associated Diseases Society, Bethesda, MD, USA.

In the research paper, the authors state that:

> *The goal of our study was to demonstrate the in-vitro susceptibility of different morphological forms of B. burgdorferi to various antibiotics using improved technical approaches in order to understand why antibiotic treatment for patients with Lyme disease could fail.*

The results of this study are fascinating, and anyone involved in Lyme disease treatment should read the full text of the article. You can find a link to the article at http://www.lymebook.com/resources. The chapter you are reading now only scratches the surface of the vast and fascinating information contained within the actual study. In the full text of the study linked above, you will also discover surprising new information about other antibiotics which are commonly used to treat Lyme disease, such as doxycycline and amoxicillin. Please, take a break from reading this book and go take a look at the full-length study!

While my discussion below will not replace the wealth of information in the study itself, I would like to summarize the points which I personally found to be most interesting and useful, and which are most helpful to the themes of this book:

1. Tinidazole is much more effective than many people had previously realized, both against the spirochete form of Borrelia as well as the "round body" form. We already know tinidazole works on the round body form (or cyst form), but we didn't know that it was also useful against spirochetes; this is a powerful discovery, since we used to view tinidazole as mainly a cyst-buster. There are few (if any) available antibiotics which can accomplish this effectiveness against both forms of Borrelia.

2. Tinidazole was significantly better at killing Borrelia than its cousin metronidazole (Flagyl).

3. The authors tested the antibiotics on free-floating, non-colonized bacteria as well as on what they refer to as "biofilm-like colonies," which are organized, densely populated groups of bacteria protected, in some cases, by a biofilm-like outer film. As expected, the antibiotics are much more effective on the free-floating bacteria than on the organized biofilm-like colonies. In the study, the authors make the following notation:

   > *Recent studies suggest that bacteria live in an environment deep within the biofilm-like colonies where diffusion of antibiotics might be difficult, and in that state, the bacteria could become 1000 times more resistant to antibiotics. This resistance could also be one of the reasons why conventional antibiotic therapy that is usually effective against free-floating bacteria becomes ineffective once a pathogen forms biofilm-like colonies.*

These two points add up to one fascinating conclusion which reinforces the message of this book: The key factor for killing Lyme disease colonies isn't just finding an effective treatment. It is also making sure that that treatment is able to reach the infections you are targeting. In other words, tinidazole is highly effective against the various forms of Borrelia when the bacteria are in their free-floating, non-colonized state, but the drug is less effective against colonized bacteria. This observation supports what we've been discussing throughout the book: Lyme disease and co-infections must be removed from the body in a similar fashion to peeling layers off of an onion; in this case, the center of the onion is the deepest layers of infection which are not penetrable by attainable antibiotic concentrations.

Lastly, if you view photos of the colonies on the second-to-last page of the study linked from the website I mentioned above, you'll note that some of the other antibiotics tested caused strange behavior and re-configuration among Borrelia colonies. Tinidazole did not cause this re-configuration; instead, it only caused shrinking and weakening of the colonies. My interpretation of this data (this is my interpretation, not the interpretation of the study authors) is that tinidazole does not activate the "Lyme disease defense mechanism," as I've called it in my previous books, while other antibiotics do activate this bacterial defense mechanism. This confirms the tremendous value of tinidazole for treating Lyme disease, since I believe that activation of the Lyme disease defense mechanism causes the bacteria to spread to new areas of the body, transform into more dormant forms, and become more entrenched and treatment-resistant. (By the way, these photos are fascinating, because we don't often get a look at the inner workings of these colonies—we are usually left to our imaginations to conceptualize these principles.)

Below are some additional thoughts I have on tinidazole as a result of the aforementioned study (remember that these points represent my own personal opinion, not that of the study authors).

What If Tinidazole Works for a While, Then Stops Working?

We can take what we've learned from the study and build on what we already know about Lyme disease to reach the following conclusion: If a person experiences tinidazole to be effective for a time but then feels decreased benefit, it may not mean that all Borrelia organisms have been eradicated, and it may not mean that remaining Borrelia organisms have become resistant to the drug. Instead, the decreasing effectiveness may indicate that the remaining Borrelia organisms are not accessible to the drug and are protected by the bacterial colony structure and its biofilms. Continued use of tinidazole when remaining bacteria are protected would likely have limited value. Even an increased dose wouldn't help. If the drug were continued under these circumstances, it is likely that increased side effects would develop simultaneously with decreased drug effectiveness.

A more prudent course of action to employ after tinidazole loses its benefit would be to rotate treatments in favor of biofilm-destroying therapies as well as therapies which target co-infections like Babesia and Bartonella (as explained throughout this book, Babesia and Bartonella have the ability to strengthen bacterial colonies and protect Borrelia from antimicrobial treatment). Sure enough, many patients note that co-infection antibiotics and antibiotic combinations do indeed show significant benefit after tinidazole loses its effect. And, after co-infection treatment and anti-biofilm treatment, it would be expected that tinidazole would again have therapeutic benefit, as the colony structure is weakened and more Borrelia become vulnerable to tinidazole. And, indeed, this expectation is confirmed via patient reports. As you can see, what is emerging here is a rotational treatment plan: when one antibiotic or anti-infective approach loses its usefulness, another is quickly substituted.

There are several potential errors a patient or practitioner may unwittingly make during the course of Lyme disease treatment if they are unaware of the above information.

1. If it is observed that tinidazole is helpful for a short period of time and then loses its benefit, patients and practitioners may discontinue the drug and never use it again, based on the belief that it can no longer be effective due to bacterial resistance, or the assumption that all of the bacteria which tinidazole targets have been eliminated. We know this would be incorrect. We know that tinidazole would again have a renewed effect later on in the recovery process, after other treatments are able to again expose Borrelia.

2. If faced with diminishing tinidazole effectiveness, patients and practitioners may come to the conclusion that the drug should be continued for a long-term period, such as months or years, to wait out the bacterial colonies and keep chipping away at bacteria that may exit the colonies and expose themselves to the drug. I believe that this course of action is not ideal. Many physicians may disagree with me, but it is my opinion, as described elsewhere in this book, that the long-term use of tinidazole (or any antibiotic for that matter) has a much less favorable cost-to-benefit ratio when compared with the use of tinidazole (or any antibiotic) on a rotational schedule as described in Chapter 3. I will certainly admit that this position is controversial and open to debate. I am simply reporting the results of my own research, personal experience, and discussion with Lyme disease patients. Using the same antibiotic long-term exposes a person to increasing side effects, and as long as the same antibiotic is used, the bacterial colony is unlikely to change its structure, so a long-term stalemate ensues.

3. Finally, when it is observed that tinidazole is losing its effect, another mistake I see often is to increase the dosage. While this may have some benefit, it likely doesn't justify the increased side effects. If tinidazole (or any drug, for that matter) stops working, it is likely not a problem with the dosage, but instead, it is time to rotate to a different treatment.

Another consideration to be aware of if and when tinidazole loses its beneficial effects is the presence of non-infectious conditions which may be protecting the bacterial colonies. At the top of the list is the presence of heavy metals in or around the bacterial colonies. Numerous studies demonstrate the ability for heavy metals to not only weaken the immune system but also protect bacteria from antibiotics. Heavy metals may be used by bacteria to help construct biofilm. As discussed throughout the book, a heavy metal detoxification program must be used heavily throughout the recovery process. Sometimes, a round of appropriate[7] heavy metal detoxification therapies can immediately render previously untreatable infections again treatable, as the metal components of the biofilm are chelated away, weakening or destroying the biofilm structure.

What If Tinidazole Appears Not to Work at All?

Maybe you aren't one of the people who first found tinidazole to be helpful and then later found that it lost its effects. Instead, maybe, you have used it and didn't notice any help at all.

Again, many doctors whose patients get no response at all from tinidazole may come to one of the following conclusions:

1. No Borrelia are present
2. The dose should be increased

While either of these conclusions may be correct, we know that a third option may also be correct: Maybe Borrelia really are present, but they aren't currently the top layer of the onion. So, maybe the correct course of action is to shelf tinidazole for a time, and then to bring it back out again after biofilm is addressed and after co-infections are treated. Then, and only then, it might be found that tinidazole has significant usefulness.

Lastly, consider the possibility that perhaps you don't even have Lyme disease if you are finding that anti-Lyme therapies aren't helping you. Do not be so fixated on the Lyme diagnosis that you are unwilling to look at other possible causes for your health problems.

---

[7] The word "appropriate" is used here because numerous heavy-metal detoxification strategies are not only inappropriate, they are also potentially harmful and can do more damage than good.

Conclusion

With this discussion in mind, I believe it to be the case that tinidazole is a very powerful and useful antibiotic. If the colony structure of these bacterial infections is considered, along with the need for co-infection treatment and treatment of the other co-factors mentioned in this chapter, tinidazole has the potential to provide unparalleled treatment coverage against Borrelia in its cyst and spirochete forms. The challenge for the patient and practitioner is to dovetail the results of in vitro, petri dish studies with the real-world, in vivo, dynamic nature of tick-borne infections. These bacteria behave quite differently inside a living body, and adequate antibiotic concentrations are difficult to achieve in vivo. Therefore, careful and well-thought out strategies must be employed to gain effective antibacterial action against these colony-forming bacteria. Mindless administration of tinidazole probably won't work; a more tactical approach must be used, which fully accounts for the configuration, strengths, and weaknesses of the infective colonies. Sometimes, the proper tinidazole protocol may require that you stay on your toes and use the drug intermittently as needed. Of course, make sure any direction you choose is undertaken only with the supervision and consent of your physician, whose advice should always be considered more accurate than this book.

Example of Tinidazole Use, With Consideration of the Above Discussion

So, what does it look like, then, to use tinidazole in an effective fashion? It must be noted that various practitioners will have various answers to this question. The example I will present here is simply based on my own experience, research, and study of this disease. Your unique needs may vary, so please consult your Lyme-literate healthcare practitioner prior to using tinidazole.

STEP 1: Initiate anti-biofilm therapy with systemic enzyme treatment, lumbrokinase/serrapeptase, heavy metal detoxification (heavy metals can be a component of biofilm), or another anti-biofilm therapy. Continue therapy for a week or two, or until Herxheimer reactions and improvement diminish.

STEP 2: Initiate anti-co-infection treatment for Babesia and Bartonella. Continue therapy until Herxheimer reactions and improvement diminish.

STEP 3: Initiate treatment with tinidazole. Continue therapy until Herxheimer reactions and improvement diminish.

STEP 4: Use rife therapy to kill any spirochetes released from the biofilm community that haven't been adequately treated yet.

STEP 5: Repeat steps 1-4. Note: it may be beneficial to delay the repeat of this cycle for 2-6 months, and in the interim, use other anti-infective therapies. See Chapter 3 for more information on rotating treatment protocols.

Admittedly, these four steps are simplistic, and your own unique circumstances will dictate a customized tinidazole protocol. The goal isn't to use a one-size-fits-all approach. The goal is to plan an intelligent treatment protocol which takes into consideration the active and ever-changing defensive activities of infective communities living in the body. Equipped with biofilm, quorum sensing, and other defense mechanisms, these infective colonies will not go quietly into the night without putting up a fight.

One final note before closing this chapter: Alinia + Tinidazole appears to be a very good combination for stubborn, treatment resistant Borrelia. However, remember what I've been repeating throughout the book: this (or any) combination will only work when Borrelia is the "top layer of the onion."

Chapter 12
Chlorine Dioxide

IMPORTANT WARNING! The FDA and other regulatory agencies have issued warnings about the dangers of chlorine dioxide. Many experts believe that chlorine dioxide (and related compounds) are toxic and should never be consumed or used by humans. Please do not use chlorine dioxide without the consent and supervision of your physician. The appearance of chlorine dioxide in this book does not indicate that I believe this treatment to be safe or advisable for use by humans. I am simply presenting research I have done, and sharing my experiences. Please do not assume that this information proves the safety of this product. I am including chlorine dioxide in the book because I have personally used it and found benefit from it. However, there are reports of chlorine dioxide causing dangerous or fatal side effects in numerous cases. It is necessary to use EXTREME caution when considering the use of chlorine dioxide. Again, this treatment should <u>never</u> be used without the consent and supervision of a licensed physician.

C chlorine dioxide has been referred to as "MMS" in the past; MMS is an abbreviation for Miracle Mineral Supplement. This substance is not new to the Lyme disease community—it has been discussed on forums for several years. However, much of the available information about this supplement is fragmented, which is why I feel that it is important to discuss in my book and share what I have learned. Furthermore, I have never shared my personal experience with this supplement, so I will do that, too, in this chapter.

First and foremost: a word about the name "MMS." Anything with "miracle" in the name immediately conjures thoughts of snake oil, quackery, slick salesmanship, and valueless products. Many researchers believe the name of the supplement has done it a significant disservice, and so have begun calling it by its chemical name, chlorine dioxide, instead of MMS.

The active ingredient in most available MMS supplements is sodium chlorite, which, when combined with an acidic activator, such as the citrus juice of lemon or lime or other chemical activators, turns into a gaseous chemical called chlorine dioxide. While there is nothing "miraculous" about chlorine dioxide, it is certainly not snake oil. It is a well-known and well-studied chemical used in many industry sanitization applications, including the sterilization of hospital equipment and even suppression of microbial life in sewer systems. In fact, many researchers cite chlorine dioxide as the most effective and reliable broad-spectrum antimicrobial chemical for use in various hospital, industrial and commercial applications. If you use Google's "Scholar" search tool to search for the words *chlorine dioxide hospitals*, you will find many references to the effective use of chlorine dioxide for sanitization of a wide spectrum of antimicrobial life.

Additionally, chlorine dioxide is not expensive to produce. While many snake oil treatments are expensive and proprietary, chlorine dioxide is a basic chemical that is not patented and, therefore, less appealing to peddlers of snake oil and valueless treatments. So, while it may not be miraculous, it is a legitimate chemical with a history of many applications.

To understand why chlorine dioxide is so effective against microorganisms, one must first understand the difference between an antibiotic substance and a microbiocide substance.

Most of us know what antibiotics are. They are pharmaceutical drugs used to kill bacteria. Antibiotics use what is known as a "mechanism of action" to kill bacteria. Antibiotics interfere with a specific process in the bacterial lifecycle. For example, some antibiotics inhibit bacteria from growing cell walls. Other antibiotics inhibit bacteria from synthesizing new proteins. Yet other antibiotics interfere with the DNA of bacteria.

The problem with antibiotics is that bacteria can become resistant to them by developing or adapting new processes to maintain life, bypassing the mechanism of action of the antibiotic. This is known as bacterial resistance and is a common problem in not only Lyme disease, but many other bacterial infections. In fact, the medical industry is in a race to develop new antibiotics faster than bacteria become resistant to existing antibiotics.

The other problem with antibiotics, at least when it comes to Lyme disease, is that the organisms involved in Lyme disease aren't always bacteria. Some organisms may even be yet-unidentified hybrid organisms which combine bacterial DNA with DNA from other kinds of life.

A microbiocide, on the other hand, is quite different from an antibiotic. A microbiocide, also sometimes called a disinfectant, or antiseptic, is a substance that does not rely as heavily on a potentially changeable bacterial process in order to kill the bacteria. Microbiocides often physically destroy the bacterium itself, so changes in the bacterial lifecycle or attempts to become resistant by the bacteria are rendered fruitless. Instead of blocking a life process, microbiocides simply destroy the physical structure of the bacterium.

Examples of microbiocides include boric acid, alcohol, iodine, hydrogen peroxide, and ozone. There are two major problems with many microbiocides when it comes to treating systemic human infections. The first problem is that these substances are often unsafe and highly toxic, so they can't be ingested or used for treatment purposes. The second problem is that they are typically so reactive that they cannot remain stable in circulation in the blood long enough to actually reach infected tissue. When they come in contact with most types of human tissue, they react and lose their anti-infective qualities immediately.

Chlorine dioxide (so-called "MMS") may provide solutions to these problems. First, it is a "selective oxidant," which means that it does not react significantly with many organic substances, and hence, a lower concentration of it is needed to achieve its anti-infective properties. Researchers in many industries consider it to be superior to chlorine and ozone for this reason. In other words, it saves its reactivity for the interaction it has with more specific types of debris and micro-organisms, instead of wasting the reactivity on neutral tissues and organic material.

Second, effectiveness at lower concentrations means that smaller amounts are needed, which lessens the potential side effects of the substance. Chlorine dioxide may be safer for human consumption than other microbiocides. Please note: I am not saying that it is safe for human consumption. Many experts are adamant that it is not safe. No one should use it without first consulting a licensed physician. I am definitely not qualified to make any judgment as to whether this chemical is safe or unsafe for human use; I am simply sharing my own research. Remember that I am a layperson, not a doctor!

Chlorine dioxide falls into the category of oxidative therapies, which are therapies that utilize molecules that contain oxygen. Other oxidative therapies include ozone, hydrogen peroxide, and oxygen itself. Many people are aware of the benefits of oxidation therapy. While the specific benefits, effects, and drawbacks of oxidative therapies are beyond the scope of this book, I encourage readers to do some independent research on oxidative therapies and their various benefits.

Chlorine dioxide is a very powerful oxidative therapy because of the properties mentioned above: it is a selective, or weak, oxidizer, so the active ingredient does not break down before it reaches the targeted infection, which also means that it is effective at lower concentrations than other oxidizing agents.

However, the advantages of chlorine dioxide do not stop there. Other oxidizing agents, such as hydrogen peroxide and ozone, have lower oxidation capacities in comparison with chlorine dioxide. Oxidation capacity is the measurement of the number of electrons that an oxidizer is capable of receiving during an oxidation reaction. While ozone and hydrogen peroxide are capable of receiving only two electrons, chlorine dioxide has the ability to accept five electrons, giving it a more than two-fold higher oxidation capacity than the other two oxidative substances.

The combination of these two factors—a higher oxidation capacity and a more selective, or weaker, oxidation strength—give chlorine dioxide a very unique position among oxidative therapies. As you can see by now, the snake oil title, "Miracle Mineral Supplement," does not accurately describe this very powerful, very scientifically credible substance.

As mentioned, chlorine dioxide is primarily used in industrial and commercial applications. At the higher concentrations used in these applications, it is a very effective microbiocide. On the other hand, humans cannot tolerate the high concentrations used in those applications. Therefore, chlorine dioxide is likely not a cure for Lyme disease & co-infections. However, it appears to be quite helpful, as we will see in the user reports listed in the next section, even at low doses.

In particular, even at very low concentrations, it appears to be very useful for disrupting the biofilms that are a part of the Lyme disease complex. As we've already seen throughout the book, biofilms are a protective slime layer that bacteria are capable of synthesizing and encasing themselves within for the purpose of protection against environmental threats. Bacteria protected by biofilm account for one of the main difficulties in treating Lyme disease. When bacteria are protected by an intact biofilm layer, antibacterial substances of all different types will not reach the bacteria and will not have the desired effect. This means that people whose infections are protected by biofilm will still incur all of the financial expenses of antibacterial herbs and pharmaceutical drugs, and still experience all of their associated side effects, but will receive little or no benefit from them.

This is why the topic of biofilms has been center stage at many recent Lyme disease conferences. Once the biofilms are removed, the infections beneath them can be accessed and treated. There are many examples of scientific literature indicating the effectiveness of chlorine dioxide against biofilms, and of all the substances available for the treatment of biofilm, chlorine dioxide is among the most powerful and scientifically proven.

There is, however, one problem that arises when biofilms are addressed with chlorine dioxide. Many bacteria remain dormant or inactive when they are protected by biofilm. After the biofilm is removed, these bacteria can re-activate and resume their proliferative activity within the body. Therefore, it is necessary to be prepared with additional antimicrobial therapy during and after use of anti-biofilm treatments. In fact, one should be prepared for a renewed fight with the infections after biofilm treatment, as once-dormant infections wake up and begin causing trouble again.

I want to reiterate that I am not making any claims about the safety of chlorine dioxide. I simply do not know if it is safe for human consumption. As you will read, I have personally used chlorine dioxide, and I didn't experience any perceptible side effects. I will also share the experiences of others who have used it. However, I readily

admit that a few user experiences do not prove that a substance is safe, and I can easily acknowledge that chlorine dioxide is unproven and potentially dangerous. The FDA lists chlorine dioxide (and MMS) as dangerous supplements which should be avoided. I am not a zealot shouting from the rooftops that this substance is safe and effective. Instead, I'm a simple researcher, documenting and chronicling my own unofficial, personal experiments and experience. If your physician advises you not to use chlorine dioxide, please respect your physician's advice and consider your physician to be more authoritative than this book.

Chlorine Dioxide User Reports

Over the last year or two, I have read reports from a couple dozen Lyme sufferers who have used chlorine dioxide. Many of these reports appeared in online Lyme disease chat groups. Below, I will share my own user report, and then I will share the reports from a few other people who gave me permission to reprint their stories here.

Bryan Rosner's Chlorine Dioxide User Report

As my previous books have explained, I was able to reach a high level of wellness using, primarily, rife machine therapy. However, rife machine therapy wasn't a silver bullet, and other treatments, some of which are discussed in my past books, also helped me. Chlorine dioxide is one treatment which helped me but which wasn't included in any writing I've done previously, so I will share my experience here. For me, chlorine dioxide was one of the few treatments that was able to penetrate the biofilm within my body and provide access to the most entrenched, dormant microbes. In this way, it was one of the rare treatments that actually allowed me to accelerate the process of peeling layers off the onion.

But let me back up for a minute and provide some background. Looking back now, I believe that I was living with some quantity of dormant infection protected by biofilm, even after I regained enough health to live a normal life. As I began to live a normal life again, sometime around the year 2004, I was pleased to observe that antibacterial treatments, including rife therapy, did not produce any response—no Herxheimer reaction and no improvement. At the time I concluded that my infections were completely gone. After all, I felt great. I had returned to normal living, and I considered myself more or less recovered.

I want to convey just how protected the remaining infection was before my use of chlorine dioxide. Before its use, rife therapy, antibiotics, and antibacterial herbs would literally do nothing for me. And so, as I said, I continued to believe that my infections were all gone. At some point, though, I heard about chlorine dioxide and decided to give it a try. I assumed that my results would be similar to what I had experienced with lots of other antibacterial therapies: nothing to tell of.

Much to my surprise, when I began taking chlorine dioxide, I started to feel the presence of some old infections in my body, a presence I hadn't felt in a long time. It was quite alarming, actually. Was I relapsing? Had this chlorine dioxide supplement brought me back to square one? What had I done? Thankfully, it turns out, the quantity of remaining bacteria was small, and the new battle which was initiated by chlorine dioxide was short-lived. Still, though, I do feel that chlorine dioxide uprooted some very deeply entrenched infections which hadn't been responding to any other treatments. This experience alone led me to include chlorine dioxide in my book.

Interestingly, I noticed that the chlorine dioxide didn't seem to be killing all of the infections it released from the biofilm. It seemed to be a better biofilm-buster than it was an infection-killer. However, and equally as interesting, when I began taking chlorine dioxide, almost immediately, other antimicrobial treatments began to have tremendous impact. For several weeks, I felt very much like I did back in 2003 when my body would crave a rife session. It was as though the chlorine dioxide had forced dormant bacteria into activity, and my body remembered what that felt like, and was telling me to go use the rife machines, which I hadn't benefited from in a long time. Shockingly, after using chlorine dioxide, these rife sessions began to again produce consistent Herx reactions followed by improvement in symptoms. As I said, and much to my relief, things this time around were much easier and more encouraging. I believe that, while the remaining infections were dormant for the preceding years, they were perhaps losing virulence and strength. The new cycle of Herxheimer reactions and improvement that I was now experiencing was much more mild and short-lived than it had been years before. The Herxheimer reactions were much less pronounced, the subsequent improvement much more subtle, and the number of Herxheimer reactions much fewer. After about two months, rife therapy and other antimicrobial treatments again lost their beneficial effect. Only now, it was clear to me that the prior two months of treatment had taken me to new levels of health that would have otherwise been unachievable in the presence of the untreated biofilms. Chlorine dioxide had helped me clear a deeper layer of the onion. After this point, additional use of chlorine dioxide yielded no results to speak of.

Was I cured, finally? I probably wasn't cured in the sense that every single infectious microorganism was cleared from my body. However, I was better than I had been before using chlorine dioxide, even if only slightly, and I believe my use of chlorine dioxide provided some interesting benefits.

I do not necessarily believe that chlorine dioxide is a breakthrough treatment. However, I do believe that it can provide some biofilm degradation that is difficult or impossible to achieve with other therapies. I wonder if those who don't seem to benefit from chlorine dioxide perhaps don't have a severe problem with biofilm? I'm not sure.

An important note before I move on to other chlorine dioxide user reports: I believe that the use of chlorine dioxide without being prepared to deal with the infections that will surface after biofilms are eliminated is dangerous and can greatly prolong the healing process. In several chapters, I've talked about the importance of therapies that accelerate the process of "peeling layers off of the onion." Chlorine dioxide is one such therapy. Unlike most antimicrobial therapies that suppress the infection and cause it to become dormant and unresponsive to treatment, I believe that chlorine dioxide does the opposite and renders dormant infections more vulnerable and susceptible to other antimicrobial treatments. In many ways, this is a good thing. However, if you do not have those antimicrobial treatments ready to go, I believe the infection could spread and become much worse. Similarly, if you aren't ready to deal with a deeper layer of the onion, use of chlorine dioxide could render a person much sicker.

How I felt during my use of chlorine dioxide, and the idea that it can activate dormant layers, may be experienced by some people as a relapse. However, in this particular case, this relapse occurs when dormant bacteria are activated, and the situation presents an opportunity to remove bacteria that were otherwise unreachable by most of our available treatments. However, this kind of relapse can also spell trouble if it is not dealt with properly, and, if the bacteria are allowed to again proliferate.

Furthermore, I believe that rife therapy, specifically, is an important tool to have available when using chlorine dioxide. In my opinion, rife therapy is one of the best available treatments for combating the active, spirochete form of Lyme disease. It was my experience that the use of chlorine dioxide activated a large number of spirochetes from dormancy, and the use of rife therapy during this time brought me the fastest and most productive benefit.

Lastly, even though I am now at risk of being repetitive, I want to again reiterate the important disclaimer with regard to chlorine dioxide. This substance has never been proven to be safe for human consumption, and in fact, the FDA has issued a warning against using it for human consumption. My use of chlorine dioxide was admittedly experimental and potentially dangerous or life-threatening. This was a decision I was personally comfortable with, however, one that I would not ever recommend for someone else. Please discuss any treatment decisions with a licensed health care practitioner, and please remember that I am not a licensed health care practitioner; I am not qualified to advise on medical treatment. I share with you my own story, and I don't ask that you follow in my footsteps.

Other Chlorine Dioxide User Reports

Here I will list several other reports from people who have posted their experiences with chlorine dioxide on various Lyme disease support communities. The names of these people will not be included, in order to protect their privacy. These reports have also not been edited, in order to preserve their authenticity and accuracy.

CHLORINE DIOXIDE USER REPORT #1

I was on Salt/C for 18 months which helped. I stopped this protocol and started taking the chlorine dioxide. I took it for 4 months. It was hell. I felt like I was going through a mild chemotherapy process. The end result is I am 80% well. Chlorine dioxide gave me so much of my life back. After 4 months my body said no more. This was a couple of years ago. It was the only protocol that worked.

It was so difficult to tell if I was getting better while taking the chlorine dioxide cause of the most intense Herx I went through for 4 months. I was so focused and completely overwhelmed by the most intense nausea and bouts of diarrhea it was impossible to tell. Once I stopped and all the Herx stopped is when I noticed I was so much better.

A couple of months ago I did take it again. I was able to work up to a high dose quickly. I stayed on it for a couple of weeks but stopped because of the nausea. Once I stopped, I did not notice any further improvement. I don't know if chlorine dioxide will get me to 100%. I feel I have killed off the Lyme and now I am dealing with healing the damage left behind. I would love to be at 100%.

CHLORINE DIOXIDE USER REPORT #2

I started taking 3-4 doses of chlorine dioxide daily beginning October 2010 and built up to taking a higher dose. I have been taking this dose for about 3 weeks.

I noticed sudden and enooooooormous improvement in brain fog and physical energy in the last 3 weeks or so. Quite miraculous (as the name suggests!). It is wonderful to feel like I have my head and my energy back—I'm catching up with years of back log of chores and tasks, clearing my desk, sorting stuff out—it's great!!—I can think clearly again, and get things done!

I have been ill—chronic fatigue, fibromyalgia, arthritis, chronic pain syndrome, Sjorne's syndrome, IBS, underactive thyroid, to name but a few—since I was 14, 38 years ago. I am beginning to feel better than I have ever felt. Without a doubt, chlorine dioxide is the major reason for this.

Other symptoms I have struggled with for years—like an irritated bladder, and feeling hungry all the time, sugar cravings etc—have also just disappeared—it's amazing!

I have just started using a rife machine last week. I have found that I Herx after 2 mins for Borrelia—mostly feel achy and some pain in my limbs --- but the Herx is very manageable and I actually feel generally better. I think the chlorine dioxide has really helped so that the rifing is not having to do all the work and the Herxing is less than I have heard others describe.

I am by no means completely well, but have started to cut out some previously essential supplements.

No time to write more but will add—EVERYONE, GIVE CHLORINE DIOXIDE A TRY—you have nothing to lose but your symptoms! It is also very affordable—which is another major plus.

CHLORINE DIOXIDE USER REPORT #3

I have had very strange twirlings, stabbings, burnings, drillings mostly in my legs. I also started with a feeling of my eyelashes twisting. I know this sounds bizarre, but although I had a bulls eye rash, the Lyme test I had came back negative. I had an oral antibiotic at the time. These strange sensations I describe, came later, so I entertained the thought that probably they are co-infections.

Thus, I began the chlorine dioxide last May. The eyelash-twisting disappeared almost immediately. The stabbings, burnings, drillings have abated and mostly have disappeared.

I NOW find that if I take a lower dose (whenever I get any return of weird sensations) it does the trick.

I'm amazed at how long the chlorine dioxide lasts for such a small amount of money. To me that says that they are not out there for the money--the ones who sell it are there to help.

CHLORINE DIOXIDE USER REPORT #4

I took chlorine dioxide for about 3 months. I really liked it. I found that it helped my Lyme symptoms and gave me increased energy. Unfortunately, I have a tendency to build up intolerances to supplements and even vitamins and some foods. This happened with chlorine dioxide and I began getting migraines from it. Once in a while if I get the sniffles, I'll take a small dose and it seems to help without causing me too many problems. I wish I could still take a higher dose of chlorine dioxide because that is the best I felt with my Lyme for a long time.

Conclusion

Chlorine dioxide is an interesting, albeit experimental, compound. I hope we can attain more substantial information about this treatment in the future, especially safety-related information. In the meantime, please seek professional advice from a licensed physician before you consider using chlorine dioxide, and please note that the FDA and various other health regulators have issued warnings about the danger of chlorine dioxide.

I will not be providing dosages for chlorine dioxide, nor will I provide sources for purchasing it. Because it has potential safety issues, I will leave this information out of the book. There are many free sources of information on chlorine dioxide, including websites and online discussion forums.

Chapter 13
Medsonix®

Introduction

Recently, several Lyme disease sufferers have posted on their blogs that Medsonix® has helped them in their recoveries. After some investigation, I was able to validate their stories, and I personally visited the main Medsonix® facility in Las Vegas, NV to investigate this new treatment.

This new machine is based on sonar technology originally used in military applications. The Medsonix® machine was invented by Alphonse Cassone, who, according to the Medsonix® website, "used to serve as a Plant Manager and Chief Transducer Designer for a subcontractor of the military for anti-submarine warfare applications." The Medsonix® website (www.medsonix.com) tells us more about Mr. Cassone's background:

> *Mr. Cassone's duties included acoustic engineering, general management, and production and oversight responsibilities in the production of piezoelectric products. Several years*

with hands on work provided valuable experience and insight into manufacturing detail, logistics and liaison between government and industry.

Mr. Cassone left his previous employment at Piezo Sona Tool Corporation (PST) and Undersea Transducer Technology (UTT) as Chief Transducer designer to pursue his own projects, resulting in the creation of the Cassone Transducer. This transducer was patented and Mr. Cassone started researching new uses in the field of low frequency sound. He has devoted over fifteen years in research and development using low-frequency acoustics for various applications. Mr. Cassone received three medical patents using acoustics in the healthcare market.

Medsonix® technology is registered with the FDA and has patents for Body Tissue Disorders, Circulatory Disorders, and Blood Disorders. The University of Las Vegas (UNLV) has confirmed that the machine is effective for these conditions as well as related conditions. In a discussion I had with Mr. Cassone during my visit to Las Vegas, he told me that while many Lyme patients benefit from his machine, the vast majority of people he helps are non-Lyme patients.

There are some very interesting user reports from Lyme sufferers who have undergone Medsonix® treatment—some in the form of YouTube videos and some in the form of blogs and forum posts. I suggest doing a Google search for *Medsonix® Lyme Disease* and reading the results. I also suggest reading one blog in particular, where a Lyme disease patient describes her own recovery using Medsonix®: www.LymeSucks.org. She attributes the first 65-70% of her recovery to intravenous antibiotics, and the remaining portion of her recovery to Medsonix®.

At first glance, Medsonix® may seem to be similar to rife technology. However, Medsonix® is actually quite different. The mechanisms of action of the two treatments share very little in common, which is why I believe that Medsonix® is a breakthrough set apart from rife therapy.

In fact, I believe Medsonix® may be one of the most important new treatments I've discovered since the writing of my last book, *The Top 10 Lyme Disease Treatments.* The high-pressure acoustic sound waves generated by Medsonix® devices are very different from the electromagnetic frequencies generated by rife machines. Medsonix® treatments appear to disrupt the infectious colonies in the body better than many or most other treatments, leading to Herxheimer reactions and improvement that bring some people to the next level of healing.

Whereas rife therapy only narrowly targets certain kinds of microorganisms which are susceptible to the frequencies used, Medsonix® appears to have a broader, wholesale effect on the body and on entire colonies of Lyme disease bacteria, biofilm, and co-infections. This is why Medsonix® holds such an important place in Lyme disease recovery. Especially toward the later phases of healing, it is apparent that the problems associated with Lyme disease go much further than a simple infection with tick-borne organisms. Problems like tissue disorders, circulation abnormalities, and entrenched, complex bacterial colony structure plague Lyme patients as they get further along in their recovery process. Circulation problems can prevent blood from reaching parts of the body, especially the brain, as well as the extremities (hands and feet). Rife therapy likely has little effect on these kinds of issues.

Medsonix® seems to alleviate many of the symptoms related to these kinds of issues, and seems to restore cognitive function and circulation throughout the body. It is unclear whether Medsonix® is attacking the infections directly, or possibly breaking up and loosening diseased tissue throughout the body, allowing blood to reach those areas so that healing can take place. The acoustic sound waves created by Medsonix® machines appear to have the ability to simply blast through diseased tissue (and possibly even biofilm), disrupting and disorganizing long-standing bacterial colonies which have been successfully using their complex and carefully constructed structures to promote survival. One thing's for sure:

whatever it is that Medsonix® is doing, it appears that no other treatment on the planet can mimic its effects.

One simple analogy we can use to understand the difference between Medsonix® therapy and rife therapy would be the following: Let's pretend that Lyme disease bacteria are ants living in an anthill. Rife therapy might be likened to drenching the anthill, or nest, of the ants with poison. Doing this will certainly kill a lot of ants, but it will also leave the structure of their home intact, so that the ants unreached by the poison can continue to undertake their survival activities. On the other hand, Medsonix® therapy can be compared with a strong vibration working its way through the ant hill. While this vibration may or may not have a direct killing effect on the ants (we just don't know), it can shake the ant hill so violently that the ants' home completely loses all structural integrity, and the ants are left scurrying around with no home in which to shelter themselves. This is a very difficult feat to accomplish, which is why Medsonix® provides benefits which are rarely achieved among other kinds of treatments. There are many treatments which can poison Lyme disease bacteria, including antibiotics and other targeted therapies, but very few of them can actually compromise the entrenched, complex, and hardy colony structures in which these infections live. (Of course, the analogy I use in this paragraph is not entirely accurate and is for illustrative purposes only. Furthermore, much of the information on how and why Medsonix® works for Lyme disease is speculation and theory.)

Throughout all of my writings, I've always emphasized the importance of avoiding treatments which suppress or attack the Lyme disease infection. By directly attacking the infection, you often make things much worse, as the infection goes into defensive mode and assumes much hardier, treatment-resistant forms, such as the cyst form and cell wall deficient form. The more the infection is attacked, the more entrenched it can become. Additionally, attacking the infection can drive it deeper into previously unaffected tissues as the very capable spirochete literally drills its way through body tissues in an effort to evade the attack. I believe that

Medsonix® is a very favorable treatment because it actually does the opposite of this. Medsonix® actually shakes up and loosens the bacterial colonies, and causes them to become less entrenched. In this way, it may actually be able to reverse some of the damage done by prior attack and suppression of the infection. And I will repeat: this ability—that is, the ability to have an equal and opposite effect of suppressing and attacking treatments—is very rare among Lyme disease treatments. Accordingly, Medsonix® may play a very important role in Lyme disease recovery, a role not easily filled by other available treatments. For these reasons, I am convinced that Medsonix® represents a breakthrough in Lyme disease treatment that might end up being recognized as one of the top Lyme disease treatments of the decade.

Can Medsonix® Actually Help Activate Dormant Layers of Infection?

We've just seen that rife therapy is very different from Medsonix® treatment. One of the very valuable things about rife therapy is that, unlike antibiotics, rife therapy can kill infections without suppressing those infections and causing them to retreat to dormant, entrenched, resistant forms. However, what rife therapy can't do is cause dormant layers of infection to activate. Since only activated layers are susceptible to anti-Lyme treatments, the activation of dormant layers of infection is very important for continuing recovery, and very few treatments can cause this activation. We don't want dormant layers to activate too quickly, lest we become overwhelmed. But we also don't want them to activate too slowly, lest the recovery process takes too long. Up until now, we haven't really had many ways to force the activation of dormant layers of infection. We've basically just had to wait. And wait. And wait. The process can take a very long time and can be one of the primary reasons why Lyme disease recovery takes such a long time.

While Medsonix® may not actually provide the same killing power that rife does, one thing it appears to do is cause the activation of dormant layers of infection. This ability makes Medsonix® one of the few treatments which might actually significantly shorten the duration of the recovery process. This benefit shouldn't be taken lightly, as very few available treatments can do this.

This ability also makes rife and Medsonix® a potentially great team: Medsonix® treatments can activate dormant layers of the infection, while rife therapy can help to kill the bacteria which emerge from those dormant layers. In addition to rife, other anti-bacterial treatments can be used to attack the newly active layers of infection which emerge following Medsonix® treatment.

Other Benefits of Medsonix® Treatment

Here are a few more points to consider as we evaluate Medsonix® therapy:

- Like rife therapy, Medsonix® (and other similar treatments) is non-invasive: no surgical instruments are used to penetrate your body, and no herbs or chemicals are introduced into your system and required to be processed and removed by your liver and other excretory organs. This makes Medsonix® a very attractive therapy, especially since Lyme sufferers are often inundated with herbs, pharmaceuticals, Lyme toxins, and other substances which can overburden the body.

- While we aren't sure if Medsonix® kills the infection directly, it does appear to expose the infection and allow blood circulation into areas which may have been previously "Lyme-occupied enemy territory." Once the colonies are disrupted and blood begins to circulate again, normal body functions can resume within diseased tissue, and these normal functions can rapidly clear out infections and toxins. The immune system and various types of blood cells can get in and re-establish a healthy bioterrain. In other words, even in the absence of rife and other killing therapies, Medsonix® can help to heal diseased, infected tissue, thus allowing the body itself to do its work and clear out the infections. The body is your best healer. Medsonix® allows your blood—your body's healer—to get where it needs to go. Here's a quick analogy to drive this point home. Let's go back to our ant story. Imagine an ant colony in an old, rotten piece of wood. Now consider the same ants living instead on a smooth plate of stainless steel. We can clearly see that the ants on the smooth piece of stainless steel would be much more vulnerable to outside threats. The ants' actual bodies aren't stronger or weaker when they are in the wood; it's the environment that is more advantageous to their survival. In the same way, healing our body's bioterrain can cause the environment where infections are living to be less hospitable to those infections, and in turn, the infections become weaker and more easily attacked and eliminated. In a metaphorical sense, Medsonix® can help turn our bioterrain into a piece of smooth stainless steel, instead of a piece of rotted wood in which the infections can protect themselves and hide.

- Medsonix® treatment probably won't result in bacterial resistance because its main effect isn't to kill bacteria but, instead, to break up bacterial colonies—including biofilm. This junk located in tissues prevents circulation and blocks blood from reaching the diseased tissue. So, eliminating the colony structure and biofilm with Medsonix® can be done without triggering bacterial resistance. Some bacterial adaptation may occur, but resistance isn't a concern with Medsonix®.

- In my past books, I've always advocated staying away from expensive, inconvenient, unsustainable treatments, and instead favored affordable, sustainable, convenient treatments, such as those which can be done in the privacy of your own home, on your own schedule. I've noted that fancy clinics—such as those which require you to visit for a few weeks, spend thousands of dollars, and then return home—are not ideal. The reason these types of clinics are not ideal is that the recovery process typically takes months or years, and so sustaining the kind of financial expense and travel required to visit specialty clinics for such a long period of time can be difficult or impossible. However, I'd like to point out an exception in the case of Medsonix®. While Medsonix® devices are currently not available for in-home use, and while traveling is typically necessary in order to use Medsonix® treatment, I believe that such travel and inconvenience may be warranted if, and only if, the treatment in question can provide some kind of permanent, long-term change in direction in the recovery process. Unfortunately, many kinds of fancy clinics don't offer this. They make you feel a little better, but when you go home, you back-track to your prior state. However, I believe that Medsonix® treatments, because of their ability to disrupt entrenched bacterial colonies and even activate dormant colonies may have long-term impact on the recovery process, and hence, a finite number of Medsonix® treatments may pay dividends for a long period of time after the therapy is discontinued. Therefore, Medsonix® treatment is an exception to my rule that preferred treatments must not include the requirement of travel and inconvenience.

When Should This Treatment Be Used?

Any time during the recovery process and as needed. Medsonix® therapy may cause a fundamental change in the bacterial colonies and may allow other treatments to work differently and/or better. However, due to its ability to activate dormant layers of infection, it may also require that you stand ready with other anti-bacterial therapies after undergoing

Medsonix® treatments. Please use this therapy only under the care of a licensed physician.

Medsonix® therapy may also be useful when you find yourself in a stalemate with your disease. Medsonix® therapy seems to be like pushing the reset button for many Lyme sufferers, allowing you to get back on track with other treatments.

Additional Information

At the present time, Medsonix® units are not available for in-home use. Therefore, to use them, a person needs to travel to one of the several Medsonix® treatment facilities throughout the country. A few facilities have come and gone. At the time of this writing, there is one in Las Vegas, NV (www.Medsonix.com) and one in Los Angeles, CA (www.Medsonixla.com). While travel to these locations may be inconvenient, for some people, the expense and inconvenience may be worth it. I believe that some percentage of Lyme sufferers may find Medsonix® to be indispensable to their recoveries.

Because Medsonix® therapy facilities are still few and far between, those interested in bringing a Medsonix® unit to their local area should contact Medsonix® via www.medsonix.com.

There are still many things we don't know about Medsonix® and its impact on Lyme disease. The information in this chapter should not be considered 100% accurate and reliable; instead, it should be viewed as experimental and a work in progress. User reports from Lyme patients using Medsonix® are still relatively few. So, if you do end up trying Medsonix®, I would encourage you to share your results with the Lyme disease community so we can continue to build a user experience database for this treatment.

Chapter 14
Yeast and Candida

M ost people who find themselves reading this book are probably already yeast experts. Yeast overgrowth (also called Candida overgrowth) has been well-known and well-documented throughout the alternative health community for decades. Lyme sufferers, in particular, are typically very aware of the dangers of yeast because the heavy antibiotic protocols used to combat Lyme disease can cause severe, extensive yeast infections. This occurs due to an unwanted side effect of the antibiotics; that is, the depletion of good bacteria from the intestinal tract and its replacement by bad, or pathogenic, yeast species.

Numerous strategies exist for combating yeast, including, but not limited to, carbohydrate restrictive diets, prescription antifungals, herbal/natural antifungals, probiotic supplementation, and more.

Because the topic of yeast overgrowth is extensively covered in dozens of other books, I will not provide in-depth treatment of the topic here. However, I will spend some time addressing a few important developments on this topic, and some treatment strategies which I believe to be very important. If you are new to the topic of yeast overgrowth, please do not rely on this chapter as your sole source of study.

Don't Underestimate the Influence of Yeast in Your Current Symptom Picture

One of the most important things to understand about yeast overgrowth is just how intertwined its symptoms are with the symptoms of Borrelia and co-infections. Many people assume that the absence of intestinal symptoms is a reliable indication that a severe yeast problem is not present. And, in some cases, this may in fact be true, especially for the general population. However, Lyme disease is unique in that people with Lyme often have systemic yeast (that is, yeast that lives throughout the body, outside of the intestinal tract). This yeast can live in close quarters with, and be nestled within the bacterial colonies of, Borrelia and its co-infections. As a result, the symptoms produced by a systemic yeast infection can be very similar to the symptoms produced by those other infections. This means that the treatment of yeast should be a high priority even if intestinal symptoms are absent.

You Can't Remove Yeast Without Clearing Out Mercury

Mercury and yeast are synergistic problems. It is often said that they will exist in the body in similar quantities. Where you find lots of yeast, you will also find lots of mercury. And where you find lots of mercury, you also find lots of yeast. Trying to remove one without addressing the other is futile. A very influential article was written over a decade ago which likened mercury to the fuel which powers candida's flame.

Mercury detoxification is one of the most dangerous journeys on which you will ever embark. Improper detoxification methodology can result in severe and long-term mercury redistribution. I have covered this topic extensively in my past books (*The Top 10 Lyme Disease Treatments,* and *Lyme Disease and Rife Machines)*. I also highly recommend the book *Amalgam Illness: Diagnosis and Treatment,* by Andrew Hall Cutler, PhD. I strongly advise you not to attempt Mercury detoxification until you have studied the principles set forth in these books.

Helpful Tools for Killing Yeast

There are two types of anti-yeast treatments: Those which are not absorbed and primarily target yeast in the intestinal tract, and those which are absorbed and fight systemic yeast. While I did just say in an earlier paragraph that Lyme sufferers deal with systemic yeast, it is also a fact that these same people often experience tremendous improvement when using treatments which do not leave the intestinal tract. Therefore, both kinds of treatments (systemic and intestinal) should be considered.

Nystatin is the common intestinal treatment used. It is a pharmaceutical product and requires a prescription. It has very few side effects, and can be very effective. It does not get absorbed from the intestinal tract, and is therefore available to clear the intestinal tract of yeast. A little known cousin of Nystatin is Amphotericin-B, which, when taken orally, is also very useful for intestinal yeast. Amphotericin-B has earned a bad reputation because, when it is given intravenously, it has terrible side effects and even goes by the nickname, "Ampho-Terrible." However, when given orally, it is not absorbed and has very few side effects. Amphotericin-B requires a prescription and is available from some compounding pharmacies. Amphotericin-B has been estimated to be 10 times more effective than Nystatin.

Systemic pharmaceutical anti-yeast treatments include fluconazole (sometimes sold under brand name Diflucan), and itraconazole (sometimes sold under brand name Sporanox). These treatments can have significant side effects and should only be used under the care of a licensed physician.

Finally, many over-the-counter, alternative anti-yeast treatments are available. Results vary depending on who you ask. A time-tested option and one of my favorites is Formula SF722 made by Thorne Research. It contains 10-Undecenoic Acid, and has been considered very useful for over a decade. It seems to work for both intestinal and systemic yeast. In my opinion, it should be considered at the top of the list of anti-yeast interventions, especially because it has a relatively mild side effects profile.

Probiotics and Repopulating the Gut With Good Bacteria

In addition to killing yeast, you can also consume supplements or foods which are rich in good bacteria. These products are known as "probiotics."

Saccharomyces boulardii is a fantastic yeast treatment, and it stands alone in its treatment category. Saccharomyces boulardii is actually a yeast supplement. Yes, you heard me right… it is a supplement comprised of yeast, which people with candida overgrowth take orally. Why would someone with a yeast overgrowth consume more yeast? Because Saccharomyces boulardii is a non-colonizing yeast. It competes with the dangerous kind of candida, attempts to push it out, and then Saccharomyces boulardii itself easily leaves the intestinal tract when it is no longer supplemented. Saccharomyces boulardii is also documented to prevent and help treat C. diff infections. Saccharomyces boulardii is one of my favorite yeast treatments.

Of course, you should also use a good probiotic supplement which contains the more traditional lactobacillus acidophilus and bifidobacterium strains.

Lastly, don't forget about plain old yogurt, which is high in protein and rich in probiotic strains.

I consider the above three tools (Saccharomyces boulardii, probiotic supplements, and yogurt) to be a fantastic trio for repopulating the gut with good microorganisms. This trio can be used alongside the yeast-killing options discussed in the prior section.

Summary

I realize that this chapter is brief and skips over important information on yeast. The topic of yeast is covered thoroughly in many different books; I did not feel the need to reinvent the wheel here. I hope that this short chapter has given you some new information that you haven't seen in other resources.

Yeast therapy can be useful throughout the recovery process, but especially during and after treatment with pharmaceutical antibiotics. Yeast-killing therapies as well as therapies which repopulate the gut with good bacteria should be used during and after every single course of pharmaceutical antibiotics, in order to prevent or address yeast overgrowth, as well as prevent the dangerous C. diff infection from occurring.

Chapter 15
Liver Support

L yme disease and co-infections are conditions that are very hard on the liver. These infections, along with parasites, may even colonize liver tissue. Also, the toxins released by these infections further stress the liver. If the liver is stressed and sluggish, which it almost always is in Lyme disease, the biotoxins released by bacteria during their regular lifecycle will continue circulating throughout the body instead of being processed and removed. These biotoxins are also neurotoxins which make you feel horrible. Systemic toxicity is further compounded during anti-bacterial treatment, when biotoxins are released in large quantities from dying organisms. If the liver is overwhelmed, detox processes come to a halt, and you feel sick a lot longer than you should. Sluggish liver processes alone can account for a huge portion of Lyme disease symptoms.

Pharmaceutical drugs and even herbal preparations used by Lyme sufferers also must be processed by the liver, adding to the burden of this already-overtaxed organ. Some of the pharmaceuticals used to treat Lyme disease and co-infections are extremely toxic to the liver, and can even cause liver failure.

And the burden placed on the liver doesn't even stop there. Heavy metals, as well as other environmental toxins, tend to accumulate in the bodies of people with Lyme disease. These additional toxins make the picture even worse for our poor livers.

A sluggish liver can lead to imbalanced hormones, weight gain, chronic fatigue, indigestion, and a host of other problems. So, taking care of your liver is important not just because the liver is the primary detox organ in the body, but also because a healthy liver can make you feel much better, quickly! When the liver is restored, it can start doing its job again, and circulating toxins can be more effectively removed. Symptoms like brain fog, fatigue, depression, anxiety, agitation, and confusion can disappear almost instantly.

Below, we will talk about supplements which support the liver. But it's important to note that a liver-care program must go far beyond supplements. Taking proper care of your liver is a lifestyle. The following behaviors can enhance liver health: occasional fasting, avoidance of overeating and obesity, getting a good night's sleep, eating lots of fruits and vegetables (especially greens and bitters), and exercise. Taking extended breaks from pharmaceuticals is also important, to give the liver a rest. Supplements are helpful, but they are not an excuse for neglecting the above behaviors.

Here is a list of liver-supporting supplements I have found to be most helpful. To learn more about how these supplements help the liver, hop over to PubMed (www.pubmed.com) and do a search for the supplement's name along with the word "liver," or "hepatoprotective."

Herbs and Supplements That Support The Liver

- Milk Thistle. This is one of the most powerful and well-established liver herbs. It is often recommended by Lyme physicians to be used during and after pharmaceutical treatment. Note, though, that it can conflict with some medications; check with your doctor before using it.

- Dandelion

- Artichoke

- Schizandra (in addition to liver protection, this herb is also an adaptogen, which can greatly improve mood, energy, calmness, and alertness)

- Licorice

- Curcumin (this substance, derived from turmeric, is also one of the top substances for fighting various types of cancer and reducing body-wide inflammation. It also has many other broad applications, and may even be useful against Babesia.)

- Alpha Lipoic Acid (use with care, this item also mobilizes mercury and can cause serious problems in mercury toxic people—read Andrew Cutler's book, *Amalgam Illness* for more information)

- N-Acetylcysteine

- Hepar Compositum, made by Heel (a homeopathic drainage remedy)

- apo-HEPAT, made by PEKANA (a homepathic drainage remedy)

- Bupleurum Liver Cleanse by Planetary Herbals. One of my favorites, this fantastic formulation is one of the most powerful available for cleansing and restoring the liver. It works so well that it often leaves the user with an enhanced sense of well-being and vitality.

I have personally used all of the above supplements and have found them to be very helpful. I suggest purchasing them (when available) from iHerb.com, which offers low prices, free shipping, customer reviews for various brands, and good customer service. Your results may vary with each of the above products. Eventually, you'll figure out which ones are most helpful to you, and you should keep them on hand at all times, along with other supportive therapies that are essential to Lyme patients, such as probiotics. Numerous other liver supplements exist; the above list is not exhaustive.

As with most treatments, all of the above liver support supplements have their limitations and can exhaust their benefit after a period of time. Therefore, these supplements can be rotated over time.

Drinking plenty of water is also important, as is eating a diet high in fat to ensure that the liver is consistently producing new bile to flush out fat-soluble toxins. Drinking lemon water can also help detox the liver, as can water with added minerals (I recommend the product "ConcenTrace" for this purpose).

Taking care of your liver can be rewarding in so many ways, the most immediate of which is feeling a lot better, quickly! Please note that this information is not comprehensive liver care instructions; many other important steps are required to care for your liver. However, the above information can greatly help those dealing with Lyme disease and co-infections and can reduce the stress the liver experiences during illness.

PART 3

The New Individual Treatments

In this part of the book, we will examine new individual treatments. Read the Information For The Reader near the beginning of the book to understand how the treatment protocols described in Part 2 differ from the individual treatments described here, in Part 3.

Part 3 of the book doesn't give guidelines on how to use the individual treatments; those guidelines are contained in Part 1 of the book. Part 1 describes the treatment template which dictates how various treatments should be conceptualized and used.

Chapter 16
Introduction to the
Individual Treatments

What are "Individual" Treatments?

Y ou may find it strange that this section of the book has the word "individual" in it. What does that mean? Do these treatments somehow stand independently from the rest of the book? You can find the answer to this question in the beginning of the book, located in the section titled, "Information for the Reader." Also, in the following paragraphs, we will take a closer look at why we refer to the treatments in this chapter as "individual" treatments.

Let's start with a review of the information we've already covered. There are two very important steps involved in a successful anti-Lyme treatment campaign. Both of these factors must be present in order to experience success.

First, you must decide which treatments to use, and you should choose many treatments, not few. Here's why. The treatments you use will only be effective for a short period of time. The longer you use any given treatment, the more likely it is that the particular treatment will not only become less effective, but also have increasing side effects. The solution to this problem is that you need to have as many treatments as possible available at your fingertips, so that as a treatment loses its effectiveness, you can replace that treatment with a new treatment. So, Step 1 involves picking which treatments you will be using and choosing as many as possible. It is Step 1 which is addressed here, in the part of the book you are reading now on the individual treatments. This chapter contains a list of individual treatments which you can choose from, to add to your treatment arsenal.

(There are other valuable reasons for having a large number of treatments available to you. For example, everyone is different, especially when it comes to Lyme disease. There are vast differences in how different people respond to the same treatments. One person's miracle treatment may be another person's waste of time. It is for this reason that so many treatment choices are needed—the more treatments you can try, the more likely it is that you'll find some that really work for you. Also, in the last 10% of healing, we have a harder time isolating exactly what is going on in the body, so a larger assortment of available treatments renders our trial and error approach more productive.)

Second, after you've figured out which treatments to use, Step 2 is understanding how to use them. This means you need to know if they should be combined or rotated. You also need to know how long to use each treatment, and which health problems to treat for at any given time. This is the step which I believe is most lacking from the many available Lyme disease books on the market. Lots of good books will offer you a list of the top treatments, but they do not tell you how and when to use them. So, Step 2 is figuring out how and when to use the treatments you selected in Step 1, and Step 2 was the focus of Part 1 of the book; specifically, Chapter 3, which looked at the Antibiotic Rotation Protocol.

(Note that Step 1 and Step 2 don't always occur in this order; Step 1 could be done last and Step 2 could be done first. In real life situations, you will typically find that these steps are an ongoing process, as you discover new treatments over time and discover new strategies for using them on an ongoing basis. The important thing is that both steps happen one way or another—that you eventually have a long list of available treatments and that you eventually know how to incorporate these treatments into your treatment plan).

Now that you understand these two steps, you can see why we call the treatments in this chapter, individual treatments. This chapter is designed to help you complete Step 1; that is, it offers you new treatments to add to your arsenal. It doesn't go into great detail about how and when the treatments should be used. They are called individual treatments because they can stand independently from each other and be dragged-and-dropped anywhere into your treatment template as you see appropriate, based on the strategy you developed in Part 1 of the book.

Be aware that the discussion of each treatment in this chapter isn't intended as comprehensive coverage of that particular treatment. The goal of this chapter is to introduce you to these new treatments, so you can do your own research and, if they seem right for you, integrate them into your own rotation protocol. Because the process of actually selecting new treatments requires some thought and analysis, throughout this chapter I will provide you with some of the basic reasoning I used to ascertain that each particular treatment is special and worth including in the book. Of course, my list of individual treatments is limited and you can select many more throughout your healing journey.

Which Treatments Are Included in This Chapter, and Why?

The treatments in this chapter include anti-infective treatments as well as supportive therapies and nutritional supplements.

The exclusion of any particular treatment from this chapter does not mean that the treatment is ineffective or not recommended. There are literally hundreds of useful treatments, and this chapter will expand your arsenal, but it isn't the final word. Remember, understanding how, when and why to use a given product is the really challenging thing. After you've learned that, you'll be able to personally evaluate new treatments and determine whether they have a place in your treatment protocol.

To discover other helpful treatments, I recommend that you read other Lyme disease books. The books I recommend are listed at www.lymebook.com. For example, one of my favorite books is *Insights Into Lyme Disease Treatment*, which is based on interviews with thirteen Lyme disease doctors. That book has a tremendous number of treatment options since you are getting not one, but thirteen doctors' protocols.

Of course, past books don't offer you new and up-and-coming treatments. One of the cornerstones of successful Lyme disease therapy, and something which this book can't offer you, is a steady stream of new treatments—treatments which are invented or discovered after this book—and other books—are written. The timeless wisdom in this book (such as the principles we've established for figuring out how to construct your overall treatment plan) will probably still apply to future treatments, but since new treatments become available quite frequently, you'll need to stay up-to-date on what is happening in the world of Lyme disease research. It is helpful to develop a system for discovering new treatments. For example, implement a weekly ritual which includes reading summary notes from recent Lyme disease conferences, checking the various online forums, and keeping up with Lyme disease publications. Also, sign up on my website to receive treatment updates at www.lymebook.com/updates.

For those who have read my past books, an important note: this chapter was written only to include relatively new treatments that I haven't covered in my prior books; I will not be repeating treatment information that appeared in those books. The absence of a treatment which appeared in my prior books does not mean that it is no longer valuable or recommended; it simply means that I have already written about it.

The Right Treatment at the Right Time

We've already seen that Step 1 is to select which treatments to use, and Step 2 is to figure out how and when to use those particular treatments. I would like to expand on Step 2 briefly. As part of your strategy for deciding how to use each particular treatment, remember that even an excellent treatment may not be useful unless it is used at the right time. When used at the appropriate time—when the layer of the onion which is susceptible to a given treatment is exposed—the given treatment can be very valuable. When used at the wrong time, the same treatment can be worthless. The process of determining when the right time occurs is more of an art than a science, and can't be standardized for you by a doctor or a generic treatment plan. It has to be determined by you, after you know what's going on in your body. The treatments in this chapter are tools, but they only work when applied correctly. Trial and error can be an important guide. Another useful tool is what we call "energetic testing," that is, various forms of asking the body what it needs. Numerous resources are available which explain what energetic testing is and how to use it.

The key point is: don't write off a treatment forever, even if you use it with no benefit. It may actually be a fantastic treatment, and if you use it again in six months, you may get wonderful results, as different layers of the infection are exposed over time. This is one of the hardest lessons to learn, because it is human nature to discard a treatment if it isn't working, and it is counter-intuitive to re-visit that treatment at a later date.

When building your treatment plan, remember that what really makes the treatments in this book valuable isn't their use individually, but instead, their use together, as part of a coordinated, consistent offensive against the disease. It is this symphony of combined and rotated treatments which constitutes an ideal treatment program. The whole is greater than the sum of its parts.

Without further adieu, here are the individual treatments, which you can drag-and-drop into your treatment template as needed.

Chapter 17
The New Individual Treatments

Neem

The neem tree is a legendary medicinal tree in India. According to the Neem Foundation, it is one of the most researched trees in the world. Every part of the tree that grows above the ground has been used to treat a variety of ailments. However, the bark, flowers, leaves and seeds are generally the only parts used medicinally.

The bark is used for malaria, pain and skin conditions. The flower is used for intestinal worms, excessive phlegm and bile reduction. The leaves have traditionally been used as a blood purifier, an antibacterial, antiviral, antifungal and anti-parasitic. The seed and seed oil are used to eliminate intestinal worms.

There are studies that substantiate some of the medical claims surrounding the neem tree. In vitro research shows that neem leaf extract is effective against certain bacteria such as staph and *E. coli*. According to the Neem Foundation, the gum of the bark possesses anti-spirochaetal properties, as well.

Based on both research and tradition, neem can justifiably be used for Babesia, Borrelia and Bartonella. And, since it is difficult to find a single herb which has activity against so many different kinds of infections, neem is a potentially great asset for Lyme sufferers who have co-infections.

As with many treatments for tick-borne illness, results can vary. Susan Bowes, owner of Tattva's Herbs blogged about her experience with neem and Lyme disease:

> "I started taking about 2,500 mg. a day. It took 3-4 months, but gradually my symptoms started going away. After 6 months I reduced my dose to 1,000 mg. a day. By that time I had just some swelling in some of my joints- but nothing like before. Since that time I have put it to the test by taking breaks from it, and after two or three weeks of being off the Neem, my symptoms will return."
> (source: http://blog.tattvasherbs.com/tag/neem-extract/)

Safety Concerns

Certain parts of the neem tree, in certain strengths, can be highly toxic and dangerous. Do not use neem products that aren't intended for human consumption. Do not overdose on neem. Do not use for extended periods. And most importantly, use only under the supervision of a physician.

Children: Neem is not safe for children. Neem has been known to cause seizures, diarrhea, vomiting, coma and death in children and infants.

Pregnancy and breastfeeding: Do not use neem if you are pregnant or nursing. It can cause miscarriage. Neem is also unsafe for infants.

Diabetes: Neem can lower blood sugar levels; therefore, levels should be closely monitored if you have diabetes.

Neem may have other side effects not listed here. Consult your physician before use.

Additional Information

If you decide to try neem, you can find organic neem supplements on Amazon.com. It is important to be patient, as with any herbal treatment, and be aware of the above safety concerns.

Alkaline Water

Various machines marketed in the alternative medicine community claim to change the pH of drinking water into a more alkaline state. These machines are available from numerous brands. The machines range in price from relatively affordable to very expensive. In my experience, alkaline water definitely has powerful biologic effects on the body. Many people report improvement in numerous health conditions.

When Should This Treatment Be Used?

For Lyme disease specifically, alkaline water may have several different benefits, including detoxification. You have probably heard by now that Lyme disease creates an acidic, toxic environment within the body and that eating alkaline foods, such as green leafy vegetables, can combat this acidic condition. Alkaline water may be a powerful treatment for aiding in the alkalinization of the body.

However, there is another use for alkaline water which appears to be very interesting. Some have reported that alkaline water stirs up or activates deeper layers of the onion. If you are currently experiencing a plateau in your healing process and you want to push the fast forward button, alkaline water may help you do just that. Although alkaline water can be an effective tool for this, be careful: Make sure you are ready to deal with whatever gets uncovered in your next layer of healing. It could be one or more infections that were dormant, or heavy metals, or other issues. While you may ultimately end up making great progress as a result of exposing these deeper problems, you will most likely face a battle of some type while you are fighting them. Remember, there is no rewind button. Once you've activated deeper layers of your healing onion, you'll have no choice but to rise to the occasion and figure out how to deal with them. Still, though, treatments which are capable of activating layers of the onion are rare, which makes alkaline water a potentially valuable therapy.

Additional Information

For more information on alkaline water, visit: http://www.enagic.com.

Immunocal®

Immunocal® first came to my attention when a fairly well-known Lyme disease patient and advocate began sharing information about the product on a Facebook group. The single ingredient of the product is "whey protein isolate." I was skeptical that this ingredient could have any real immunological benefits because I, and many others, have used whey protein for health and muscle development, and I wondered how different this stuff could really be in comparison with plain old whey protein. However, after using the product myself and hearing many reports from Lyme sufferers, I have become convinced that Immunocal® has significant benefits, specifically for the immune system, and above-and-beyond what regular whey protein can accomplish. In fact, the Facebook group and product website contain links to many independently verified scientific studies about the protein contained in Immunocal®. According to www.immunocal.com,

> *Immunocal® is an all-natural non-prescription health product available worldwide. This special protein holds many national and international patents and is medically recognized in the Physicians' Desk Reference ("PDR" U.S.A.) and Compendium of Pharmaceutical Specialties ("CPS" Canada). It has undergone over 30 years of research and has been taken safely and effectively by millions of individuals.*

Like many things with Lyme disease, the rhetoric of product manufacturers is much less important than actual reports from real people using the product. In the case of Immunocal®, some have reported intense Herx reactions and subsequent improvement from infection-related symptoms.

When Should This Treatment Be Used?

One of my favorite things about Immunocal® is that it works by strengthening and building up the immune system, as opposed to many Lyme disease treatments which have toxic effects and ultimately weaken the body (such as pharmaceuticals). While I think pharmaceuticals (especially antibiotics, anti-protozoals, and anti-parasitics) are absolutely necessary for maximum healing from the infections associated with Lyme disease, long breaks from these treatments are essential. It is during these breaks that I advocate using treatments that build up the body. Immunocal® appears to not only build up the body, but also modulate the immune system to better combat the infections. So, Immunocal® can be implemented as part of your Rotation Protocol during phases of treatment when you are not using pharmaceuticals. I believe it would be counterproductive to use it at the same time pharmaceuticals are used, since the two types of treatments have opposite effects and would likely cancel each other out, to some degree.

Additional Information

For more information on Immunocal®, visit www.immunocal.com. You can also visit the Facebook group which discusses this product: https://www.facebook.com/groups/getyourglutathioneup/

IgG 2000 DF™

IgG is shorthand for Immunoglobulin G. IgG is an antibody isotope, or in layman's terms, an important constituent of the immune system. Your body is supposed to make IgG and other types of antibodies, but in chronically ill people, IgG levels are often very low, leading to delayed recovery from infections and a number of other problems and symptoms. Many alternative health care practitioners choose to administer supplemental IgG to their patients intravenously, and such an approach has been found to be quite helpful. In fact, Dr. Burton Waisbren, MD, who wrote *Treatment of Chronic Lyme Disease* (a book published by BioMed Publishing Group, the same company that publishes the book you have in your hands), used intravenous IgG in almost all of his Lyme disease patients and reported that he had great results.

Of course, intravenous treatments can be expensive, inconvenient, and unsustainable over the long term, for numerous reasons. Therefore, various supplement manufacturers have attempted to formulate oral products containing IgG. One such product is "IgG 2000 DF™," manufactured by Xymogen®. While possibly not as effective as its intravenous counterpart, oral formulations offer affordability, convenience, and according to many reports, at least some level of benefit. IgG 2000 DF™ has been used by a number of Lyme disease sufferers who report that it seems to help their immune systems fight the infections. Hence, I recommend it as a part of your overall treatment protocol.

When Should This Treatment Be Used?

The explanation for when and how this treatment should be used is almost identical to the explanation for the product mentioned previously in this chapter, Immunocal®. Please reference the section on Immunocal® entitled, "When Should This Treatment Be Used." While Immunocal® and IgG 2000 DF™ are similar, they are different enough that they are not redundant, and certain people may find better results with one or the other. Additionally, when one begins to lose its effect, the other may be rotated in for a new, fresh benefit.

Additional Information

See https://www.xymogen.com. The product can also be ordered from various online retailers including, at the time of this writing, Amazon.com

Note: This product may have been discontinued and replaced with a similar product called IgG 2000 CWP™ Capsules.

Boron and Related Compounds

Boron is a chemical element contained in the Periodic Table of the Elements, with symbol "B" and atomic number 5. It also exists as a mineral and is often one of the ingredients in multi-mineral supplements. Boron has a number of health benefits, but most interestingly, it has been shown to have immuno-modulatory effects as well as the ability to kill infectious microorganisms. Products containing boron are often formulated into insecticides, fungicides, and antiseptics, a fact that demonstrates boron's ability to kill not only small microorganisms, but potentially also larger pests like insects. Any compound used for antiseptic purposes generally has a very broad spectrum effect, which further demonstrates the power and versatility of boron. Some evidence also shows that boron can be anti-parasitic against worms and other parasites commonly found in the Lyme disease complex. Boron also has many other promising uses, including benefits for arthritis, lupus, hormone balancing, allergies, and more.

Boron can be purchased in various chemical forms. Many forms of boron are toxic and very dangerous when consumed orally. Great care must be taken when using boron as a supplement, and you should NEVER use a boron product which is not intended for human consumption. You can find supplements which contain boron and which are intended for human consumption on various websites such as iherb.com and amazon.com. Boron should only be used under the care of a licensed physician.

Some websites and patients have noted very positive results from consuming boron supplements. There are even reports of improvement or remission from difficult and often "incurable" health conditions. Many such experiences and websites can be accessed with a simple Google search for *boron taken internally*, or similar phrases.

PLEASE NOTE: Boron and related compounds can cause severe sickness and death in humans when taken in large quantities! The many toxic effects include testicular toxicity: even in low doses, boron compounds can cause impotence and lesions to form on the testicles. Therefore, use boron only under the care of a licensed physician, and only in products which are formulated for use in humans.

When Should This Treatment Be Used?

This book recommends ONLY consuming boron supplements which have been formulated for human consumption; any experimentation outside of such products should be considered dangerous and potentially fatal. Boron supplements should be used only under the care and direct supervision of a licensed physician. So why does this book contain information on boron, if it is so dangerous? According to WebMD and various other sources, boron is likely safe to consume in very low doses, such as those found in certain supplements. It has been my observation and experience that using boron in these safe, low doses can have some of the benefits listed in the prior paragraphs. Therefore, safe, low doses of boron can be considered one item in your arsenal of treatments.

As a mineral, boron can be taken as a nutritional supplement throughout the recovery process.

Additional Information

To learn more, do a Google search for *boron taken internally*. See also: https://www.nexusmagazine.com/articles/doc_view/226-the-borax-conspiracy

Double Helix Water®

I was initially unsure of this product until a person with Lyme disease convinced me that it was helping them. The product's website, www.doublehelixwater.com, offers information on the science behind the product. I've received reports of Herxing and improvement from people using this product. It's mechanism of action may be different enough from most other products that it may make a good asset for your treatment protocol.

When Should This Treatment Be Used?

I believe it can be used according to the standard principles of the Antibiotic Rotation Protocol.

Additional Information

www.doublehelixwater.com

Moringa Oleifera

This is a hidden gem of a treatment. Also known as the drumstick tree, or horseradish tree, supplements made from this tree have many powerful effects. Several years ago, an article was written by a person who hypothesized that Moringa oleifera might have benefit for Lyme disease patients due to its many methods of action, including, but not limited to, anti-viral, anti-bacterial, anti-inflammatory, anti-fungal, and immuno-modulatory properties. As it turns out, this person was correct, and Moringa oleifera is turning out to be beneficial, indeed.

But there's more. It turns out that Moringa oleifera also has antihelminthic activity (meaning that it kills larger parasites, including worms). If you read Chapter 7, you'll see that not only are researchers discovering that worms play a primary role in Lyme disease, but also that worms or worm-like organisms can actually migrate from the gut and join forces with Lyme disease colonies throughout the body. What's the signif-icance of this fact? It means that using effective antihelminthic therapies won't just clear your gut of intestinal worms and parasites, but it will also directly attack the synergistic infective colonies throughout the body, providing relief and healing from all kinds of Lyme disease symptoms and problems, not just those which are isolated to the gut. This is a huge breakthrough finding, and one that is changing lives. This is also what makes Moringa oleifera a very valuable treatment.

A study, published in April 2009 by an Asian research journal, cited the findings of researchers working in India and studying Moringa oleifera. Here are some excerpts from the study:

> *Ethanolic extracts of Moringa oleifera and Vitex negundo were taken for anthelmintic activity against Indian earthworm Pheritima posthuma. Various concentrations of both extracts were tested and results were expressed in terms of time for paralysis and time for death of worms. Piperazine citrate (10 mg/ml) was used as a reference standard and distilled water as a control group. Dose dependent activity was observed in both plant extracts but Moringa oleifera shows more activity as compared to Vitex negundo.*

Preliminary phytochemical screening has shown the presence of saponin, steroids, carbohydrates, alkaloids, tannins, proteins, flavonoids in ethanolic extracts of these plants. From the results it is observed that Moringa oleifera has potent anthelmintic activity.

One of the problems with treating worm and worm-like infections involved in Lyme disease is that all of the known treatments lose their effectiveness quite rapidly when used to attack the infections. This is why many anti-worm therapies are needed: When one begins to lose effectiveness due to organism resistance, another can quickly be added into the protocol. Accordingly, the more antihelminthic therapies we have available, the better. Moringa oleifera is one such treatment which should be considered highly valuable.

But the good news about Moringa oleifera doesn't stop there. Research also shows that Moringa Oleifera directly attacks biofilm. Yes, you heard me correctly. This amazing supplement attacks bacteria, viruses, fungi, worms and worm-like organisms, and it also attacks biofilm. Here is a quote from a study conducted at Rutgers University Medical School:

This study showed that [Moringa oleifera] had ... antimicrobial properties. Moringa seeds have been reported to act directly upon microorganisms resulting in growth inhibition, but to our surprise, the seed cover had a dramatic effect and thus prevented the formation of biofilm itself. These experiments were carried out using strain NJ 9709-Staphylococcus epidermidis, a strain with antibiotic resistance.

Several other studies also demonstrate this anti-biofilm capability.

As a result of the above discussion, Moringa Oleifera should be considered an extremely valuable treatment. And in fact, user reports from Lyme sufferers seem to confirm this with very encouraging early results, with some people even reporting dramatic breakthroughs in their recovery process. It should be noted that results depend on which layer of your disease process is currently "on top," or active; as with any Lyme disease treatment, the correct treatment must be matched with the correct layer of the onion. Determining which treatments to choose can be complex and require experience, trial and error, and getting to know your body in order to learn its responses and what they mean. Energetic testing and muscle testing may also be helpful.

When Should This Treatment Be Used?

Moringa oleifera can be used as part of your Antibiotic Rotation Protocol, as discussed in Chapter 3. After a period of use, the treatment will likely lose effect, but it should again become effective at some point in the future.

Additional Information

A number of sources are available from which to purchase Moringa oleifera. It is not an expensive supplement. Be sure you choose a source that does not include superfluous or undesirable ingredients. The Swanson brand has been used with good results and is very affordable.

Liposomal Vitamin C

The drug industry has long been encapsulating various drugs in "liposomes," which are lipid coatings that surround the drug in order to make it more absorbable and bioavailable.

Recently, the same has been done for non-pharmaceutical substances, including vitamin C. It turns out that "liposomal vitamin C" is in fact much more absorbable and bioavailable than other forms of vitamin C. In fact, liposomal vitamin C can be extremely valuable for Lyme disease sufferers, especially those who suffer from adrenal fatigue.

Many pioneering Lyme patients and researchers are also attempting to encapsulate other substances in liposomes. The results have been very promising. In some cases, normal Lyme supplements may have a many-fold increased effect if they are prepared using a liposomal recipe/process. One Lyme researcher I'm in contact with has experienced intense Herxheimer reactions and improvements by making a homemade product containing liposomal houttuynia (also known as HH), a treatment primarily used for Bartonella. I have also heard of some who use homemade liposomal essential oils with promising results.

When Should This Treatment Be Used?

Throughout the recovery process especially when healing from adrenal fatigue (see Chapters 5 and 6 for more on adrenal fatigue).

Additional Information

There are various brands available. One of the best, in my opinion, is Liv-On Laboratories Lypo-Spheric Vitamin C. You can purchase this and other brands from Amazon.com. Watch out, though, for other ingredients and fillers contained in commercial products: unwanted additives and fillers can end up in the product's liposomes and can be absorbed in much higher quantities in comparison with non-liposomal products!

You can go online and find recipes for making liposomal vitamin C at home. It is unclear how effective homemade liposomal vitamin C is. Some researchers believe that the homemade version isn't actually the real thing; instead, they believe it is emulsified vitamin C which could be less effective. The jury is still out on this. Personally, I have found homemade liposomal Vitamin C to be helpful, but maybe not quite as helpful as the professionally manufactured products. The homemade version certainly appears to have some significant benefits. For example, if I consume 5 grams of non-liposomal vitamin C, it can leave me with gastrointestinal side effects and other undesirable issues. If I consume 5 grams of my homemade liposomal vitamin C, I experience no side effects and the perceived benefits are much stronger.

I use the "Brooks Bradley Method" for making homemade liposomal vitamin C. Instructions for this method can be found using Google to search for the above-quoted method name. The materials and ingredients required are inexpensive and include an ultrasonic jewelry cleaner, a blender, as well as sodium ascorbate powder and sunflower lecithin powder.

When it comes to do-it-at-home healing approaches, the benefits and affordability of homemade liposomal recipes are hard to beat, even if they are slightly less effective than commercially available brands. Additionally, when making my own homemade recipes, I can leave out the fillers and preservatives contained in some commercial brands.

Eiro Super Antioxidant Juice

Don't skip over this one thinking that this product is only an antioxidant. It has shown to be much more. Many Lyme sufferers have reported direct improvement from taking it. The price of the product has also dropped significantly, making it more accessible. Some of its ingredients have been shown to have profound anti-inflammatory, immuno-modulatory, and even anti-microbial properties. The product contains several Superfruits including: Caja, Acai, Pomegranate, Acerola, Camu Camu, and Black Cherry.

When Should This Treatment Be Used?

It can be used as part of the Antibiotic Rotation Protocol.

Additional Information

Visit www.eirobrands.com. Note: the company has several other products, but the Super Antioxidant Juice is the one I am referring you to. Rumors have been circulating that the Eiro Juice product may be discontinued. If it is discontinued, similar results may theoretically be attainable by simply purchasing and using the above-listed ingredients.

Resistant Microbes® by Herbs of Light

Introduction

Herbs of Light is a quality company that makes numerous herbal products. One of their products is a blend of herbs called Resistant Microbes®. It has proven to be beneficial in both of the available forms, capsule and liquid.

When Should This Treatment Be Used?

This product can be used as part of the Antibiotic Rotation Protocol.

Additional Information

www.herbsoflight.com

Stinging Nettle

Stinging nettle, or nettles, is a popular and well-known herb which has many diverse effects. Relevant to Lyme disease sufferers, it can help to regulate hormones, especially testosterone, and it also works as a potent anti-inflammatory and anti-allergy medicine. During allergy season, it can be combined with quercetin for a potent anti-allergy therapy.

When Should This Treatment Be Used?

To address hormone dysregulation, allergies, and inflammation.

Additional Information

Nettles is manufactured by various brands.

Virapress®

A healthcare practitioner with whom I have worked extensively first turned me onto this product, telling me that it was among the most amazing products she had ever used. Its primary effect is to stimulate and modulate the immune system. Virapress® is a bovine extract containing proteins, amino acids, and salts. User reports indicate that results can be quite powerful in stimulating and balancing the immune system during Lyme disease and other infectious diseases as well as other immunological dysfunction.

When Should This Treatment Be Used?

As part of your Antibiotic Rotation Protocol; also to fight viruses, colds, flus, and other infection-based maladies.

Additional Information

www.virapress.com

Tart Cherry Extract

Tart cherry supplements have received a tremendous amount of mainstream press, research, and attention. In studies, tart cherry has been shown to have many biological effects, including anti-inflammatory, immuno-modulatory, muscle recovery, antioxidant, and more. It is used by athletes to increase peak performance and by those with psoriasis and other autoimmune disorders to calm an overactive immune system.

Because of its safety and affordability, it can be quite a valuable asset to those fighting Lyme disease. Lyme sufferers have reported decreased inflammation, increased energy, and reduced severity of Herxheimer reactions.

When Should This Treatment Be Used?

With regard to Lyme disease, tart cherry can be a fantastic agent for symptom reduction resulting from Herxheimer reactions, ongoing inflammation, and a dysregulated immune system. Of all the supplements discussed in this book, tart cherry is among the safest and most well-researched. It can be used as needed during any phase of Lyme disease recovery. As mentioned, it is also very affordable.

Additional Information

Dozens of brands are available; pick your favorite.

DMG & TMG

The word "methylation" is thrown around so much by so many doctors, patients, and researchers that you would think most people understand methylation by now and have at least some idea of the effectiveness of the various available treatments. On the contrary, most people still have no idea what methylation is and how to assist in the methylation process.

Methylation is a process that occurs in the body and which is involved in the proper functioning of many different body systems. Methylation happens when a methyl group (which is composed of three hydrogen atoms and one carbon atom) is donated to a reaction inside the body. Methyl groups are needed for a wide variety of bodily functions including repairing DNA, turning on and off genes, fighting cancer, eliminating infections, and removing environmental toxins. Lyme disease weakens the methylation process in numerous ways. Deranged methylation leads to lots of different types of health problems, including fatigue, fibromyalgia, the inability to detox heavy metals, behavioral problems and addictive behavior, insomnia, mental illness, and many others.

For proper methylation, a number of conditions must be ideal inside the body. Since these conditions are rarely ideal, and furthermore, are usually quite compromised in someone with Lyme disease, methylation defects can plague many modern citizens, but especially those suffering from Lyme disease.

How to correct methylation is a very broad topic, far too large for the scope of this book. Some of the most important steps you can take include supplementing critical nutrients which are required for the methylation pathway to function properly. These nutrients include, but are not limited to:

- Zinc
- B2/riboflavin
- Magnesium
- B6/pyridoxine
- B12/methylcobalamin
- Folate (from food or folinic acid)

When these nutrients are present, methylation is facilitated. Doctors and researchers have many different approaches to improving methylation, and the topic is hotly debated. It is such a broad topic, in fact, that an entire book could be written on it; and in fact, books have been written.

Here, though, instead of addressing the topic thoroughly, I will simply share some useful tips. To improve methylation, it is helpful to use supplements known as "methyl donors," i.e., supplements which can be broken down in the body and give up their methyl groups to be used during the methylation process.

Two methyl donors which have been very helpful to many Lyme disease sufferers are Dimethylglycine and Trimethylglycine. Trimethylglycine (TMG) is the more powerful of the two, but can also be too much for some people, causing insomnia, overstimulation, and other side effects. Dimethylglycine (DMG) is often better tolerated. However, the best choice between the two varies widely between individuals based on individual biochemistry and body composition. Both TMG and DMG are found in certain food sources but can also be purchased in supplement form. While these substances will not cure the underlying causes of methylation defects, they can offer great relief and increased function by supporting the methylation process. People who do in fact suffer from true methylation defects often find TMG and DMG to be incredibly helpful for dozens of symptoms. DMG and TMG have also been quite helpful to people with other chronic health problems, including those with autism-spectrum disorders.

When Should This Treatment Be Used?

Throughout the recovery process, as needed, under the care of a physician. Side effects can include overstimulation, insomnia, and hyperactivity.

Additional Information

Many different brands of DMG and TMG are available; pick your favorite. I also recommend the book entitled *Building Wellness with DMG: How a Breakthrough Nutrient Gives Cancer, Autism & Cardiovascular Patients a Second Chance at Health*, by Roger V. Kendall.

Supplemental Creatine

Most of us have heard of creatine in the context of bodybuilding: we see flashy, cheesy advertisements for sugar-laced creatine supplements that promise to "bulk you up" or "increase your strength by tenfold in just a few weeks!"

So, you must now forget everything you know about creatine, or at least, be willing to take a fresh look at this stigmatized substance. It turns out that creatine is also very useful in some kinds of chronic disease. Creatine levels are often low in people with chronic disease and infection, and raising these levels can lead to all kinds of improvement in symptoms, such as energy levels, mental clarity, sleep, strength (and the ability to perform much-needed daily exercise), and more. Some chronically ill people have extremely low creatine levels and can benefit tremendously from supplemental creatine.

When Should This Treatment Be Used?

Throughout the recovery process; especially to sharpen mental clarity and reduce cognitive symptoms as well as to increase exercise tolerance and the ability to perform strength-training exercise.

Additional Information

Some brands and manufacturing processes produce inferior creatine. I suggest using products which contain the Creapure® brand of creatine. This type of creatine is manufactured in a special GMP facility in Germany. The best kind of creatine is creatine monohydrate, and the brand I like most is Jarrow Formulas. Make sure the product you purchase isn't loaded with artificial flavors and sweeteners.

Low-Dose Naltrexone (LDN)

Naltrexone, a pharmaceutical drug, is an opioid receptor antagonist used primarily in the management of alcohol dependence and opioid dependence. As an off-label use, and in very low doses, it has also gained quite a reputation for mitigating the effects of chronic inflammatory disease. Specifically, it has been shown to have powerful anti-inflammatory effects and immuno-modulatory effects.

For some Lyme disease sufferers, LDN is a lifesaver and can both decrease regular, ongoing disease symptoms as well as the symptoms of Herxheimer reactions, allowing patients to tolerate more aggressive treatment. For other Lyme sufferers, LDN may be moderately helpful but may not be quite as profound.

One thing is for sure: many Lyme doctors are adopting the use of LDN to help their patients deal with the inflammatory symptoms associated with Lyme disease.

LDN is believed to have a very low side effect profile. It is also very inexpensive (although it does require a prescription).

The major drawback to LDN is that it can cause insomnia, and in some cases, severe insomnia. For some people, this side effect can be too severe to justify use of this treatment.

As a precaution, I would like to note that some Lyme sufferers and researchers believe that too much LDN can cause some impairment of the immune system and cause Lyme disease to become worse. Many practitioners may disagree with this statement. However, I've seen enough evidence for the validity of this warning that I feel it is important to present here.

When Should This Treatment Be Used?

Throughout the recovery process to balance the immune system, decrease inflammation, and increase the ability to tolerate Herxheimer reactions.

Additional Information

A great resource to learn more about LDN is: www.lowdosenaltrexone.org. LDN can be purchased from various sources, including compounding pharmacies, and is relatively inexpensive.

Pyloricin® by Pharmax®

This is a high-quality supplement which contains oregano oil, clove oil, ginger oil, and wormwood oil (artemesia absinthium—there are several types of wormwood with different functions). These ingredients are known to target many types of parasites as well as Lyme disease co-infections. Although other products have similar ingredients, people who have used this product have noticed that it is much more powerful and effective than other products containing the same ingredients; this is likely due to the combination and potency of these ingredients.

When Should This Treatment Be Used?

Use this product by itself or in combination with other co-infection treatments. Pyloricin® appears to be quite useful against Bartonella and Babesia. Note, though, that it can cause inflammation and significant Herxheimer reactions, so be ready to complement the treatment with appropriate anti-inflammatory treatment options.

Additional Information

Many retailers only sell this product to health care practitioners, but there are a few who also sell direct to consumers. A Google search can yield these retailers.

Mild Hyperbaric Oxygen Therapy (MHBOT)

For years now, Lyme disease sufferers have been aware of Hyperbaric Oxygen Therapy (HBOT). Hundreds of scientific studies prove the healing benefits of HBOT, especially with respect to neurological injuries and conditions. HBOT is available in many locations across the country, in both alternative as well as conventional medical clinics.

HBOT is not a new treatment for Lyme disease, and a great deal of information is available online about this therapy. Therefore, I won't spend much time going into details here.

However, what many people do not know is that a "mild" form of HBOT (MHBOT) is available. In this form, less pressure is used to pressurize the chamber, and as a result, MHBOT has less potential risks and is easier to administer. In fact, portable MHBOT chambers are available for a fraction of the cost of standard HBOT chambers, and many people own and use MHBOT chambers in their homes. Affordability and accessibility are huge advantages for MHBOT: even if regular HBOT helps you, the cost, and inconvenience of traveling to receive treatment, can render standard, full-pressure HBOT to be impractical for many people.

Furthermore, some evidence exists to show that MHBOT may actually have different effects on the body in comparison to regular HBOT, effects which may even be more beneficial in Lyme disease treatment when compared with standard HBOT. This aspect of the therapy is relatively controversial, so I'm not making any claims here about which type of HBOT is more effective.

In any case, dozens of Lyme sufferers on the various internet chat groups have experienced a renewed interest in HBOT due to the advent of the mild form of treatment, which is more affordable and accessible. Many of these people now own and use MHBOT chambers daily and have reported substantially positive results from their use. Some people are reporting amazing benefits from the treatment, and a few are even reporting complete recoveries. One of the standard observations seems to be that it takes some time to see results; daily use for periods of weeks or months might be required before a person can come to any conclusions about the treatment.

Some readers may be wondering about my opinion on the topic of HBOT given what I've said about it in my past books. In short, I've made statements in my past books that HBOT only leads to temporary results, and furthermore, that it may cause suppression and dormancy of bacteria instead of actually killing the bacteria. Well, the introduction of MHBOT takes care of my first objection: the reason that past results have been temporary is that, in the past, people were required to travel to HBOT clinics and pay high prices for a series of treatments. After the series concludes, the patient goes back home and hopes and prays that the results last. In most cases relapses took place weeks or months after the treatments were terminated. However, now that MHBOT is available and recognized as helpful to Lyme sufferers, home use is possible which allows continued therapy. This is really a significant development for HBOT therapy and solves the problem of only attaining temporary results with this therapy.

Now, let's look at the second objection I put forth in my prior books, namely, that HBOT causes suppression of bacteria instead of eradication. I still believe that this concept may hold true for early cases of Lyme disease, when there is a high population of free-swimming spirochetes that hasn't yet become entrenched deeply within tissue. For people with early Lyme, HBOT may in fact drive the infection deeper. However, I think the situation may be somewhat different for people with late-stage Lyme. These folks have already tried everything, and have likely already undertaken many different kinds of suppressive therapies, including many different kinds of antibiotics. For those with late-stage Lyme, it is likely that the remaining bacteria in the body are entrenched and sequestered in tightly-packed, dense colonies of bacteria, surrounded by biofilm. Other treatments may no longer provide any benefit, and a person may feel like they are at a complete stalemate with the disease. HBOT might be able to chip away at the integrity of these deeply entrenched colonies. Some studies show that the oxidative effects of HBOT actually destroy biofilm. And, HBOT also supercharges the immune system, increases wound healing, and even stimulates stem cell production. So, for those with late-stage Lyme, I believe that HBOT, including MHBOT, may be a more favorable treatment selection than for those with early stage Lyme disease.

The topic of treating Lyme with MHBOT is broad and extensive. This information isn't intended to be exhaustive, but instead, it is intended to introduce the reader to this treatment modality. If you feel that this treatment may be beneficial to you, it is easy to conduct additional research by searching Google for *mild hyperbaric oxygen Lyme disease.*

When Should This Treatment Be Used?

As part of a Lyme disease recovery program to stimulate the immune system, attack infections, and promote tissue healing.

Additional Information

OxyHealth makes very reputable and affordable hyperbaric chambers; see www.oxyhealth.com.

Earthing

Earthing, or grounding, is connecting with the Earth's energy, either by walking barefoot on the ground or in sea water, or by using a grounding mat, pad or rod when indoors. When a person engages in "Earthing," they are doing nothing more than simply creating an electrical connection between themselves and the ground, in a similar fashion to how electrical circuits are "grounded" to release excess and unwanted positive charges. This kind of therapy (if you can call it that) has become increasingly popular among Lyme disease patients in recent years, and there are now books, blogs, and websites dedicated to the topic.

Humans used to be connected to the Earth's energy in many of our daily activities, but today we are removed from that energy as we spend comparatively more time inside. Also, materials in the shoes we wear, like rubber and vinyl, are non-conductive, so they create a barrier between the Earth's electric field and us.

Not only are we disconnected, but we are also bombarded by environmental electromagnetic frequencies of approximately 50-60 Hertz. These frequencies can destabilize and excite the body's electrons, increasing free radicals. The cells in our body have a positive charge, while Earth is a huge reservoir of negatively charged electrons. Earthing pairs the Earth's negatively charged electrons with the positively charged cells in our body, creating stability and shielding us from the harmful effects of electromagnetic fields (EMF's).

A number of studies have demonstrated the benefit of Earthing, such as the following: *Ober, A. Clinton, ESD Journal, "Grounding the Human Body to the Earth reduces chronic inflammation and related chronic pain." 2003*
http://www.groundology.com/us/scientific-research [Jan 8, 2014]

Earthing is as easy as going outside, taking off your shoes and socks, and walking, sitting or lying down on the grass or the beach. The human body is 60-70% water, and therefore, a good conductor of electrons, as long as there is direct contact with the ground. Walking in dewy grass or in seawater also maximizes conductivity. Alternatively, you can ground yourself while inside, using any one of the many Earthing products available: grounding mats, pads, blankets, patches, rods and more. Mats, pads and blankets allow you to ground while sitting at your computer, watching TV, or sleeping. Special footwear allows you to be grounded while moving around and doing your daily activities.

How can Earthing help Lyme patients specifically? One theory is that "the frequencies from Earthing might cause the entrenched cyst form of Borrelia, such as those in the joints, to open and go into the bloodstream," says Dr. Stephen Sinatra, founder of grounded.com, in an interview with Alix Mayer in November 2010. Another possibility is that "the blood thinning aspect of Earthing allows other treatments to reach deeper tissues." Finally, it's possible that "increased blood oxygenation due to Earthing has a detrimental effect on spirochetes."

Still other explanations are possible, such as the potential detoxing benefits of Earthing. And, studies demonstrate the many positive benefits of negative ions when used for health purposes.

Earthing can possibly help specific symptoms associated with Lyme disease and co-infections, like chronic inflammation, pain, and elevated or depleted cortisol. From a study by A. Clinton Ober, co-author of the book, *Earthing*, "When the human body is grounded, induced body voltage is significantly reduced; cortisol, a well known biomarker for stress and inflammation, normalizes and test subjects experience a significant reduction in chronic inflammation and related chronic pain…"

As an adjunctive therapy for Lyme disease treatment, Earthing's blood thinning effect can be beneficial to Lyme patients as they often have hyper-coagulated blood. Because Earthing may also improve detoxification pathways for Lyme patients, it is advised that you start out slow to avoid an intense Herxheimer, or healing, reaction. For more information on Earthing and detoxification effects, read Alix Mayer's excellent article on her personal experience.

http://earthinginstitute.net/earthing-for-lyme-patients-go-slow/
(Mayer is the co-founder of spirochicks.com).

Earthing may also improve blood sugar, blood pressure and thyroid function.

If your doctor isn't familiar with Earthing, it is recommended that you have a conversation with him or her prior to use, as Earthing can have physiological effects on the body. Earthing doesn't require a prescription, but a doctor's supervision should be sought before experimenting with this therapy. Make sure to discuss any medication or other healing modalities you may be using, to be sure there won't be any interactions or related issues.

As a precaution, when grounding outside with bare feet, take all precautions against exposure to ticks and mosquitoes.

Additional Information

For more information on Earthing, see the following resources:

www.grounded.com
www.earthing.com
www.groundology.com
http://products.mercola.com/earthing-mat/
http://earthinginstitute.net/

Blog Posts on Earthing and Lyme Disease

http://www.spirochicks.com/2010/11/earthing-overlooked-electroceutical.html—Part 1
http://www.spirochicks.com/2011/02/earthing-lyme-hypotheses.html—Part 2
http://knowlyme.wordpress.com/2011/07/05/natural-lyme-remedies-that-are-working-for-me-part-1/

Published Papers & Studies on Earthing

http://www.groundology.com/us/scientific-research

Books on Earthing

Earthing: The Most Important Health Discovery Ever? by Clinton Ober, Stephen T. Sinatra and Martin Zucker (Apr 9, 2010)

Get Grounded, by Christopher Logan, (Feb 27, 2013)

A book for children: *From the Ground Up*, Laura Koniver, MD (December 4, 2012)

Documentary on Earthing

"The Grounded" Documentary by Director Steve Kroschel

Curcumin

Curcumin is a constituent of the well-known spice, turmeric. There are many herbs and substances mentioned in this book which help decrease inflammation and help to regulate the immune system. Curcumin is at the top of that list of substances, and is a great asset in the fight against Lyme disease. In fact, according to one top LLMD, curcumin may be the single most helpful herb available in the fight against inflammation and immune system issues!

Many experts believe that chronic inflammation itself can be the problem which keeps Lyme sufferers sick, and which allows their Lyme disease to become chronic in the first place. The further along a person is in the recovery process, the more important it becomes to address chronic inflammation: in the beginning of the recovery process the bacterial load may be so high that addressing inflammation may yield only small improvements in symptoms. However, if you are near the end of the recovery process and chronic inflammation is keeping you sick even after your infectious load has been greatly reduced (I believe many Lyme sufferers fall into this category), then addressing this inflammation can yield leaps and bounds of symptom improvement, as quickly as overnight!

Curcumin has many other benefits, as well, including anti-cancer properties, the ability to help with skin diseases, and beneficial effects in a plethora of diseases such as Alzheimer's, colitis, ulcers, high cholesterol, scabies, diabetes, HIV, uveitis, and viral infections.

Because of its many benefits, few side effects, and affordability, curcumin is a great asset to people with Lyme disease and other chronic diseases.

When Should This Treatment Be Used?

It can be used throughout the recovery process or as needed to address immune system issues and chronic inflammation.

Additional Information

There are various brands available, I prefer the NOW Foods brand.

Venus Fly Trap (Dionaea Muscipula)

This plant extract has been used widely in the Lyme disease community and appears to have anti-Borrelia activity. It appears to be among the more effective herbals for Borrelia.

When Should This Treatment Be Used?

It can be used as an anti-Borrelia herbal preparation, according to the guiding principles of the Antibiotic Rotation Protocol.

Additional Information

There are various brands available.

EGCG and Green Tea Extract

Each infection in the Lyme-group targets specific areas of the body for infection. Some infections, including Bartonella, adhere to endothelial and epithelium cells. Green tea and its extracts are particularly helpful for these infections. The effectiveness of green tea as a treatment for Bartonella is a result of the catechins contained in the supplement.

Green tea contains about 30% catechins, whereas black teas contain only 4%. EGCG is a type of catechin contained in many types of teas, but found in high levels in green tea. EGCG can be purchased as a supplement and has potent anti-Bartonella activity especially against Bartonella dwelling in endothelial cells.

Stephen Buhner's work shows that the EGCG extract of green tea helps endothelial cells and red blood cells affected by Bartonella through the reduction of inflammatory responses Bartonella causes in the body.

Due to the complicated nature of testing for Lyme-group infections, EGCG may be used as soon as general evidence of Bartonella symptoms occurs, even if test results are negative for Bartonella. Because EGCG has so few side effects, its use can be justified even when unsure of the presence of Bartonella.

Additional Information

Treatment with a natural green tea extract, or EGCG supplement, does not require a prescription. The trusted Now brand of EGCG Green Tea Extract® is available from iherb.com. For further information on the use of EGCG for Bartonella, consult the books written by Stephen Buhner.

Sarsaparilla Root

Sarsaparilla root (Smilax officinalis) has been used medicinally all over the world for centuries for a variety of ailments, including, but not limited to psoriasis, syphilis, leprosy, rheumatism, acne, gonorrhea, digestive disorders, menopause and impotence. Despite the broadness of its use, the herb is universally known as an excellent blood purifier and detoxifier.

Long used as a flavoring agent in foods, beverages and pharmaceuticals, sarsaparilla is a member of the lily family and grows as a brambled, woody vine in tropical and temperate parts of the world. There are over 350 species and its name comes from the Spanish word zarza (bramble or bush), parra (vine) and illa (small). Many sarsaparilla species are cultivated to form impenetrable thickets called catbriers or greenbriers as the vines are covered in pricklies. Only the root is used medicinally.

Sarsaparilla root works as a blood cleanser and detoxifier, an immunomodulator (selectively reduces overactive immune cells), an anti-bacterial, anti-parasitic, anti-inflammatory, hepatoprotective (protects the liver), analgesic, antioxidant, antimutagenic (cellular protector), anti-fungal, kidney-stimulator, hormonal regulator, diuretic (increases urination), appetite improver, a fatigue fighter, and it enhances the bioavailability of other herbs and drugs.

It seems especially effective at stimulating the removal of accumulated waste products from the cells, blood and lymph. This action is attributed to the herb's varied quantity of chemical compounds called "saponins," which are common in plants with immune-enhancing actions. Saponins reportedly bind with endotoxins in the blood and even cross the blood brain barrier.

There is some clinical evidence suggesting its effectiveness in the treatment of spirochete infections. It was used to treat syphilis by French physician Nicholas Monardes in 1574 before the advent of antibiotics, and the Chinese have also used a species called "Tu fu ling" (Smilax glabra) to treat several types of spirochete infections.

So, Lyme sufferers can use sarsaparilla root as a Herx reliever and an anti-spirochete treatment. It is also currently utilized by some Lyme disease practitioners as an effective neurological cleanser. They report that it assists Lyme sufferers with the neurotoxic effects of the disease. As you can see, sarsaparilla has a broad range of uses and can be a very helpful supplement when treating Lyme disease.

When Should This Treatment Be Used?

Sarsaparilla root can be used during the recovery process as needed.

Stomach irritation is the most commonly reported side effect of the herb, although Stephen Harrod Buhner, who included sarsaparilla root in his book, *Healing Lyme,* warns of a possible interaction with aloe. Because it is an effective catalyst for other treatments, it is advisable to proceed cautiously when taking the herb at the same time as other herbs and medicines.

Some of the saponins in sarsaparilla root are considered plant steroids and have been marketed to athletes as a substitute for anabolic steroids. There is no evidence suggesting that plant steroids can be converted into anabolic steroids, and sarsaparilla root contains no testosterone, despite what some of the sales-oriented internet noise might suggest.

Although there have been complaints of kidney irritation and even temporary damage when ingesting large quantities of the herb, no permanent kidney damage has been clinically demonstrated. If you have kidney disease, it is recommended that you either refrain from using sarsaparilla root or consult with your doctor as the effect of the herb on individuals with kidney disease has not been reliably documented.

Additional Information

No prescription is necessary for sarsaparilla root but, when shopping, be sure to pay attention to the species and origin of the herb you are purchasing. There is a sarsaparilla from India which belongs to an entirely different plant family (Asclepiadaceae) and which is referred to as false sarsaparilla, as it does not contain the same saponins and other properties found in the Smilax species originating in tropical America.

The brand recommended by Buhner is Nature's Way which is available from iHerb.com.

You can find more information about sarsaparilla root from the following sites:

http://www.rain-tree.com/sarsaparilla.htm
http://buhnerhealinglyme.com/resources/herb-source-list/#smilax
http://www.rain-tree.com/reports/sarsaparilla-techreport.pdf

Haritaki Fruit (Terminalia Chebula)

A 17-year old student in Mississippi discovered that an ancient Ayurvedic herb called Terminalia chebula (TC for short, and also known as Haritaki Fruit) was able to penetrate biofilm and kill the pseudonomas bacteria involved in cystic fibrosis. Other studies confirmed this discovery. After the discovery, pioneering Lyme sufferers figured that maybe a similar benefit could be seen in Lyme disease, since Lyme disease also involves bacteria which hide behind biofilm.

Lo and behold, it turns out that TC does, in fact, have a significant benefit for Lyme disease patients, complete with Herxheimer reactions (often quite profound reactions) and subsequent improvement. In fact, this little-known Lyme disease remedy may be one of the most important new discoveries of the last several years; for some Lyme sufferers, TC appears to be a game changer—not a silver bullet, but a very helpful addition to the arsenal.

Other fascinating research has been conducted on TC, research that makes this treatment even more promising for Lyme disease. One study at a university in India found that TC can inhibit the quorum sensing abilities of bacteria which live in colonies. If you aren't familiar with quorum sensing, it is the fascinating and advanced ability for bacteria living together in colonies to communicate with one another and respond to threats (such as antibiotics) in an organized, unified fashion. One way to understand quorum sensing is to imagine that each of the millions of Lyme disease bacteria inhabiting the body has its own walkie-talkie and can communicate with all of the other bacteria, essentially creating a much more advanced survival plan than could be achieved if all of the bacteria were acting independently. The stuff of science fiction, it is believed that quorum sensing is one of the primary reasons why Lyme disease bacteria are so stubborn and difficult to kill. Furthermore, this communication can even take place between different kinds of infections: Borrelia can communicate with Babesia, and Babesia can communicate with Bartonella, etc.

The study done by the Indian university is entitled: *Ellagic Acid Derivatives from Terminalia chebula Downregulate the Expression of Quorum*

Sensing Genes to Attenuate Pseudomonas aeruginosa PAO1 Virulence. Here is an excerpt from the study:

> *Burgeoning antibiotic resistance in Pseudomonas aeruginosa has necessitated the development of anti pathogenic agents that can quench acylhomoserine lactone (AHL) mediated Quorum Sensing (QS) with least risk of resistance. This study explores the anti quorum sensing potential of T. chebula Retz. and identification of probable compounds(s) showing anti QS activity and the mechanism of attenuation of P. aeruginosa PAO1 virulence factors....*
>
> *This is the first report on anti QS activity of T. chebula fruit ... which down regulate the expression of lasIR and rhlIR genes ... causing attenuation of its virulence factors and enhanced sensitivity of its biofilm towards tobramycin.*

Note that TC isn't only good at defeating quorum sensing, but it also causes bacterial biofilm to be more susceptible to antibiotics (in this case, tobramycin). Some studies even show that it can actually degrade bacterial biofilm.

Sure, the above study is in reference to pseudomonas bacteria, not Lyme disease bacteria, but empirical evidence indicates that at least some of the same processes are also happening when Lyme sufferers use this treatment. Quorum sensing and biofilm formation are two of the very stubborn, difficult problems associated with Lyme disease, so a treatment which can have at least some impact in these two areas should not be overlooked. As with so many of the most effective Lyme treatments, the formal research specific for Lyme disease just isn't there yet. So, you have a choice: ignore these treatments until double-blind studies have been done, or use them based on clinical evidence and take the chance that they may not work as well as you had guessed. As long as the side effects of the treatment are not significant, it has always been my position that I am much better off to experience the potential benefits of these treatments before double-blind studies are conducted, because in many cases, such studies are decades away or more likely, may never even be completed. While Lyme-specific studies are often rare, most herbs have a large amount of available information with regard to generalized side effects, so even if the benefits of a particular treatment aren't proven, as long as the treatment is safe, why not give it a try? One of the only side effects I was able to find for TC is the potential lowering of blood sugar levels. However, other side effects may be possible, so use this treatment only under the care and supervision of a licensed physician.

Don't pass up TC in your Lyme disease treatment campaign—it can make quite a difference in the healing process.

When Should This Treatment Be Used?

As needed throughout the recovery process to combat quorum sensing and biofilm associated with the infectious organisms and co-infections which cause Lyme disease.

Additional Information

A very well-known and often-used Ayurvedic combination product known as Triphala contains several ingredients, one of which is Terminalia chebula (TC). However, results with Triphala seem to be inferior to results attained when using TC alone in a stand-alone product. Furthermore, I prefer using pure TC powder, not processed versions of TC which may be sold in capsule form. A product which I believe to be high quality and which has some track record is "Organic Haritaki Fruit Powder®" made by Banyan Botanicals. It is inexpensive and can, at the time of the writing of this book, be purchased from Amazon.com. It contains 100% pure TC powder with no other ingredients.

Elderberry

Elderberry is a fantastic supplement with many broad applications. It stimulates and balances the immune system, shortens the duration of the flu and other illness, alleviates allergies, stimulates the cardiovascular system, is anti-inflammatory, anti-infective, and can help sinus and respiratory congestion. It can also decrease healing time for various physical traumas and wounds. Elderberry has been used for hundreds of years as a medicinal plant and has many other benefits not listed here.

Lyme sufferers notice that it can boost their immune response and make them feel better. Elderberry is not a core supplement for Lyme disease, but it can be helpful as an adjunct during the recovery process. It is one of those powerful herbal supplements that almost everyone should know about and have in their cabinet.

When Should This Treatment Be Used?

During the recovery process as a supportive intervention for various health challenges; may also be useful in Lyme disease to strengthen the body and reduce symptoms; especially helpful when fighting colds and flus.

Additional Information

Many good brands of Elderberry are available; pick your favorite online or bricks-and-mortar store to shop.

Noni

Belonging to the coffee family, noni trees (scientific name: Morinda citrifolia) are found in a number of geographic locations around the world and are known for possessing many medicinal properties. Unfortunately, noni is often overlooked because it has been over-hyped and is commonly associated with faddish, unsubstantiated medical claims. However, noni is one of the most powerful substances available to us in the fight against Lyme disease and co-infections, especially Babesia.

When Should This Treatment Be Used?

There are many published scientific studies which verify noni's effectiveness against protozoan parasitic infections such as Malaria and Babesia. Additionally, noni possesses anti-inflammatory, immuno-modulatory, and other beneficial properties. Because noni supplements are generally very affordable and non-toxic, this treatment has a very favorable risk-to-reward ratio. Noni should be a part of your Babesia treatment protocol.

Additional Information

The brand of noni I've used and like is Now Foods.

Coptis

Coptis (Huang Lian, also called goldenthread or canker root), a genus of flowering plant with between 10-15 different species, is a foundational herb used in Traditional Chinese Medicine (TCM). In addition to the flowering plant, its root system is composed of rhizomes and contains berberine (a powerful alkaloid used for many gastrointestinal applications), palmatine, hydrastine and coptisine. This rhizome system looks very similar to ginger root, which, when dried, can be steeped into a tea or made into a tincture that is used for numerous medicinal purposes.

Although there are many types of coptis, not all are used for medical applications. The two major types that have been used are Coptis teeta and Coptis chinensis. Originally, Coptis teeta was found in the eastern Himalayas and, due to deforestation and over-collection of the plants, is now an endangered species. The local people used the collection and sale of Coptis teeta as a source of income, so it has been over-harvested for some time. Efforts to grow it in a controlled environment have not been very successful. It was commercially marketed in the 1950's and 1960's in Canada to be used for its anti-microbial and anti-inflammatory properties. The roots were dried and then steeped into a bitter tea which was then swabbed on areas of thrush (candidiasis). It was also used for dyspepsia and insomnia.

The second type of coptis, which is now used in medical treatments, is Coptis Chinensis. It is native to China and one of the 50 fundamental herbs used in TCM. Coptis chinensis was made popular following the research and protocol created by two very well known physicians who are experts in Chinese Medicine and is the herb primarily used for the treatment of Lyme disease. According to TCM, it is considered a "cooling" herb and, therefore, treats conditions that are associated with heat, such as insomnia, irritability and inflammation (heat in TCM means diseases of activity, not necessarily temperature). The cooling aspect can also help with high fevers and delirium. The berberine found in the Coptis chinensis root is primarily useful for gastrointestinal issues, so it treats: diarrhea, vomiting, bacterial dysentery, abdominal cramps, acid reflux, ineffective or painful bowel movements, bloody stools, chronic gallbladder inflammation and the pain of irritable bowel syndrome.

Coptis helps with conditions of the heart, liver, stomach and large intestine. As the name "canker root" suggests, it has also been effective on canker sores, tongue ulcers and swollen gums. It even has properties that will help clear up skin issues such as acne, boils, carbuncles, burns or infected cuts. Due to its antibiotic properties, gargling with a diluted tincture can help ease a sore throat.

Additional Information

Coptis chinensis plays a role in the treatment of Lyme disease due to its anti-microbial effects, anti-fungal properties, small molecular weight, potential to cross the blood brain barrier, ability to be taken long-term, limited side effects, use in cases of thrush or other oral sores, and aid to the gastrointestinal system that has likely been damaged by years of western antibiotic use. The supplement does not require a prescription, but as always, it should only be used under the supervision of your physician. One of my favorite brands is the Plum Flower brand, and the product is called "Coptis Teapills®."

PART 4

Parting Words

In this final section, we will examine some tips for success and also look at where to find additional updates in the future.

Chapter 18
Tips for A Faster Recovery

N ow that you're nearing the end of my book, I would like to leave you with some tips for recovery to help you along the path of healing from Lyme disease.

How Lyme Doctors Can Help During the Recovery Process

Over the years, I've been asked if I advocate self-treatment instead of treatment under the care of a licensed, experienced Lyme disease doctor. In a word, the answer is: NO! I believe that every Lyme disease sufferer should be under the care of the best Lyme doctor available. In fact, I think this is essential to getting well in most cases.

However, what I do believe is that Lyme patients should not abdicate all responsibility for their healing to a Lyme doctor. Inversely, no Lyme patient should be arrogant and self sufficient to the degree that they feel they don't need a Lyme doctor. These two courses of action are extremes;

in one extreme, a person refuses to get to know their own body and relies solely on an expert, and in the other extreme, a person rejects outside wisdom and takes matters entirely into their own hands. Each extreme can have disastrous consequences. Relying only on a doctor's input denies you the progress you can make by getting to know your own body so that you can carefully consider your doctor's advice and determine if it matches up with your own unique needs. And on the other hand, being overly self-sufficient denies you the tremendous wisdom and experience of Lyme disease practitioners.

Here's the ideal scenario, in my opinion: During the periods of time between doctor's appointments (and these periods of time can be long; some doctors only see their Lyme patients every 4-12 weeks) a person should be actively engaged in their healing process. They should be taking notes, learning their body, doing their own research, experimenting with new treatments (with their doctor's permission), and gaining as much knowledge and wisdom as possible. This way, when it comes time for the appointment, the patient can present the physician with an enormous amount of useful information about their particular case, to help the physician determine the best steps for healing. It is this partnership—this team mentality—that leads to treatment success.

This approach to healing is only possible when you are working with a physician who is open-minded and who respects your authority as a patient. Doctors who prescribe one-size-fits-all treatment plans, and who are unwilling to listen to your experiences and unique needs, should be avoided.

Lastly, it is not a guarantee that the doctor you are seeing will have the right tools to heal you. Each doctor has been educated differently, and has had different patients, and different experiences. All you have to do in order to see this is interview a dozen different Lyme doctors—you'll notice that each of them takes a different approach in fighting Lyme disease. This is one reason why it is so important to stay engaged in your own recovery process. Your doctor will help you, but he or she won't have all the answers for you. (I've actually been part of a book project in which we really did interview more than a dozen Lyme doctors, and I was shocked by how differently each of them look at this condition! The book is titled, *Insights Into Lyme Disease Treatment: 13 Lyme-Literate Healthcare Practitioners Share Their Healing Strategies*).

Keep an Open Mind

The world of Lyme disease is strange, and many seemingly ridiculous treatments may actually work. I was skeptical for a long time. I passed up many good treatments. Be less skeptical and try new things. I'm not saying to be a brainless consumer ready to fork over your hard-earned cash to swindlers—do your homework and make smart decisions. But, just because you haven't heard of a new treatment before or you aren't familiar with how it works, don't assume it is not a valid form of treatment. 90% of the treatments I was skeptical about turned out to be valid and some of them turned out to be very important. Remember, the experts of Western medicine will often ridicule treatments that come from other parts of the world, other cultures, and other medical paradigms. Don't listen to these so-called experts. Listen to the patients who actually use the treatments; ask them if they've received help. Ideally, you can also rely on clinical studies, but for the vast majority of Lyme disease treatments, such studies aren't available.

Don't Become Hyper-Focused on Any Particular Infection or Health Problem

Don't wear blinders. If you start treating Bartonella, for example, and you feel better fast, the tendency is to hyper-focus on Bartonella even after all available Bartonella treatments result in a continued plateau in progress. The plateau probably doesn't mean you need to try even more Bartonella treatments, instead, it probably means another infection or issue has taken dominance and it's time to move on to treating that problem. After we experience improvement from one particular kind of treatment, it's far too easy for us to subconsciously reach the conclusion that all future progress will in some way be tied to that particular treatment, or treatment strategy. We must be able to shift gears and move on when a particular treatment has run its course.

So, If you hit a plateau, it is time to change things up. Think outside the box and move to a new treatment approach.

What to Expect When Treating Lyme Disease

Many Lyme sufferers notice a general pattern in their recovery. This pattern doesn't apply equally to everyone, but if you can learn to recognize the parts of the pattern that apply to you, your recovery process can be much smoother.

The phases of recovery move you from being really sick to being much better. Here's what the experience can feel like.

1. When really sick, everything is out of control and you have dramatic Herxheimer reactions to almost any treatment. Symptoms cycle randomly and it's very hard to know whether you are moving forward or backward. This part of the illness can be the most confusing, frustrating, and difficult.

2. Eventually, you get to the point where you have some pattern, or cycle, of Herxing and improvement. You can correlate cause and effect with the treatments you are using, and you don't feel like the entire recovery process is pure chaos. Things are still hard at this point, but the sense of order can lead to a feeling of control and continued progress. This is the phase when you may begin to recognize the presence of co-infections, because your symptoms will begin to become defined and differentiated, and you'll be able to recognize specific symptoms of the different co-infections.

3. Finally, the last phase of healing involves two primary features:

    a) The infections will finally calm down, and any remaining organisms are tough, entrenched, and difficult to treat. In this phase, you must get creative and strategic in order to expose and kill the last of the infections. This is the phase of recovery that this book is most targeted toward. While symptoms during this phase are often not completely overwhelming and debilitating, they are extremely persistent and non-responsive to treatment. Only the correct treatments applied at the correct time will help move you forward.

    b) As the infections calm down and symptoms of infections decrease, there is more time and energy available to figure out what else might be making you sick, and which supportive therapies should be used. Various parts of this book are intended to help address this particular phase. Examples of treatments which focus on this area of recovery include the KPU protocol, dietary recommendations, rebuilding the adrenal glands, etc.

Note that in the final phases of recovery, the pace of change within the body can accelerate, and you must stay three steps ahead and have new treatment options ready to go at all times. As you get to the deepest layers of the onion, you'll be facing the most difficult problems which didn't respond to all your prior treatments. This is where you'll make the biggest leaps of improvement, but also find the most stubborn enemies.

Find a Healthy Balance Between Living Life and Treating Lyme Disease

If all you do is try to live your life and ignore your infections, you may continue to get sicker and sicker, and the reversal of your illness may become more and more difficult. On the other hand, if all you do is focus on treatment, you may miss the present moment and you may defer all enjoyment of life until a later date. Neither of these extremes is ideal; instead, seek a balance between treatments and enjoyment of life. Obviously the illness will impede your enjoyment of life to some degree, but there are still many ways you can enjoy the world, and people around you, even when sick.

Pharmaceutical Antibiotics Can Help You or Hurt You

Some pharmaceutical antibiotics will just get along with your body. They will energize you, decrease excessive inflammation, kill your infections, and make you feel great. Other drugs will drain you, sicken you, cause horrible side effects, and be rejected by your body. Of course, sometimes these bad reactions can be beneficial Herxheimer reactions. But, other times, these reactions may simply be your body rejecting the treatment. Learn to use the drugs which help you the most, and avoid the drugs which don't get along with you. A doctor can't always figure this out for you since he or she can't predict the unique ways in which your body will respond to treatment. Everyone is different.

The Yin and Yang of Lyme Disease Treatment

If Yin and Yang are opposites, so are the two different parts of Lyme disease recovery: the "tearing down" part, and the "building up" part. Yes, you need to spend time attacking the infections, killing them with aggressive treatments, and taking no prisoners. But you also need to spend time taking breaks from aggressive treatments, so you can build up the body and allow it to heal. You need a lot of both kinds of approaches. Don't focus too heavily on either one.

The Natural Approach to Lyme Disease May Delay Recovery

A prolific author and friend called me and told me she thought she had Lyme disease and wanted to fight it naturally, at all costs, avoiding pharmaceuticals. I told her the story of another friend I had, a person who had been sick with chronic fatigue syndrome for two decades and had also tried to avoid pharmaceutical treatments at all costs. Finally, a doctor convinced this friend with chronic fatigue syndrome to try pharmaceutical antibiotics. He was repulsed by the idea of putting such toxic chemicals into his body, but since he was so desperate, he agreed to try the drugs.

To his surprise, the antibiotics started helping him, and he got better and better. After about 6 months of heavy duty pharmaceutical treatment, he had is life back. He now travels the world and even participates in large, organized athletic events. He lost the 50 pounds he had gained while sick, he took control of the family business, got his finances back in order, and he regrets all the time he wasted before he tried the antibiotics.

The desire to use natural treatments is certainly understandable. But sometimes, the infections are stronger than our bodies. Sometimes, people die without antibiotics. And sometimes, Lyme sufferers don't experience real progress until they incorporate pharmaceuticals into their protocols.

There is a fine line to walk. Some doctors prescribe too many drugs, for too long, and keep using them after they have lost effectiveness. The proper balance is to use them powerfully and effectively when they can do good, and then take breaks from them during which time you use restorative, natural therapies, as well as herbs. It's a balance, but avoiding drugs completely may just be sentencing yourself to a life of unnecessary misery.

Keep Your Supplements Organized

"I haven't had a Babesia flareup in years," you may be thinking to yourself. "Man, I forget which herbs worked for me back then."

Don't let this happen to you. Keep your supplements organized. Keep lists on paper, or on your computer, to remind yourself of which supplements have helped you with which problems. Use Tupperware or other containers to separate Babesia treatments from Bartonella treatments, and adrenal therapies from probiotics.

It can be difficult to stay organized when your brain isn't working, but it's important to do the best you can. Unfortunately, lack of organization during the recovery process can be a major cause of delayed progress.

There's No Silver Bullet Lyme Disease Treatment (at least, not yet)

You should never believe someone who says, "this is the best treatment for Lyme disease, period!" It may be a great treatment, but remember that Lyme disease is a complex illness with dozens of underlying dysfunctions and contributing factors. Why is this realization important? Because, it changes the question you should be asking. Instead of asking, "what are the best treatments in the world for Lyme disease"? (a question that can send you on a wild goose chase and set you up to succumb to wild marketing claims), you should be asking, "what layer of the onion am I currently dealing with, and what treatment should I use for that layer?" One is a pie-in-the-sky, silver bullet seeking question... the other is a logical question that demonstrates understanding of your situation and a desire to apply the correct solution. I'm not saying that a silver bullet treatment will never be developed. Maybe one day, we'll be able to modify human DNA so that we are no longer susceptible to all of these environmental and infectious attacks. But until that day, we need to be realistic and clear-minded.

When Infections Are Present, True Progress Won't Occur Until They Are Addressed

All the Yoga, green smoothies, and multi-vitamins in the world aren't going to eliminate Borrelia and co-infections. While some people claim that these kinds of therapies have cured their Lyme disease, I've just never seen it happen. In my opinion, lifestyle adjustments, nutrition, and other similar approaches aren't enough. You have to address the infections in order to get well.

What is Energy Testing?

Energy testing is a means for determining what is going on inside your body, and which treatments your body needs. While energy testing isn't something I've chosen to explain thoroughly in this book, I strongly believe that it is a useful tool in the recovery process, and I encourage you to learn more about it and pursue it. I've spoken with many Lyme sufferers who say they wouldn't be well if it weren't for energy testing.

Focus on Sustainability in your Treatment Program

Because Lyme disease typically requires months or years to recover from, it is very difficult to sustain ongoing treatments which are cost-prohibitive and highly inconvenient, or which require extensive travel. Build a sustainable treatment program. Try to preserve your financial health as much as possible. Many treatments which are administered at physicians' offices can be used elsewhere, or even in the privacy of your own home, for a fraction of the cost. Try to focus on the long haul. Intensive programs at specialized clinics can drain your bank account but only provide temporary remission of symptoms. It is the sustainable treatments which lead to ongoing improvement.

To drive this point home, here is a conversation I had with a friend via text messaging. This friend is a very important, high-ranking medical official, and even he was at a loss for how to handle Lyme disease.

> **Friend**: *Hello Bryan. Hope you have had a great Christmas season. Do you know if the [expensive medical clinic in city XYZ] has a good reputation for treatment of Lyme disease? Or is there a better center within driving distance you'd recommend? I have a friend whose husband is suffering from Lyme disease. Thanks and best wishes!*

> **My response**: *First of all, please note that I am not a doctor, so I can't offer you medical advice. However, I'll do what I can to share what I know. This is a complex question. I spent $15,000 at the clinic you mention back in 2002. I spent that in 10 days! It was an intensive program. It didn't work. It made me feel better for a little while. The reason it didn't work is that any successful Lyme treatment MUST be done for long periods of time (except in early Lyme, when an adequate course of antibiotics may be effective). In long standing Lyme, treatments must be long term and therefore, expensive fancy clinics are impractical. Several months after I left that clinic, I still had my Lyme disease but I didn't have my $15,000 anymore, which limited the treatment options I could pursue later. Home based treatments which can be managed by a local or remote doctor are the best options. This is true regardless of whether you choose pharmaceutical or alternative means. By the way, the CDC this summer upped their estimated number of new Lyme cases per year from 20k/yr to 300k/yr!*

I'm not sure if my friend listened to my thoughts or not, but I hope he at least considered them. Money is usually limited when debilitated by Lyme disease, so it should only be spent carefully, on sustainable treatment programs which provide long-term results.

Don't Overlook the Importance of Exercise

You really can't expect to get better if you don't exercise. Even if only a small amount of exercise can be tolerated, it is better than nothing. Exercise is critically important to the recovery process for many reasons. It helps detoxification, keeps muscle tone, stimulates the production of hormones, and allows the body to renew itself. There's no substitute for exercise. Cardiovascular exercise should be undertaken with caution for those who are very sick. Resistance training provides many benefits and is often more tolerable, especially to those with adrenal issues.

Lyme Disease and Brain Healing

Lyme disease can have incredibly diverse effects on the brains of different people. Some people notice difficulty thinking, remembering things, and calling up vocabulary words. Other people experience extreme emotional volatility. And, of course, many people experience all of the above. It shouldn't surprise us that this kind of brain dysfunction occurs. After all, the brain is a physical organ, and when it is damaged, it can malfunction, just like all of our other organs. It is for this reason that it is so sad to see Lyme sufferers (and others with mental illness) persecuted as if their brain dysfunction was somehow related to their character. Psychosomatic issues are often no more voluntary than an upset stomach.

But you probably already know all of this. What you may know less about are the mechanisms behind the roller coaster ride you experience as your brain heals from Lyme disease. You don't just wake up one morning with a normal brain. As you get better, brain functions come back online in fits and starts, and the whole experience can be quite bizarre. I recall a time during the year 2004 when I started having crazy flashbacks to the time and place when I first got sick. I would wake up in the middle of the night and literally believe that I was living in the house I had lived in when I got Lyme disease. I could smell the old carpet, I could hear the sounds, I could sense the layout of the house. Only, I wasn't actually in that old house, it was just a flashback. I believe my brain was associating the newfound health it was experiencing with the last time it had experienced that health when I lived in the previous home. Strange, indeed.

Something else that can happen as your brain recovers: the brain can end up in a kind of no-man's land. At some point, the brain may actually have the capacity to recover but it will not do so without help. This is why people who have experienced traumatic brain injury require therapy in order to regain the mental functions they have lost. The brain can recover, but it needs training. Learning new things, doing puzzles, reading books, and engaging in other mentally challenging activities can speed the process of recovery.

Interestingly, emotions may need to be retrained just like other mental functions. It can be important to remind yourself how you used to feel about life, certain activities, and even yourself. This is one of the reasons why I believe it is so difficult for people to recover from mental illnesses which they have had since birth, such as autism. These people don't have a past frame of reference from which to rebuild their sense of normal. They can't remind themselves of what normal felt like, and they can't choose to embrace normal feelings while rejecting unhealthy feelings. Those of us who got sick later in life have the advantage that we know what we are trying to return to; we know what it was like to feel normal. Accordingly, we can train our brains to go in the right direction.

An easy way to remind your brain of what normal feels like is to start participating in activities that you used to love before you got sick. Allow yourself to become immersed in these activities, and gently open the door for past emotions to come rushing back into your consciousness. I think this is one big reason why I enjoy mountain biking so much (that's me on the cover of the book!). Before I got sick with Lyme disease, mountain biking was an emotional lifeline for me; it cleared my mind and renewed my spirit. After having had Lyme disease, I found that mountain biking was actually more than just a fun hobby—it was like therapy, training my brain to start to work like it had worked before the disease. Some of my mental and emotional healing came not from Lyme treatments, but from activities like this, which reminded my brain to start working again like it had worked before.

Practicing normal brain function may cause headaches and discomfort because you are forcing electrical signals through parts of your brain that have been damaged or dormant for years. If thinking was your weakness when you were sick, try to help your brain to think, but be prepared for some discomfort as your brain turns on areas which haven't been used in a long time. Likewise, if your feelings have been most affected, expect that certain healthy feelings might cause headaches as your brain is used in ways it hasn't been used in years.

The areas where your brain will need the most help will be unique and different from other Lyme sufferers. Your brain may have been hit hardest in a different area than the brain of the Lyme sufferer who sits across from you in your doctor's waiting room.

Many Lyme sufferers notice that getting back in touch with their souls is the last thing they achieve in recovery, and this is why Lyme disease is so hard—the most important healing step doesn't come until the end, which means you have to fight, and live, for years, with your innermost self missing. One of the reasons that this deep sense of self, or soul, may have the hardest time returning is simply that it requires the most fine-tuning and normal functioning inside the brain. Although I am personally a believer in the spiritual side of life, I can still acknowledge that our brains are our window through which we experience our lives and through which we experience the planet around us. If you cut off my leg, I'm still me. If you take away my hands, I'm still me. But if you take away my brain, I'm no longer me. Of course, this kind of conversation can take us down philosophical roads which I will reserve for people who are much smarter than me. The point is that the brain is very important when it comes to how we feel, and the feelings of peace and calm which used to define us before illness won't return until the brain hasn't just healed a small amount, but has healed almost completely. So, patience is required during the final phases of recovery. It takes time for the brain to return to this normal state.

Lastly, top Lyme experts have contended that unresolved emotional conflict can prevent complete brain healing. Although I was skeptical of such a seemingly outlandish claim for a long time, I am now a believer in this concept. The kinds of unresolved conflict you may be holding onto include diverse and broad areas, such as past romantic relationships, perfectionism, guilt, co-dependency, regret, fear, worry, insecurity, and many others. For some reason, these unhealthy feelings and memories become co-mingled with the chronic dysfunction that occurs in the physical brains of Lyme sufferers, and complete healing only occurs when the physical is healed in tandem with the emotional. This is, for sure, one of the most mysterious and fascinating aspects of Lyme disease recovery. However, again, it shouldn't really surprise us, because we know that the brain is a complex and delicate organ that controls how we experience the world around us.

This discussion of brain healing only scratches the surface. It is not intended to be a complete discussion, but I hope that it has provided you with some new perspective on how your brain heals, as well as some tools for a speedier recovery.

Why We Can't Find Simple Solutions to the Problem of Lyme Disease

This is a topic which we've addressed various times throughout the book, but I want to make some final comments on the problem of Lyme disease, and why it is so difficult to cure.

Many minor ailments can easily be healed with simple solutions. For example, blurry vision can be taken care of with prescription glasses, so the person with blurry vision never seeks deeper healing and correction of lifestyle issues or other problems. While obesity can be a stubborn problem, diet and exercise work in many cases of obesity, so the problem of obesity can be treated without a deep understanding of why the interventions are working. A bruised knee is another example of a problem we know how to deal with, and which has a straightforward solution.

Lyme disease is much different. To really recover you have to heal deeply, and this requires a huge paradigm shift that impacts all parts of your life including your work, diet, recreation, finances, emotional outlook, priorities, and more. OK, so you've heard me say these things already, but why are they true and important?

One of the reasons that Lyme disease requires such deep healing is that this disease takes advantage of deep weaknesses in your physical being and your mental state. Each of us have different weaknesses due to our genetics, experiences, and environment. Tick-borne infections take up residence in the parts of our bodies that are the weakest. Therefore, we won't get completely well until we address these weaknesses. Yet, these weaknesses can be the most difficult health challenges we have, because they have been in the making for decades of our lives. It has taken a lifetime for the weaknesses to manifest, so it can take a lifetime, or at least a long time, for them to be healed.

And, before we can even begin to address these weaknesses, we have to stop them from progressing further. We have to halt whatever conditions were present to cause them to happen. And since these conditions can infiltrate our entire lives, they can be very difficult to reverse. We aren't talking about what brand of pants we wear, we are talking about deep factors which include how we think, how we live, what we eat, where we live, which activities we pursue, which toxins we are exposed to, and which genetic issues we've been given by our ancestors. We are even talking about our emotional, spiritual, and mental challenges and how those have affected our health over the years.

Consider this example. Imagine an out-of-control car speeding down a hill. It is your job to safely bring that car to a stop, and then get it back up the hill where it came from. You will have many tasks to do in order to get it slowed down and going back up the hill, including the following steps:

1. You have to stop it from continuing to accelerate. Your body or environment or both, for whatever reason, predispose you to getting worse, not better, in terms of infections and toxicities. You have to arrest this trend of worsening. This stops our out-of-control car from accelerating further.

2. Once you have arrested the worsening, you actually have to start doing things that get you better. This starts slowing the car down. The car won't actually stop until you are doing as much to get better as you are to get worse.

3. Once you have gotten the car to a complete stop, you have to start using treatments, lifestyle changes, and healing approaches which outweigh the negative physical, mental and genetic influences in your life. If you can accomplish this, the car will start reversing its course and moving back up the hill. And things now become even harder since these changes must become permanent; if they are temporary, the car can start to backslide. Hence, you have to make lasting and deep changes to almost every aspect of your life.

4. As you push the car back up the hill, the challenges change as you encounter different layers of the onion, and if you don't adapt, the car can easily slip and start sliding down again.

Yes, I can acknowledge that our healing journeys aren't perfectly represented in this car analogy. The car example is just intended to illustrate that the recovery process is challenging and requires sustained discipline and effort. It also requires deep understanding, and a willingness to explore mental and spiritual issues. It is much more involved than healing a bruise, correcting poor vision, or dieting and exercising. And this is why there are no simple solutions to the problem of Lyme disease.

Also, in order to get well you have to use the right treatments at the right times and avoid the wrong treatments. The right treatments are often obscure, not commonplace, not known to most health care practitioners (and remember, you don't usually have health care practitioners on your side anyway, which is why it is so important to have a good Lyme doctor!). The victim of a broken leg (a relatively simple health problem) being treated at a local hospital has access to the best medical resources commanded by the best doctors and facilities, all targeted at helping him or her. In contrast, the victim of Lyme disease (a complex and deeply rooted health problem) often has very few, overworked medical professionals helping him or her, and often requires little-understood, complex treatment modalities administered in the proper chronological order and with accurate monitoring. Here you see another reason why simple answers to the problem of Lyme disease are elusive.

Lastly, another difference between Lyme disease and many other common health problems is that acute illness and trauma screams loudly, "Here I am, I need to be fixed now." These acute problems are easily found on tests, and their consequences are clear and defined. So, the best and brightest minds in medicine are waiting for you to arrive at the hospital or doctor's office as you seek help for something like a broken leg, pneumonia, or a heart attack.

Chronic illness on the other hand whispers softly, "I'm confusing, I'm not easy to test for, I'm not easy to fix, no two cases of me are alike, my existence may be due in part to socially acceptable activities like overconsumption of sugar or living near electromagnetic radiation, my cure isn't commonly found in Western Medicine, I may require a couple dozen interventions to be healed, and improvement in my symptoms may take weeks, months, or years to see." Lyme disease further whispers, "My cause is elusive bacteria which are hard to test for and diagnose and which may survive antibiotic therapy, rendering me a stealthy, poorly understood problem that most doctors will overlook or even deny exists."

See the difference? The odds are stacked against Lyme disease patients in almost every possible way.

Please note that I am not continuing to talk about the difficulty in healing from Lyme disease to discourage my readers. Instead, I talk about this so that Lyme disease might gain the attention and alarm that it deserves, and so that those who suffer from it can be given the compassion and help that they deserve. It is quite possible that throughout all of medical history, there's never been another disease which has been subject to this level of disparity between the seriousness of the disease and the seriousness of the medical response. On a scale from 1 to 10, Lyme disease is a 10 in terms of the devastation it is inflicting on society. Yet, to date, the urgency put forth by the medical community to find a solution to Lyme disease has been a 1 on a scale from 1 to 10. It's time to educate the world about Lyme disease, and change this disparity. Lyme disease demands the best that medicine has to offer. It is do or die. Those suffering from this disease need the truth to be known.

Feeling Good Can be a Delicate Condition

Early in the recovery process, you are so sick that your body can rarely, or never, maintain equilibrium, and therefore, you feel bad most or all of the time. It may even seem like doing the right things doesn't matter: you can eat gluten-free and sugar-free, get enough rest, and do all the right things, and you always feel bad. So why bother? During this phase of recovery, your only consolation will be this: there is a light at the end of the tunnel, and you are getting closer to it!

When you finally get close to the light at the end of the tunnel, the experience changes. Eventually, as your body becomes less burdened by infections and toxins, it will be within your control to feel better more and more often. All of those lifestyle choices that seemed to have no impact, will start to have impact. By making healthy choices and staying away from the things that make you feel bad, you'll be able to feel good much of the time. In this way, feeling good is possible, but it can be a delicate condition. It is easy at this point to lapse back into feeling poorly, if you don't do what it takes to help your body maintain its newfound yet delicate equilibrium.

The moral of the story here is that self control will keep you feeling good. Avoiding sugary desserts, getting enough sleep, and making other good decisions—these aren't easy challenges. But succeeding in these challenges is worth it, because feeling healthy is so much more rewarding than the temporary indulgences that can throw you off track.

Where to Buy Supplements

I think it is important to save as much time, energy and money as possible when recovering from Lyme disease, so that these precious resources can be reserved for essential applications during the recovery process. Purchasing supplements online usually saves time because you aren't driving to and from stores, and money because online prices often beat prices of brick-and-mortar stores.

You can also read user reviews for supplements online, to make sure you are buying the best brands. The websites I prefer due to their abundant user reviews, low prices, and speedy shipping, are Amazon.com and iHerb.com. At the time of the writing of this book, I recommend an Amazon Prime membership which entitles you to free 2-day shipping. If you need a supplement fast, 2-day shipping can really make the online purchasing option realistic, whereas a 5-7 day shipping window would be impractical.

Lastly, purchasing supplements online can give you access to a broad selection. Local stores are limited to carrying hundreds or thousands of products while online stores can offer hundreds of thousands or millions of choices.

Who is the Best Lyme Doctor? What is the Best Lyme Treatment?

I can't count the number of times I get asked these questions. There are no simple answers to these questions. Let's start with the "best Lyme doctor." Of the many great Lyme doctors, each treats Lyme slightly (or dramatically) differently. For example, doctor A may use lots of antibiotics, while doctor B may use lots of herbs, and doctor C might do lots of hormone testing. Well, if a person has a lot of messed up hormones, doctor C would be best. If a person can't tolerate pharmaceutical antibiotics, but has a high infection load that is susceptible to herbs, doctor B would be best. And if a person has a high tolerance for pharmaceutical drugs, maybe doctor A would offer a fast track to recovery. So, yet again, we come down to the individual and unique needs of Lyme patients. The actual best doctor for you is the doctor who can best address your specific health challenges. This is another reason why it's so important to pay close attention to your body. You won't be able to identify the "best doctor" for you if you don't know what your unique challenges are!

The same logic can be applied to the "best Lyme treatment" question. Can you tolerate pharmaceuticals? Are your main problems infections, or other underlying issues? Does your body need to be rebuilt, or inundated with anti-infective treatments? Which co-infections do you have? Which have already been treated? What genetic weaknesses and strengths do you have? The "best treatment" will be different depending on your answers to these questions. And, just like we saw in the previous paragraph, paying attention to your body and discovering how your unique situation differs from the situations of other Lyme sufferers, is the first step to identifying which treatments will be best for you.

This logic is the core philosophy of this book. Instead of writing a book which provides endless details on the thousands of available treatment options, I've decided to write a book which provides strategies for developing a unique treatment protocol that's right for you.

Keeping up with the Latest Lyme Disease Treatment Information

Because Lyme disease information is changing so rapidly, I will start sharing future treatment updates in a newsletter instead of in books (as long as my audience—you—provide feedback that this change in format is acceptable...initial survey results indicate that many of my readers are excited to receive more frequent updates from me in newsletter form).

Even if you already receive my email newsletter, you will not automatically be subscribed to my new, subscription-based treatment updates which will contain my latest research and findings. If you would like to subscribe to the new updates, please visit:

www.lymebook.com/updates

In the future, I will be putting a great deal of time and energy into bringing you breaking news on new, cutting-edge treatments, via this newsletter, so be sure to check it out!

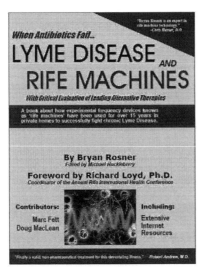

Book • $35

When Antibiotics Fail: Lyme Disease And Rife Machines, With Critical Evaluation Of Leading Alternative Therapies

By Bryan Rosner
Foreword by Richard Loyd, Ph.D.

There are enough books and websites about what Lyme disease is and which ticks carry it. But there is very little useful information for people who actually have a case of Lyme disease that is not responding to conventional antibiotic treatment. Lyme disease sufferers need to know their options, not how to identify a tick.

This book describes how experimental electromagnetic frequency devices known as rife machines have been used for over 15 years in private homes to fight Lyme disease. Also included are evaluations of more than 25 conventional and alternative Lyme disease therapies, including:

- Homeopathy
- IV and oral antibiotics
- Mercury detox.
- Hyperthermia / saunas
- Ozone and oxygen
- Samento®
- Colloidal Silver
- Bacterial die-off detox.
- Colostrum
- Magnesium supplementation
- Hyperbaric oxygen chamber (HBOC)
- ICHT Italian treatment
- Non-pharmaceutical antibiotics
- Exercise, diet and candida protocols
- Cyst-targeting antibiotics
- The Marshall Protocol®

Many Lyme disease sufferers have heard of rife machines, some have used them. But until now, there has not been a concise and organized source to explain how and why they have been used by Lyme patients. In fact, this is the first book ever published on this important topic.

The Foreword for the book is by Richard Loyd, Ph.D., coordinator of the annual Rife International Health Conference. The book takes a practical, down-to-earth approach which allows you to learn about*:

> "This book provides life-saving insights for Lyme disease patients."
>
> **- Richard Loyd, Ph.D.**

- Antibiotic treatment problems and shortcomings—why some people choose to use rife machines after other therapies fail.
- Hypothetical treatment schedules and sessions, based on the author's experience.
- The experimental machines with the longest track record: High Power Magnetic Pulser, EMEM Machine, Coil Machine, and AC Contact Machine.
- Explanation of the "herx reaction" and why it may indicate progress.
- The intriguing story that led to the use of rife machines to fight Lyme disease 20 years ago.
- Antibiotic categories and classifications, with pros and cons of each type of drug.
- Visit our website to read FREE EXCERPTS from the book!

Disclaimer: *Your treatment decisions must be made under the care of a licensed physician. Rife machines are not FDA approved and the FDA has not reviewed or approved of these books. The author is a layperson, not a doctor, and much of the content of these books is a statement of opinion based on the author's personal experience and research.*

Paperback book, 8.5 x 11", 203 pages, $35

The Top 10 Lyme Disease Treatments: Defeat Lyme Disease With The Best Of Conventional And Alternative Medicine

By Bryan Rosner
Foreword by James Schaller, M.D.

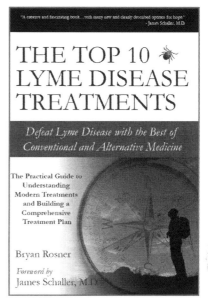

"A concise and fascinating book...with many new and clearly described options for hope."
- James Schaller, M.D.

THE TOP 10 🦟
LYME DISEASE
TREATMENTS

Defeat Lyme Disease with the Best of
Conventional and Alternative Medicine

The Practical Guide to
Understanding
Modern Treatments
and Building a
Comprehensive
Treatment Plan

Bryan Rosner

Foreword by
James Schaller, M.D.

Book • $35

This information-packed book identifies ten promising conventional and alternative Lyme disease treatments and gives practical guidance on integrating them into a comprehensive treatment plan that you and your physician can customize for your individual situation and needs.

The book was not written to replace Bryan Rosner's first book (*Lyme Disease and Rife Machines*, opposing page). It was written to complement that book, offering Lyme sufferers many new foundational and supportive treatment options, based on the author's extensive research and years of personal experience. Topics include*:

- Systemic enzyme therapy, which helps detoxify tissues and blood, reduce inflammation, stimulate the immune system, and kill Lyme disease bacteria.
- Lithium orotate, a powerful yet all-natural mineral (belonging to the same mineral group as sodium and potassium) capable of profound neuroprotective activity.
- Thorough and extensive coverage of a complete Lyme disease detoxification program, including discussion of both liver and skin detoxification pathways. Specific detoxification therapies such as liver cleanses, bowel cleanses, the Shoemaker Neurotoxin Elimination Protocol, sauna therapy, mineral baths, mineral supplementation, milk thistle, and many others. Ideas to reduce and control herx reactions.
- Tips and clinical research from James Schaller, M.D.
- A detailed look at one method for utilizing antibiotics during a rife machine treatment campaign.
- Wide coverage of the Marshall Protocol, including an in-depth discussion of its mechanism of action in relation to Lyme disease pathology. Also, the author's personal experience with the Marshall Protocol over 3 years.
- An explanation of and new information about the Salt / Vitamin C protocol.
- Hot-off-the-press information on mangosteen fruit (not to be confused with mango) and its many benefits, including antibacterial, anti-inflammatory, and anti-cancer properties.
- New guidelines for combining all the therapies discussed in both of Rosner's books into a complete treatment plan. Brief and articulate for consideration by you and your doctor.
- Also includes updates on rife therapy, cutting-edge supplements, political challenges, an exclusive interview with Willy Burgdorfer, Ph.D. (discoverer of Lyme), and much more!

"Bryan Rosner thinks big and this new book offers big solutions."
- James Schaller, M.D.

"Another ground-breaking Lyme Disease book."
- Jeff Mittelman, moderator of the Lyme-and-rife group

"Brilliant and thorough."
- Nenah Sylver, Ph.D.

Do not miss this top Lyme disease resource. Discover new healing tools today! Bring this book to your doctor's appointment to help with forming a treatment plan.

Paperback book, 7 x 10", 367 pages, $35

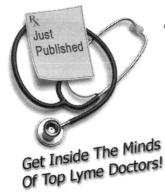

Get Inside The Minds Of Top Lyme Doctors!

13 Lyme Doctors Share Treatment Strategies!

In this new book, not one, but thirteen Lyme-literate healthcare practitioners describe the tools they use in their practices to heal patients from chronic Lyme disease. Never before available in book format!

**Insights Into Lyme Disease Treatment:
13 Lyme Literate Health Care Practitioners
Share Their Healing Strategies**

**By Connie Strasheim
Foreword by Maureen Mcshane, M.D.**

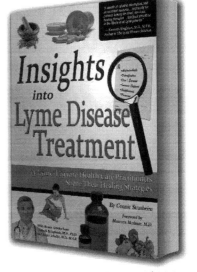

If you traveled the country for appointments with 13 Lyme-literate health care practitioners, you would discover many cutting-edge therapies used to combat chronic Lyme disease. You would also spend thousands of dollars on hotels, plane tickets, and medical appointment fees—not to mention the time it would take to embark on such a journey.

Even if you had the time and money to travel, would the physicians have enough time to answer all of your questions? Would you even know which questions to ask?

Paperback • 443 Pages • $39.95

In this long-awaited book, health care journalist and Lyme patient Connie Strasheim has done all the work for you. She conducted intensive interviews with 13 of the world's most competent Lyme disease healers, asking them thoughtful, important questions, and then spent months compiling their information into 13 organized, user-friendly chapters that contain the core principles upon which they base their medical treatment of chronic Lyme disease. The practitioners' backgrounds span a variety of disciplines, including allopathic, naturopathic, complementary, chiropractic, homeopathic, and energy medicine. All aspects of treatment are covered, from anti-microbial remedies and immune system support, to hormonal restoration, detoxification, and dietary/lifestyle choices. **PHYSICIANS INTERVIEWED:**

- Steven Bock, M.D.
- Ginger Savely, DNP
- Ronald Whitmont, M.D.
- Nicola McFadzean, N.D.
- Jeffrey Morrison, M.D.
- Steven J. Harris, M.D.
- Peter J. Muran, M.D., M.B.A.

- Ingo D. E. Woitzel, M.D.
- Susan L. Marra, M.S., N.D.
- W. Lee Cowden, M.D., M.D. (H)
- Deborah Metzger, Ph.D., M.D.
- Marlene Kunold, "Heilpraktiker"
- Elizabeth Hesse-Sheehan, DC, CCN
- Visit our website to read a <u>FREE CHAPTER</u>!

Paperback book, 7 x 10", 443 pages, $39.95

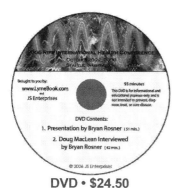

DVD • $24.50

Rife International Health Conference Feature-Length DVD (93 Minutes)

Bryan Rosner's Presentation and Interview with Doug MacLean

The Official Rife Technology Seminar Seattle, WA, USA

If you have been unable to attend the Rife International Health Conference, this DVD is your opportunity to watch two very important Lyme-related presentations from the event:

Presentation #1: Bryan Rosner's Sunday morning talk entitled *Lyme Disease: New Paradigms in Diagnosis and Treatment - the Myths, the Reality, and the Road Back to Health*. (51 minutes)

Presentation #2: Bryan Rosner's interview with Doug MacLean, in which Doug talked about his experiences with Lyme disease, including the incredible journey he undertook to invent the first modern rife machine used to fight Lyme disease. Although Doug's journey as a Lyme disease pioneer took place 20 years ago, this was the first time Doug has ever accepted an invitation to appear in public. This is the only video available where you can see Doug talk about what it was like to be the first person ever to use rife technology as a treatment for Lyme disease. Now you can see how it all began. Own this DVD and own a piece of history! (42 minutes)

Lymebook.com has secured a special licensing agreement with JS Enterprises, the Canadian producer of the Rife Conference videos, to bring this product to you at the special low price of $24.50. Total DVD viewing time: 1 hour, 33 minutes. We have DVDs in stock, shipped to you within 3 business days.

Price Comparison (should you get the DVD?)

Cost of attending the recent Rife Conference (2 people):
Hotel Room, 3 Nights = $400
Registration = $340
Food = $150
Airfare = $600
Total = $1,490

Cost of the DVD, which you can view as many times as you want, and show to family and friends:
DVD = $24.50

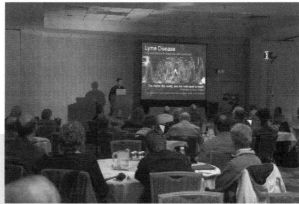

Bryan Rosner
Presenting on
Sunday Morning
In Seattle

DVD
93 Minutes
$24.50

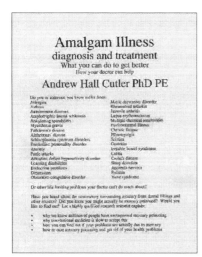

Amalgam Illness
diagnosis and treatment
What you can do to get better
How your doctor can help

Andrew Hall Cutler PhD PE

Book • $35

Amalgam Illness, Diagnosis and Treatment: What You Can Do to Get Better, How Your Doctor Can Help

By Andrew Cutler, PhD

This book was written by a chemical engineer who himself got mercury poisoning from his amalgam dental fillings. He found that there was no suitable educational material for either the patient or the physician. Knowing how much people can suffer from this condition, he wrote this book to help them get well. With a PhD in chemistry from Princeton University and extensive study in biochemistry and medicine, Andrew Cutler uses layman's terms to explain how people become mercury poisoned and what to do about it. The author's research shows that mercury poisoning can easily be cured at home with over-the-counter oral chelators – this book explains how.

In the book you will find practical guidance on how to tell if you really have chronic mercury poisoning or some other problem. Proper diagnostic procedures are provided so that sick people can decide what is wrong rather than trying random treatments. If mercury poisoning is your problem, the book tells you how to get the mercury out of your body, and how to feel good while you do that. The treatment section gives step-by-step directions to figure out exactly what mercury is doing to you and how to fix it.

"Dr. Cutler uses his background in chemistry to explain the safest approach to treat mercury poisoning. I am a physician and am personally using his protocol on myself."

- Melissa Myers, M.D.

Sections also explain how the scientific literature shows many people must be getting poisoned by their amalgam fillings, why such a regulatory blunder occurred, and how the debate between "mainstream" and "alternative" medicine makes it more difficult for you to get the medical help you need.

This down-to-earth book lets patients take care of themselves. It also lets doctors who are not familiar with chronic mercury intoxication treat it. The book is a practical guide to getting well. Sections from the book include:

- Why worry about mercury poisoning?
- What mercury does to you – symptoms, laboratory test irregularities, diagnostic checklist.
- How to treat mercury poisoning easily with oral chelators.
- Dealing with other metals including copper, arsenic, lead, cadmium.
- Dietary and supplement guidelines.
- Balancing hormones during the recovery process.
- How to feel good while you are chelating the metals out.
- How heavy metals cause infections to thrive in the body.
- Politics and mercury.

This is the world's most authoritative, accurate book on mercury poisoning.

Paperback book, 8.5 x 11", 226 pages, $35

Hair Test Interpretation: Finding Hidden Toxicities

By Andrew Cutler, PhD

Hair tests are worth doing because a surprising number of people diagnosed with incurable chronic health conditions actually turn out to have a heavy metal problem; quite often, mercury poisoning. Heavy metal problems can be corrected. Hair testing allows the underlying problem to be identified – and the chronic health condition often disappears with proper detoxification.

Hair Test Interpretation: Finding Hidden Toxicities is a practical book that explains how to interpret **Doctor's Data, Inc.** and **Great Plains Laboratory** hair tests. A step-by-step discussion is provided, with figures to illustrate the process and make it easy. The book gives examples using actual hair test results from real people.

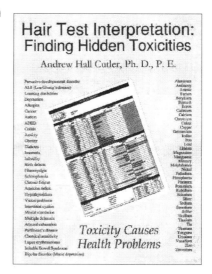

Book • $35

One of the problems with hair testing is that both conventional and alternative health care providers do not know how to interpret these tests. Interpretation is not as simple as looking at the results and assuming that any mineral out of the reference range is a problem mineral.

Interpretation is complicated because heavy metal toxicity, especially mercury poisoning, interferes with mineral transport throughout the body. Ironically, if someone is mercury poisoned, hair test mercury is often low and other minerals may be elevated or take on unusual values. For example, mercury often causes retention of arsenic, antimony, tin, titanium, zirconium, and aluminum. An inexperienced health care provider may wrongfully assume that one of these other minerals is the culprit, when in reality mercury is the true toxicity.

> "This new book of Andrew's is the definitive guide in the confusing world of heavy metal poisoning diagnosis and treatment. I'm a practicing physician, 20 years now, specializing in detoxification programs for treatment of resistant conditions. It was fairly difficult to diagnose these heavy metal conditions before I met Andrew Cutler and developed a close relationship with him while reading his books. In this book I found his usual painful attention to detail gave a solid framework for understanding the complexity of mercury toxicity as well as the less common exposures. You really couldn't ask for a better reference book on a subject most researchers and physicians are still fumbling in the dark about."
> **- Dr. Rick Marschall**

So, as you can see, getting a hair test is only the first step. The second step is figuring out what the hair test means. Andrew Cutler, PhD, is a registered professional chemical engineer with years of experience in biochemical and healthcare research. This clear and concise book makes hair test interpretation easy, so that you know which toxicities are causing your health problems.

Paperback book, 8.5 x 11", 298 pages, $35

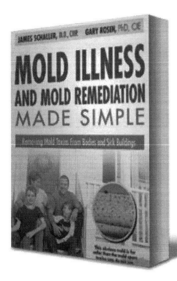

Book • $32.95

Mold Illness and Mold Remediation Made Simple: Removing Mold Toxins from Bodies and Sick Buildings

By James Schaller, M.D. and Gary Rosen, Ph.D.

Indoor mold toxins are much more dangerous and prevalent than most people realize. Visible mold in and around your house is far less dangerous than the mold you cannot see. Indoor mold toxicity, in addition to causing its own unique set of health problems and symptoms, also greatly contributes to the severity of most chronic illnesses.

In this book, a top physician and experienced contractor team up to help you quickly recover from indoor mold exposure. This book is easy to read with many color photographs and illustrations.

Paperback book, 8.5 x 11", 140 pages, $32.95
Also available on our website as an eBook!

Go online to **www.LymeBook.com** to learn more about these new books, just released!

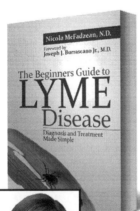

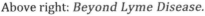

Don't miss these great new resources by authors Connie Strasheim and Nicola McFadzean, ND. Above left: *The Beginner's Guide to Lyme Disease.* Above right: *Beyond Lyme Disease.*

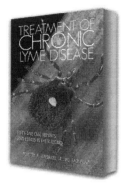

Book • $24.95

Treatment of Chronic Lyme Disease: 51 Case Reports and Essays In Their Regard

By Burton Waisbren Sr., MD, FACP, FIDSA

DON'T MISS THIS BOOK! A MUST-HAVE RESOURCE. What sets this Lyme disease book apart are the credentials of its author: he is not only a Fellow of the Infectious Diseases Society of America (IDSA), he is also one of its Founders! With 57+ years experience in medicine, Dr. Waisbren passionately argues for the validity of chronic Lyme disease and presents useful information about 51 cases of the disease which he has personally treated. His position is in stark contrast to that of the IDSA, which is a very powerful organization. **Quite possibly the most important book ever published on Lyme disease, as a result of the author's experience and credentials.**

Paperback book, 6x9", 169 pages, $24.95

**Bartonella:
Diagnosis and Treatment**

By James Schaller, M.D.

2 Book Set • $99.95

As an addition to his growing collection of informative books, Dr. James Schaller penned this excellent 2-part volume on Bartonella, a Lyme disease co-infection. The set is an ideal complementary resource to his Babesia textbook (next page).

Bartonella infections occur throughout the entire world, in cities, suburbs, and rural locations. It is found in fleas, dust mites, ticks, lice, flies, cat and dog saliva, and insect feces.

This 2-book set provides advanced treatment strategies as well as detailed diagnostic criteria, with dozens of full-color illustrations and photographs.

Both books in this 2-part set are included with your order.

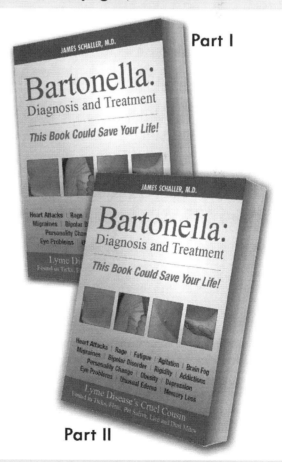

Part I

Part II

2 paperback books included, 7 x 10", 500 pages, $99.95

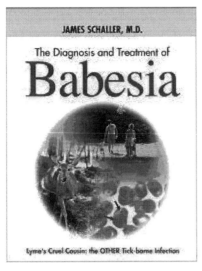

JAMES SCHALLER, M.D.

The Diagnosis and Treatment of

Babesia

Lyme's Cruel Cousin: the OTHER Tick-borne Infection

Book • $55

The Diagnosis and Treatment of Babesia: Lyme's Cruel Cousin – The Other Tick-Borne Infection

By James Schaller, M.D.

Do you or a loved one experience excess fatigue? Have you ever had unusually high fevers, chills, or sweats? You may have Babesia, a very common tick-borne infection. Babesia is often found with Lyme disease and, like all tick-borne infections, is rarely diagnosed and reported accurately.

The deer tick which carries Lyme disease and Babesia may be as small as a poppy seed and injects a painkiller, an antihistamine, and an anticoagulant to avoid detection. As a result, many people have Babesia and do not know it. Numerous forms of Babesia are carried by ticks. This book introduces patients and health care workers to the various species that infect humans and are not routinely tested for by sincere physicians.

Dr. Schaller, who practices medicine in Florida, first became interested in Babesia after one of his own children was infected with it. None of the elite pediatricians or child specialists could help. No one tested for Babesia or considered it a possible diagnosis. His child suffered from just two of these typical Babesia symptoms:

- Significant Fatigue
- Coughing
- Dizziness
- Trouble Thinking
- Fevers
- Memory Loss

- Chills
- Air Hunger
- Headache
- Sweats
- Unresponsiveness to Lyme Treatment

With 374 pages, this book is the most current and comprehensive book on Babesia in the English language. It reviews thousands of articles and presents the results of interviews with world experts on the subject. It offers you top information and broad treatment options, presented in a clear and simple manner. All treatments are explained thoroughly, including their possible side effects, drug interactions, various dosing strategies, pros/cons, and physician experiences.

"Once again Dr. Schaller has provided us with a much-needed and practical resource. This book gave me exactly what I was looking for."

- Thomas W., Patient

Finally, the book also addresses many other aspects of practical medical care often overlooked in this infection, such as treatment options for managing fatigue. Plainly stated, this book is a must-have for patients and health care providers who deal with Lyme disease and its co-infections. Dr. Schaller's many years in clinical practice give the book a practical angle that many other similar books lack. Don't miss this user-friendly resource!

Paperback book, 7 x 10", 374 pages, $55
Also available on our website as an eBook!

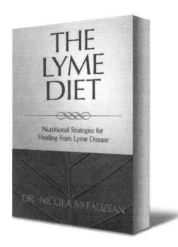

Book • $24.95

The Lyme Diet: Nutritional Strategies for Healing from Lyme Disease

By Nicola McFadzean, N.D.

We know about antibiotics and herbs. But what is the right diet for Lyme sufferers? Now you can read about the experience of Dr. Nicola McFadzean, N.D., in treating Lyme patients using proper diet.

The author is a Naturopathic Doctor and graduate of Bastyr University in Seattle, Washington. She is currently in private practice at her clinic, RestorMedicine, located in San Diego, California.

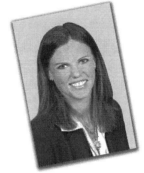

Nicola McFadzean, N.D.

This book covers numerous topics (not just diet-related):

- Reducing and controlling inflammation
- Maximizing immune function via dietary choices
- Restoring the gut & regaining healthy digestion
- Detoxification with food

- Hormone imbalances
- Biofilms
- Kefir vs. yogurt vs. probiotics
- Candida, liver support, and much more!

Paperback book, 6x9", 214 Pages, $24.95
Also available as an eBook on our website!

The Stealth Killer: Is Oral Spirochetosis the Missing Link in the Dental & Heart Disease Labyrinth? *By William D. Nordquist, BS, DMD, MS*

Can oral spirochete infections cause heart attacks? In today's cosmopolitan urban population, more than 51 percent of those with root canal–treated teeth probably have infection at the apex of their root. Dr. Nordquist, an oral surgeon practicing in Southern California, believes that any source of bacteria with resulting chronic infection (including periodontal disease) in the mouth may potentially lead to heart disease and other systemic diseases. With more than 40 illustrations and x-ray reproductions, this book takes you behind the scenes in Dr. Nordquist's research laboratory, and provides many tips on dealing with Lyme-related dental problems. A breakthrough book in dentistry & infectious disease!

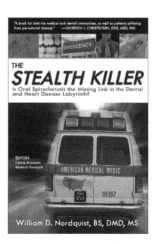

Paperback Book • $25.95

Paperback book, 6x9", 161 pages, $25.95

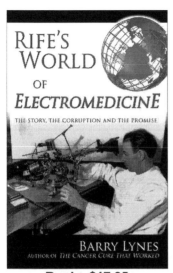

Rife's World of Electromedicine: The Story, the Corruption and the Promise

By Barry Lynes

The cause of cancer was discovered in the early 1930's. It was a virus-sized, mini-bacteria or "particle" that induced cells to become malignant and grow into tumors. The cancer microbe or particle was given the name BX by the brilliant scientist who discovered it: Royal Raymond Rife.

Laboratory verification of the cause of cancer was done hundreds of times with mice in order to be absolutely certain. Five of America's most prominent physicians helped oversee clinical trials managed by a major university's medical school.

Book • $17.95

Sixteen cancer patients were brought by ambulance twice a week to the clinical trial location in La Jolla, California. There they were treated with a revolutionary electromedicine that painlessly, non-invasively destroyed only the cancer-causing microbe or particle named BX. After just three months of this therapy, all patients were diagnosed as clinically cured. Later, the therapy was suppressed and remains so today.

In 1987, Barry Lynes wrote the classic book on Rife history (*The Cancer Cure That Worked*, see catalog page 14). *Rife's World* is the sequel.

Paperback book, 5.5 x 8.5", 90 pages, $17.95

Physicians' Desk Reference (PDR) Books (opposing page)

Most people have heard of *Physicians' Desk Reference* (PDR) books because, for over 60 years, physicians and researchers have turned to PDR for the latest word on prescription drugs.

THOMSON ™

You may not know that Thomson Healthcare, publisher of PDR, offers PDR reference books not only

"I relied heavily on the PDRs during the research phase of writing my books. Without them, my projects would have greatly suffered."

- Bryan Rosner

for drugs, but also for herbal and nutritional supplements. No available books come even close to the amount of information provided in these PDRs—*PDR for Herbal Medicines* weighs 5 lbs and has over 1300 pages, and *PDR for Nutritional Supplements* weighs over 3 lbs and has more than 800 pages.

We carry all three PDRs. Although PDR books are typically used by physicians, we feel that these resources are also essential for people interested in or recovering from chronic disease. For the supplements, herbs, and drugs included in the books, you will find the following information: Pharmacology, description and method of action, available trade names and brands, indications and usage, research summaries, dosage options, history of use, pharmacokinetics, and much more! Worth the money for years of faithful use.

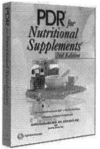

PDR for Nutritional Supplements *2ⁿᵈ Edition!*

This PDR focuses on the following types of supplements:

- Vitamins
- Minerals
- Amino acids
- Hormones
- Lipids
- Glyconutrients
- Probiotics
- Proteins
- Many more!

Book • $69.50

"In a part of the health field not known for its devotion to rigorous science, [this book] brings to the practitioner and the curious patient a wealth of hard facts."

- Roger Guillemin, M.D., Ph.D., Nobel Laureate in Physiology and Medicine

The book also suggests supplements that can help reduce prescription drug side effects, has full-color photographs of various popular commercial formulations (and contact information for the associated suppliers), and so much more! Become educated instead of guessing which supplements to take.

Hardcover book, 11 x 9.3", 800 pages, $69.50

PDR for Herbal Medicines *4ᵗʰ Edition!*

PDR for Herbal Medicines is very well organized and presents information on hundreds of common and uncommon herbs and herbal preparations. Indications and usage are examined with regard to homeopathy, Indian and Chinese medicine, and unproven (yet popular) applications.

In an area of healthcare so unstudied and vulnerable to hearsay and hype, this scientifically referenced book allows you to find out the real story behind the herbs lining the walls of your local health food store.

Use this reference before spending money on herbal products!

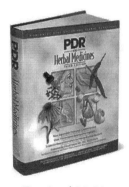

Book • $69.50

Hardcover book, 11 x 9.3", 1300 pages, $69.50

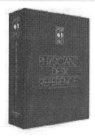

PDR for Prescription Drugs *Current Year's Edition!*

With more than 3,000 pages, this is the most comprehensive and respected book in the world on over 4,000 drugs. Drugs are indexed by both brand and generic name (in the same convenient index) and also by manufacturer and product category. This PDR provides usage information and warnings, drug interactions, plus a detailed, full-color directory with descriptions and cross references for the drugs. A new format allows dramatically improved readability and easier access to the information you need now.

Book • $99.50

Hardcover book, 12.5 x 9.5", 3533 pages, $99.50

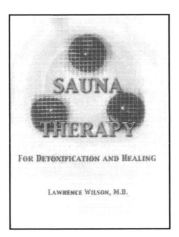

Book • $22.95

Sauna Therapy for Detoxification and Healing

By Lawrence Wilson, MD

This book provides a thorough yet articulate education on sauna therapy. It includes construction plans for a low-cost electric light sauna. The book is well referenced with an extensive bibliography.

Sauna therapy, especially with an electric light sauna, is one of the most powerful, safe and cost-effective methods of natural healing. It is especially important today due to extensive exposure to toxic metals and chemicals.

Fifteen chapters cover sauna benefits, physiological effects, protocols, cautions, healing reactions, and many other aspects of sauna therapy.

Dr. Wilson is an instructor of Biochemistry, Hair Mineral Analysis, Sauna Therapy and Jurisprudence at various colleges and universities including Yamuni Institute of the Healing Arts (Maurice, LA), University of Natural Medicine (Santa Fe, NM), Natural Healers Academy (Morristown, NJ), and Westbrook University (West Virginia). His books are used as textbooks at East-West School of Herbology and Ohio College of Natural Health. Go to www.LymeBook.com for free book excerpts!

Paperback book, 8.5 x 11", 167 pages, $22.95

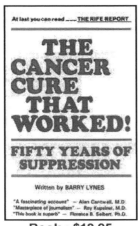

Book • $19.95

Over 50,000 Copies Sold!

The Cancer Cure That Worked: Fifty Years of Suppression

At Last You Can Read... The Rife Report

By Barry Lynes

Investigative journalism at its best. Barry Lynes takes readers on an exciting journey into the life work of Royal Rife. **We are now the official publisher of this book. Call or visit us online for wholesale terms.**

"A fascinating account..." -Alan Cantwell, MD

"This book is superb." -Florence B. Seibert, PhD

"Barry Lynes is one of the greatest health reporters in our country. With the assistance of John Crane, longtime friend and associate of Roy Rife, Barry has produced a masterpiece..." **-Roy Kupsinel, M.D., editor of *Health Consciousness Journal***

Paperback book, 5 x 8", 169 pages, $19.95

Rife Video Documentary
2-DVD Set, Produced by
Zero Zero Two Productions

Must-Have DVD set for your Rife technology education!

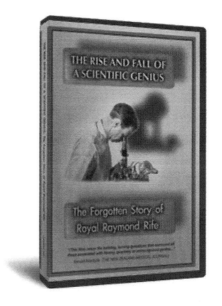

In 1999, a stack of forgotten audio tapes was discovered. On the tapes were the voices of several people at the center of the events which are the subject of this documentary: a revolutionary treatment for cancer and a practical cure for infectious disease.

The audio tapes were over 40 years old. The voices on them had almost faded, nearly losing key details of perhaps the most important medical story of the 20th Century.

But due to the efforts of the Kinnaman Foundation, the faded tapes have been restored and the voices on them recovered. So now, even though the participants have all passed away...

2-DVD Set • $39.95

...they can finally tell their story.

"These videos are great. We show them at the Annual Rife International Health Conference."
-Richard Loyd, Ph.D.

"A mind-shifting experience for those of us indoctrinated with a conventional view of biology."
-Townsend Letter for Doctors and Patients

In the summer of 1934 at a special medical clinic in La Jolla, California, sixteen patients withering from terminal disease were given a new lease on life. It was the first controlled application of a new electronic treatment for cancer: the Beam Ray Machine.

Within ninety days all sixteen patients walked away from the clinic, signed-off by the attending doctors as cured.

What followed the incredible success of this revolutionary treatment was not a welcoming by the scientific community, but a sad tale of its ultimate suppression.

The Rise and Fall of a Scientific Genius documents the scientific ignorance, official corruption, and personal greed directed at the inventor of the Beam Ray Machine, Royal Raymond Rife, forcing him and his inventions out of the spotlight and into obscurity. **Just converted from VHS to DVD and completely updated.**

Includes bonus DVD with interviews and historical photographs! Produced in Canada.

Visit our website today to watch a FREE PREVIEW CLIP!

2 DVD-set, including bonus DVD, $39.95

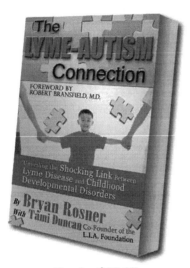

Book • $25.95

The Lyme-Autism Connection: Unveiling the Shocking Link Between Lyme Disease and Childhood Developmental Disorders

By Bryan Rosner & Tami Duncan

Did you know that Lyme disease may contribute to the onset of autism?

This book is an investigative report written by Bryan Rosner and Tami Duncan. Duncan is the co-founder of the *Lyme Induced Autism (LIA) Foundation*, and her son has an autism diagnosis.

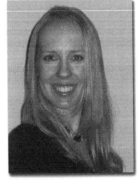

Tami Duncan, Co-Founder of the Lyme Induced Autism (LIA) Foundation

Awareness of the Lyme-autism connection is spreading rapidly, among both parents and practitioners. *Medical Hypothesis*, a scientific, peer-reviewed journal published by Elsevier, recently released an influential study entitled *The Association Between Tick-Borne Infections, Lyme Borreliosis and Autism Spectrum Disorders*. Here is an excerpt from the study:

> *"Chronic infectious diseases, including tick-borne infections such as Borrelia burgdorferi, may have direct effects, promote other infections, and create a weakened, sensitized and immunologically vulnerable state during fetal development and infancy, leading to increased vulnerability for developing autism spectrum disorders. An association between Lyme disease and other tick-borne infections and autistic symptoms has been noted by numerous clinicians and parents."*

—**Medical Hypothesis Journal.**
Article Authors: Robert C. Bransfield, M.D., Jeffrey S. Wulfman, M.D., William T. Harvey, M.D., Anju I. Usman, M.D.

Nationwide, 1 out of 150 children are diagnosed with Autism Spectrum Disorder (ASD), and the LIA Foundation has discovered that many of these children test positive for Lyme disease/Borrelia related complex—yet most children in this scenario never receive appropriate medical attention. This book answers many difficult questions: How can infants contract Lyme disease if autism begins before birth, precluding the opportunity for a tick bite? Is there a statistical correlation between the incidences of Lyme disease and autism worldwide? Do autistic children respond to Lyme disease treatment? What does the medical community say about this connection? Do the mothers of affected children exhibit symptoms? **Find out in this book.**

Paperback book, 6x9", 287 pages, $25.95

Dietrich Klinghardt, M.D., Ph.D.
"Fundamental Teachings"
5-DVD Set

Includes Disc Exclusively For Lyme Disease!

Dietrich Klinghardt, M.D., Ph.D. is a legendary healer known for discovering and refining many of the cutting-edge treatment protocols used for a variety of chronic health problems including Lyme disease, autism and mercury poisoning.

Now you can find out all about this doctor's treatment methods from the privacy of your own home! This 5-DVD set includes the following DVDs:

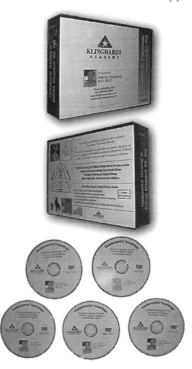

- **DISC 1**: The Five Levels of Healing and the Seven Factors

- **DISC 2**: Autonomic Response Testing and Demonstration

- **DISC 3**: Heavy Metal Toxicity and Neurotoxin Elimination / Electrosmog

- **DISC 4**: Lyme disease and Chronic Illness

- **DISC 5**: Psycho-Emotional Issues in Chronic Illness & Addressing Underlying Causes

5-DVD Set • $125

Dr. Dietrich Klinghardt is one of the most important contributors to modern integrative treatment for Lyme disease and related medical conditions. This comprehensive DVD set is a must-have addition to your educational library.

5-DVD Set, $125

Our catalog has space limitations, but our website does not! Visit www.LymeBook.com to see even more exciting products.

Don't Miss These New Books & DVDs, Available Online:

- Babesia Update 2009, by James Schaller, M.D.
- Marshall Protocol 5-DVD Set
- Cure Unknown, by Pamela Weintraub
- The Experts of Lyme Disease, by Sue Vogan
- The Lyme Disease Solution, by Ken Singleton, M.D.
- **Lots of Free Chapters and Excerpts Online!**

Don't use the internet? No problem, just call (530) 573-0190.

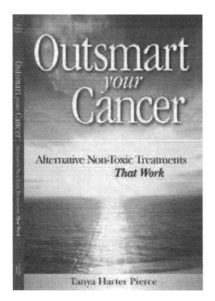

Book and Audio CD • $24.50

Outsmart Your Cancer:
Alternative Non-Toxic Treatments
That Work   By Tanya Harter Pierce

Why BLUDGEON cancer to death with common conventional treatments that can be toxic and harmful to your entire body?

When you OUTSMART your cancer, only the cancer cells die — NOT your healthy cells! *OUTSMART YOUR CANCER: Alternative Non-Toxic Treatments That Work* is an easy guide to successful non-toxic treatments for cancer that you can obtain right now! In it, you will read real-life stories of people who have completely recovered from their advanced or late-stage lung cancer, breast cancer, prostate cancer, kidney cancer, brain cancer, childhood leukemia, and other types of cancer using effective non-toxic approaches.

Plus, *OUTSMART YOUR CANCER* is one of the few books in print today that gives a complete description of the amazing formula called "Protocel," which has produced incredible cancer recoveries over the past 20 years. **A supporting audio CD is included with this book**. Pricing = $19.95 book + $5.00 CD.

Paperback book, 6 x 9", 437 pages, with audio CD, $24.95

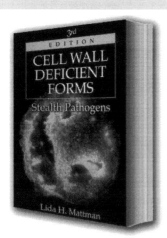

Hardcover Book • $169.95

Cell Wall Deficient Forms: Stealth Pathogens

By Lida Mattman, Ph.D.

This is one of the most influential infectious disease textbook of the century. Dr. Mattman, who earned a Ph.D. in immunology from Yale University, describes her discovery that a certain type of pathogen lacking a cell wall is the root cause of many of today's "incurable" and mysterious chronic diseases. Dr. Mattman's research is the foundation of our current understanding of Lyme disease, and her work led to many of the Lyme protocols used today (such as the Marshall Protocol, as well as modern LLMD antibiotic treatment strategy). Color illustrations and meticulously referenced breakthrough principles cover the pages of this book. A must have for all serious students of chronic, elusive infectious disease.

Hardcover book, 7.5 x 10.5", 416 pages, $169.95

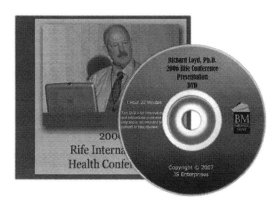

DVD • $24.50

Richard Loyd, Ph.D.,
presents at the Rife
International Health
Conference in Seattle

**Watch this DVD to gain a
better understanding of the
technical details of rife
technology.**

Dr. Loyd, who earned a Ph.D.
in nutrition, has researched and
experimented with numerous
electrotherapeutic devices,
including the Rife/Bare unit,
various EMEM machines, F-Scan,
BioRay, magnetic pulsers, Doug Machine, and more. Dr. Loyd also has a wealth of
knowledge in the use of herbs and supplements to support Rife electromagnetics.

By watching this DVD, you will discover the nuts and bolts of some very
important, yet little known, principles of rife machine operation, including:

- Gating, sweeping, session time
- Square vs. sine wave
- DC vs. AC frequencies
- Duty cycle
- Octaves and scalar octaves

- Voltage variations and radio frequencies
- Explanation of the spark gap
- Contact vs. radiant mode
- Stainless vs. copper contacts
- A unique look at various frequency devices

DVD, 57 minutes, $24.50

Under Our Skin:
Lyme Disease Documentary Film

A gripping tale of microbes,
medicine & money, UNDER OUR SKIN
exposes the hidden story of Lyme
disease, one of the most serious and
controversial epidemics of our time.
Each year, thousands go undiagnosed
or misdiagnosed, often told that their
symptoms are all in their head.
Following the stories of patients and
physicians fighting for their lives and
livelihoods, the film brings into focus a
haunting picture of the health care
system and a medical establishment all
too willing to put profits ahead of patients.

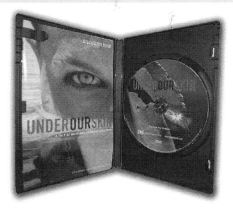

DVD • $34.95

**Bonus Features: 32-page discussion guidebook, one hour of bonus
footage, director's commentary, and much more! FOR HOME USE ONLY**

DVD with bonus features, 104 minutes, $34.95 *MUST SEE!*

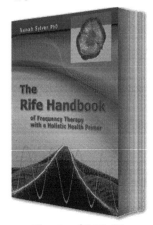

The Rife Handbook of Frequency Therapy, With a Holistic Health Primer

Revised 2011 Edition!   By Nenah Sylver, PhD

This is the most complete, authoritative Rife technology handbook in the world. A hardcover book, it weighs over 2 lbs. and has more than 730 pages. A broad range of practical, hands-on topics are covered:

- New Revised Edition released in 2011 is twice as long as original book! Now with a complete index!
- Royal Raymond Rife's life, inventions, and relationships.
- Recently discovered data explaining how Rife's original machines worked.

Book • $112.50

- Frequently Asked Questions about Rife sessions and equipment, with extensive session information.
- Ground-breaking information on strengthening and supporting the body.
- A 200-page, cross-referenced Frequency Directory including hundreds of health conditions.
- Bibliography, Three Appendices, Historical Photos, Complete Index, AND MUCH MORE!
- DVD available at www.LymeBook.com with author's recent Rife Conference presentation.

Hardcover book, 8.5 x 11", 730 pages, $112.50

Ordering is Easy!

Phone: Toll Free (866) 476-7637
Online: www.LymeBook.com

Detailed product information and secure online ordering is available on our website. Bulk orders to bookstores, health food stores, or Lyme disease support groups – call us for wholesale terms.

Do you have a book inside you? Submit your book proposal online at: www.lymebook.com/submit-book-proposal.

Join Lyme Community Forums at: www.lymecommunity.com.

Get paid to help us place our books in your local health food store. Learn more: www.lymebook.com/local-store-offer.

DISCLAIMER

This disclaimer is in reference to all books, DVDs, websites, flyers, and catalogs published by Bryan Rosner, DBA BioMed Publishing Group.

Our materials are for informational and educational purposes only. They are not intended to prevent, diagnose, treat, or cure disease. Some of the treatments described are not FDA-Approved. Bryan Rosner is a layperson, not a medical professional, and he is not qualified to dispense medical advice.

These books and DVDs are not intended to substitute for professional medical care. Do not postpone receiving care from a licensed physician. Please read our full disclaimer online at: www.lymebook.com/homepage-disclaimer.pdf.

INDEX

5-nitroimidazole, 293
10-Undecenoic Acid, 330
2,3-Dimercapto-1-propanesulfonic acid, 276

A

Abdominal cramps, 383
Acai, 358
AC Contact Machine, 410
Acerola, 358
AC frequencies, 427
Aches, 217, 252
Acid reflux, 383
Acne, 375, 383
Acoustic sound waves, 318-19
Activated charcoal, 276
Acupuncture, 197
Adrenal glands, 92, 103, 133, 147, 159-76, 182-84, 187-90, 193, 195, 199, 231-32, 234, 391
Agriculture, 128
Air Hunger, 75, 418
ALA (Alpha Lipoic Acid), 262, 267, 276, 335
Albendazole, 219, 222, 224
Alinia, 219-20, 222, 301
Alkaline water, 347
Allergies, 57, 71, 136-37, 238, 279, 352, 359, 380
Allicin, 252-53
Almonds, 129, 148, 156
Aluminum, 262, 415
Alzheimer's, 269, 373
Amalgam dental fillings, 414
Amateur body-building contests, 145
Amazon Prime, 149, 169, 177, 347, 351-52, 357, 380, 405
Ambien, 256
Amino acids, 134-36, 170, 277, 360, 421
Amoxicillin, 252-53, 294
Ampho-Terrible, 329
Annual Rife International Health Conference, 410, 423
Anticoagulant, 418
Anti-fungal, 354, 375
Antihelminthic therapies, 354-55
Antihistamine, 418
Antimutagenic, 375
Antioxidant, 134, 150, 358, 360, 375
Ants, 320, 323

Anxiety, 95, 162, 167, 181, 183-84, 188-89, 195, 197, 213, 254, 334
Anyanwu, Samuel, 293
Apo-HEPAT, 277, 335
Appetite, 81, 232, 375
Apple, 139, 145-46
Apple pectin, 276, 282
Arachidonic acid, 13, 261, 283
Arsenic, 414-15
Artemesia absinthium, 365
Artemisinin, 117
Arthritis, 283, 314, 352
Artichoke, 335
Artificial lights, 201
Asclepiadaceae, 377
ASD (Autism Spectrum Disorder), 424
Ashwagandha, 170
Asia, 120
Asparagus, 147, 153
Atkins' Diet, 141
Autism, 264, 363, 398, 424-25
Autonomic Response Testing, 118, 281, 425
Avocado, 147

B

Babesia, 42, 71, 73-75, 103, 107-8, 111, 117-18, 121, 164, 199, 211-14, 220-23, 237, 242, 292, 297, 301, 335, 346, 366, 378, 381-82, 394, 417-18
Baby carrots, 146, 155
Bacon, 130, 145, 147
Bacterial load, 373
Bacterial resistance, 90, 111, 297, 305, 323
Baked potato, 148
Bananas, 139, 150, 156
Banyan Botanicals, 380
Bartonella, 42, 58, 71, 74, 91-92, 103, 107-8, 110, 116, 120, 174-75, 210-12, 214, 221, 224, 231, 237, 242, 357, 366, 374-75, 378, 389, 394, 417
Basic Parasite Protocol, 12, 219-21, 223
Bastyr University, 419
BCA (Borrelia Clinic of Augsburg), 289
Beam Ray Machine, 423
Beginner's Guide to Lyme Disease, 38
Benicar, 252-53

INDEX

Benzodiazepines, 254
Berberine, 382-83
Berries, 139, 150
Bible verses, 199
Bile, 134, 271-73, 275, 345
Biltricide, 219, 221
Binders, 13, 134, 270-72, 280
Biofilm, 73, 77-78, 103-4, 111-12, 114, 116, 211-12, 216-17, 222-23, 226, 237-38, 241, 247, 249, 269, 291-92, 296, 298-99, 301, 307-12, 319, 323, 355, 368, 377-80
Biophotons, 13, 120, 285-90
BioRay, 427
Bioterrain, 323
Biotin, 261, 282
Biotoxins, 269, 272, 275, 277, 333
Bitter tea, 382
Black Cherry, 358
Blood, 63, 73, 131, 171, 195, 254, 265, 271, 273-74, 306, 318-19, 322-23, 345, 370-71, 374-76, 411
Blood sugar, 131, 140, 142, 144, 347, 371, 380
Blood vessel, 135, 254
Bloody stools, 383
Blueberries, 139, 147, 150
Bock, Steven, 412
Bodybuilding, 136, 142, 363
Body fat, 145, 268
Boric acid, 306
Boron, 352-53
Bowel movements, painful, 383
Bowes, Susan, 346
Bransfield, Robert C., 424
Breads, 129, 140, 144, 146
Breakfast, 137, 140, 145-47, 155
Breastfeeding, 4, 347
Breath, shortness of, 164
Broccoli, 153
Brooks Bradley Method, 358
Buhner, Stephen, 375, 377
Bulls eye rash, 315
Bupleurum Liver Cleanse, 335
Burgdorfer, Willy, 411
Butter, 130, 136-37

C

Cacao, 150
Cadmium, 262, 414
Caja, 358
Calories, 130-31, 139, 149, 153, 155

Camu Camu, 358
Canada, 229, 349, 382, 423
Canadian Pharmacies, 228
Cancer, 79, 131, 283, 286, 335, 361, 363, 420, 423, 426
  breast, 426
  kidney, 426
  late-stage lung, 426
  prostate, 426
Candida, 14, 327, 330, 382, 419
Canker sores, 383
Cantwell, Alan, 422
Carbohydrates, 130-31, 139-42, 144-45, 150, 170
Carbon atom, 361
Cardiovascular exercise, 397
Carrots, 153, 156
Casein, 136-37
Cassone, Alphonse, 317-18
Catechins, 374
Celery, 147, 153
Cell phones, 181
Chebula Retz, 379
Chemotherapy, 286
Chest congestion, 161
Chicken, 196, 231
  organic, 170
Chicken-apple sausage, 147
Chicken breast, 147
Chicken broth, 147, 170
Childhood leukemia, 426
Children, 203, 263-64, 346, 372, 418, 424
Chills, 418
China, 95, 376, 382
Chinese Medicine, 383
Chiropractic, 412
Chlamydia, 222
Chlorella, 276
Chlorine dioxide, 13, 241, 303-16
Chocolate smoothies, 150
Cholesterol, 10, 127, 132-33, 137, 145, 170, 373
Cholestyramine, 276
Chronic fatigue syndrome, 60-61, 160, 393
Cilantro, 276
Clays, 276
Coconut Cream, 147
Coenzyme Q-10, 94
Coil Machine, 234, 410
Colostrum, 410
ConcenTrace, 336

INDEX

Constipation, 273
Copper, 13, 100, 282-83, 414, 427
Coptis, 382-83
Cortisol, 171-72, 371
Coughing, 418
Counseling, 23, 166, 197, 199, 256
Cowden, Lee, 412
Crane, John, 422
Creapure, 364
Creatine, 363-64
Cucumber, 153
Curcumin, 335, 372-73
Cyst form, 222, 242, 292-94, 300, 320, 370, 410
Cystic fibrosis, 378

D

Dairy, 129, 132, 135-38, 149, 158
Dandelion, 335
DHA, 132, 134
Diabetes, 131, 347, 373
Diarrhea, 313, 346, 383
Diethylcarbamazine, 224, 232-33
Dimercaptosuccinic acid, 276
Dimethylglycine, 362
Dinner, 133, 140, 147-48, 156-57, 189
Dionaea Muscipula, 15, 374
Discontentment, 183, 191
DMG, 361-63
DMPS, 267-68, 276
DMSA, 267-68, 276
DNA, 211-12, 214, 305, 361, 394
DNP, 412
Doctor's Data, 415
Dove Press, 293
Doxycycline, 116, 294
Dreams, 198, 232
Dried fruit, 148
Duncan, Tami, 424

E

Earthing, 369-72
Eastern Himalayas, 382
Ecclesiastes, 199
Edlow, Jonathan A., 1
EDTA, 276
EGCG and Green Tea Extract, 15, 374-75
Eggs, 130, 132, 135, 145-46, 196, 231
Egg yolks, 132

Ehrlichia, 107
Eiro Juice, 358
Elderberry, 380-81
Electrical circuits, 369
Electrical signals, 399
Electric field, 243, 369
Electricity, 206, 208
Electric light sauna, 422
Electromagnetic fields, 370
Electromagnetic frequencies, 319, 369
Electromagnetic radiation, 404
Electrons, 307, 369-70
Electrosmog, 425
Ellagic Acid Derivatives, 378
EMEM Machine, 410
Emotional conflict, unresolved, 11, 162-63, 188-89, 193-97, 199, 400
Emotional trauma, 58, 76
Endocrine abnormalities, 238
Endothelial, 374
Espresso, 208
Ethanolic extracts of Moringa oleifera, 354
Ethylenediaminetetraacetic acid, 276
Eucalyptus trees, 203
Exercise, 16, 59, 76, 133, 141, 145, 163, 165, 174, 184-85, 192, 217, 231, 233, 252, 334, 364, 397, 410

F

Facebook, 3, 26, 31, 348, 350
Fancy clinics, 324, 396
Fat
  animal, 185
  healthy, 130
  hydrogenated, 132
Fatigue, 95, 101, 104, 141-42, 160, 163, 171, 210, 233, 334
Feces, 134, 271, 273, 417
Fermentation, 138
Fever, 75, 81, 285, 383, 418
Fiber, 138-39, 150, 153-54, 158, 273
Fibromyalgia, 314, 361
Finances, 244, 255, 308, 324, 393, 401
Fish, 123, 130, 133-35
Fish-free DHA supplements, 134
Flagyl, 64, 291, 295
Flashbacks, 194, 397-98
Flax, 133-34, 150, 152
Fluconazole, 329
Flus, 279, 285-86, 360, 380-81

INDEX

Folate, 362
Food allergens, 82, 158
Formula SF722, 330
F-Scan, 427

G

Gallbladder, 272
Glandulars, 171-72
Glutathione, 134
Gluten, 10, 76-77, 82, 143-44, 147
Glyconutrients, 421
Google, 25-26, 28-31, 132, 146, 152, 158, 189, 221, 229, 284, 290, 304, 318, 352-53, 358, 366, 368
Grains, 10, 129, 132, 140, 142-46
Great Plains Laboratory, 415
Greek yogurt, 146
Green tea, 374
Grocery stores, 140, 157
Grounding, 197, 369-71
Guilt, 165, 185, 188-89, 197, 400
Gut binders, 267, 271-73, 275-77, 282
Gym, 145, 192-93, 251

H

Hair Mineral Analysis, 415, 422
Half & Half, 137, 149
Haritaki Fruit, 377
Harris, Steven J., 412
Harvard Medical School, 1
Harvey, William T., 424
HBOT (Hyperbaric Oxygen Therapy), 366-68
HBOT therapy, 366-68, 410
Headaches, 101, 233, 399, 418
Heart, 33, 91, 106, 154, 274, 383
Heart attacks, 79, 283, 403, 419
Heart pounding, 233
Heavy Whipping Cream, 136-37, 149, 151-52
Heel, 277, 335
Hepar Compositum, 277, 335
Hepatitis, 223
Hepatoprotective, 224, 334, 375
Hesse-Sheehan, Elizabeth, 412
HH, 357
HIV, 286, 373
Homemade liposomal products, 357
Homeopathic drainage remedies, 277
Homeopathic nosodes, 287
Homeopathy, 95, 252, 287, 410, 421

Huang Lian, 382
Humaworm, 225
Humic acid, 276
Hydrogen atoms, 361
Hydrogen peroxide, 306-7
Hydrophilic, 274
Hyperactivity, 363
Hyperbaric Oxygen Therapy. See HBOT
Hypercoagulation, 196
Hyperthermia, 410
Hypnotherapy, 197
Hypoglycemia, 131
Hypotension, 253

I

IBS, 314
Ice, 150-51
Ice cream, paleo, 152
ICHT Italian treatment, 410
IgG, 254, 350-51
IgM, 254
Immunocal, 348-51
Immunomodulator, 224, 351, 358, 360, 364, 375, 381
Impotence, 352, 375
India, 229, 345, 354, 377-78
Indian and Chinese medicine, 421
Indigestion, 334
Infants, 346-47
Insecticides, 351
Insecurity, 165, 194-95, 400
Insomnia, 184, 254, 361-63, 365, 382-83
Insulin, 131, 140, 142, 144
Intestinal flora, 95, 116, 329-30
Intestinal parasites, 71, 209, 214, 221
Intestinal symptoms, 209, 214, 328
Intestinal tract, 71, 99, 134, 210, 271, 273, 282, 327-30
Intestine, large, 383
Intravenous antibiotics, 62, 248, 254, 318
Intuition, 232
Iodine, 262, 306
Irritability, 210, 213, 383
ITIRES, 277
Itraconazole, 329
Ivermectin, 219-22, 225
Ixodes dammini tick, 1

J

INDEX

Jarrow Formulas, 149, 169, 364
Journal of Infection and Drug
    Resistance, 293
Juice, citrus, 304
Juicing, 153

K

Kale, 153
Kefir, 419
Kendall, Roger V., 363
Ketosis, 140
Kidneys, 99, 160, 273, 375, 377
Kinnaman Foundation, 423
Kunold, Marlene, 412
Kupsinel, Roy, 422

L

Lactose, 136-38
Lam, Michael, 176-77, 185
Las Vegas, 317-18, 325
LDN (Low-Dose Naltrexone), 364-65
LEDs, 287
Lemon, 154, 304
Lethargy, 141-42
Lettuce, 147, 153
L-glutamic acid, 134
Licorice, 171, 335
Lipophilic, 225, 274
Liposomal houttuynia, 357
Liposomal recipe/process, 356-58
Liposomal vitamin c, 169, 356
Liposomes, 356-57
Lithium orotate, 411
Logan, Christopher, 372
Low-Dose Naltrexone. See LDN
Loyd, Richard, 410, 423, 427
Luecke, David F., 293
Lumbrokinase/serrapeptase, 301
Lunch, 140, 147, 152, 155, 204
Luxuries, 28, 182-83
Lynes, Barry, 420, 422

M

MacLean, Doug, 413
Macronutrients, 127-28, 134, 149-50,
    152, 154-55
Magnesium, 261-62, 362
Magnetic field, 238, 243

Magnetic pulsers, 427
Malaria, 345, 381
Manganese, 261, 282
Marra, Susan L., 412
Marschall, Rick, 415
Marvelous Paleo Smoothie, 148, 151-
    52
Materialism, 191
Mayer, Alix, 370-71
McFadzean, Nicola, 38, 412, 419
Meat, 129-30, 147-48, 156
Mebendazole, 222, 224
Medsonix, 13, 247, 317-25
Memory loss, 210, 213, 418
Mental clarity, 364
Mental illnesses, 361, 397-98
Mepron, 111, 199, 229
Mercola, Joseph, 131
Methylation, 361-63
Methyl donors, 362
Metronidazole, 291
Metzger, Deborah, 412
MHBOT (Mild Hyperbaric Oxygen
    Therapy), 15, 366-68
Migraines, 316
Mild Hyperbaric Oxygen Therapy. See
    MHBOT
Milk thistle, 94, 335, 411
Mimosa Pudica, 225-26
Mineral baths, 411
Mineral deficiency, 262, 264
Mini-crashes, 185-86
Mini-relapse, 73
Miscarriage, 347
Mold, 52, 60, 82, 103, 416
Monotherapy, 62
Morinda citrifolia, 381
Moringa Oleifera, 226, 353-56
Mountain biking, 4, 184, 192, 398
Moxidectin, 225
Multiple Systemic Infectious Diseases
    Syndrome, 86
Multivitamin, 94, 169, 395
Muran, Peter J., 412
Muscle aches, 220
Muscle mass, 145
Muscle recovery, 360
Muscle tone, 144, 397
Mycoplasma, 71, 107
Myers, Melissa, 414

N

INDEX

N-Acetylcysteine, 335
Naltrexone, 364
Nap, 202-3
Nasal congestion, 279-80
Nausea, 313-14
Neem, 345-47
Neti pot, 280
Nettles, 359
Neurological injuries, 366
Neurotoxins, 333, 425
Neurotransmitters, 135
New York Times, 143, 227
Nitazoxanide (also called Alinia), 222-23
Noni, 381
Nordquist, William D., 419
Nutrient deficiencies, 57-58, 100-101, 262
Nystatin, 329

O

Oatmeal, 144-45
Ober, Clinton, 370-72
Obesity, 130-31, 139, 141, 157, 283, 334, 401
Oils, 147, 357
   clove, 365
   coconut, 130, 132, 146, 156
   ginger, 365
   oregano, 365
   wormwood, 365
Olive Leaf Extract, 30
Omega-6 fatty acid, 283
Omega fatty acids, 94, 133, 150
Onchocerca cervicalis, 221
Onchocerca volvulus, 221
Online pharmacies, 228-30, 428
Opioid receptor antagonist, 364
Organic groceries, 217
Organic neem supplements, 347
Outdoors, 11, 182, 200-201
Overeating, 145, 334
Oxford's Journal of Antimicrobial Chemotherapy, 222
Oxygen, 252, 306, 369, 410
Ozone, 252, 306-7, 410

P

Pantethine, 169
Pantothenic acid, 169

PAO1 Virulence, 379
Parastroy, 225
Pastries, 129, 140
Past romantic relationships, 400
Past wounds, 194
Peanut Butter, 147, 156
Pecans, 147-48
Pekana, 277, 335
People Pleasing, 11
Perfectionism, 11, 187-88, 197, 400
Pharmax, 365
Physique, 142, 144-45
Phyto-chemicals, 155
Piezo Sona Tool Corporation, 318
Piperazine citrate, 354
Planetary Herbals, 335
Plants
   flowering, 382
   medicinal, 381
Plasma tubes, 243
Plateau in progress, 62, 75, 87-88, 110, 117, 122, 348, 389-90
Plum Flower, 383
Poem, 189-90
Poesnecker, Dr., 176-77
Pomegranate, 358
Potato chips, 129, 148-49
Poultry, 130, 135
Pregnancy, 347
Pregnenolone, 132, 171
Probiotics, 14, 63, 94, 116, 330-31, 336, 394, 419, 421
Protein
   animal, 135, 170
   high, 150
   high-quality, 132
   milk, 136
   pea, 170
   vegetable, 135
Protozoan parasites, 214, 222, 381
Pseudonomas, 377, 379
Psoriasis, 360, 375
Psychiatric manifestations, 79
Psychologist, 188
Psychosomatic issues, 397
Pulse Therapy, 120
Pyloricin, 365-66
Pyrantel pamoate, 219, 222

Q

QS. See Quorum Sensing
Quackery, 281, 304

INDEX

Quorum Sensing (QS), 116, 237, 301, 378-80

R

Rages, 231
Raisins, 147-48
Red meat, 135
    even, 130, 135
Refined carbohydrates, 71, 131, 142, 146, 152
Relapses, 74, 88, 120, 248, 312, 368
Relaxation, 59, 83, 163, 181, 202, 205-6, 252
Remission, 51, 73, 352, 396
RENELIX, 277
Resistant Microbes, 14, 359
RestorMedicine, 419
Rhodiola, 170
Rice, 132, 139-40, 144
    brown, 142, 144
Rice bread, 144
Rice noodles, 144
Rice tortillas, 144
Rifampin, 64, 108, 116
Rife therapy, 12, 103-5, 119, 121, 235-51, 253, 255-57, 310-12, 318-23, 411, 413, 422-23, 427-28
Root, ginger, 382
Rosen, Gary, 416
Rossi, Michael, 293
Rutgers University Medical School, 355

S

Saccharomyces boulardii, 330-31
Salad, 147-48, 153
Salt/C Protocol, 252, 313
Salt water, 280
Samento, 410
Sandwich, 144, 147
Sapi, Eva, 293
Saponins, 355, 376-77
Sarsaparilla, 375-77
Satiety, 131, 137, 148-49
Saturated fats, 127, 132-33, 137, 145, 149, 170
Savely, Ginger, 412
Scalar octaves, 427
Schizandra, 335
Schizophrenia, 136, 195
Sedentary office work, 182

Seibert, Florence B., 422
Seizures, 79, 346
Self-acceptance, 188, 192
Self control, 187, 195, 405
Self-employment, 255
Self-navigate, 115
Self-perception, 198
Sero-negativity, 1
Shortness of breath, 164
Sierra Nevada Mountain Range, 231
Silver, colloidal, 119, 410
Simplicity, financial, 191
Sinatra, Stephen, 370, 372
Sine wave, 427
Sinus cavities, 280
Sinus infection, 280
Sjorne's syndrome, 314
Skeptics, 98, 281
Skin conditions, 345, 373, 383
Sleep, 82, 163, 173, 189, 192, 233, 253-54, 257, 334, 364, 405
Smilax glabra, 376
Smilax officinalis, 375
Smoothies, 137-38, 147-55, 395
Snacks, 10, 139-40, 146, 148, 151-52, 155
Snow, 214
Sodium ascorbate powder, 358
Sodium chlorite, 304
Solar plexus, 281, 287
Solidago compositum, 277
Soup, 147, 196
Spaghetti, 46
Spark gap, 427
Staphylococcus epidermidis, 222
STARI (Southern tick-associated rash illness), 1
Steak, 148
Steroids, 355, 376-77
Stevia, 150-52, 154
Stinging Nettle, 359
Strasheim, Connie, 239, 412
Strawberries, 139
Strep throat, 37
Stressful jobs, 190
Suicidal ideation, 79
Sun, 182, 191, 201
Sunflower lecithin powder, 358
Surgical instruments, 322
Swanson brand, 356
Sweats, 75, 418
Swollen gums, 383

Syphilis, 375-76

T

Tai Chi, 252
Tapping, 199
Tart cherry, 15, 360-61
TC (Terminalia chebula), 377-80
Tea, 374, 382
Terminalia Chebula, 377-78, 380
. *See* TC
Testosterone, 359, 377
Thorne Research, 330
Thrombotic stroke, 283
Thrush, 382-83
Tick bite, 424
Ticks, 72, 200, 210, 371, 410, 417-18
Tinnitus, 253
TMG, 362-63
Tobramycin, 379
Trees
  drumstick, 353
  horseradish, 353
Trimethylglycine, 362
Triphala, 380
Turmeric, 335, 372
TV, 201-2, 370

U

Ubichinon compositum, 277
Ulcers, 373, 383
Ultrasonic jewelry cleaner, 358
Unforgiveness, 189
Unhealthy feelings, 181, 188, 205, 398, 400
University of Las Vegas (UNLV), 318
Unprocessed foods, 129

V

Vanilla extract, 152
Veganism, 134-35
Vegetables
  dietary, 153-54
  green leafy, 347
  raw, 153-54
Vegetarianism, 135
Venus Fly Trap, 15, 374
Vigorous exercise, 59
Virapress, 360
Vitamin B5, 169
Vitamin B6, 261, 263-64, 267-68, 282

Vitex negundo, 354
Voltage, 427
Vomiting, 346, 383

W

Waisbren, Burton, 417
Walkie-talkie, 378
Water, 137, 150-52, 201, 272, 278, 336, 370
  alkaline, 347-48
  distilled, 354
Weight lifting, 251-52
Weight loss, 130, 154
Westbrook University, 422
Wheat toast, 145
Whey protein, 10, 135-37, 149, 151, 170, 277, 348
WI-FI signals, 202
Wilson, Lawrence, 422
Wine, red, 150
Wobenzym, 112
Worms, 12, 71, 209, 211-14, 221, 224, 345, 352, 354-55
Wulfman, Jeffrey S., 424

X

Xymogen, 350

Y

Yahoo, 250
Yale University, 426
Yale University Press, 1
Yeast, intestinal, 14, 71, 139, 327-31
Yoga, 217, 395
Yogurt, 138, 146, 148, 331, 419

Z

Zucker, Martin, 372

Also by Bryan Rosner

When Antibiotics Fail: Lyme Disease and Rife Machines, With Critical Evaluation of Leading Alternative Therapies

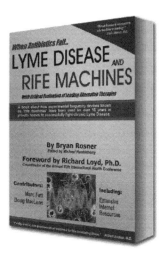

The Top 10 Lyme Disease Treatments: Defeat Lyme Disease With The Best Of Conventional and Alternative Medicine

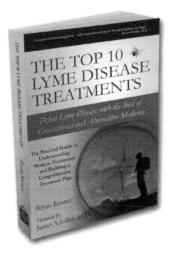

(No picture shown) The Lyme-Autism Connection: Unveiling the Shocking Link Between Lyme Disease and Childhood Developmental Disorders

Learn more about Bryan's books at www.LymeBook.com